BONNIE STERN

HEART SMART™

The Best of HeartSmart™ Cooking

RANDOM HOUSE
CANADA

HEART
AND STROKE
FOUNDATION
OF CANADA

Finding answers. For life.

www.randomhouse.ca

Library and Archives Canada Cataloguing in Publication

Stern, Bonnie
        HeartSmart / Bonnie Stern.

Includes index.
"Heart and Stroke Foundation of Canada".

ISBN-13: 978-0-679-31412-7
ISBN-10: 0-679-31412-1

        1. Heart—Diseases—Diet therapy—Recipes. 2. Low-fat diet—
Recipes. I. Heart and Stroke Foundation of Canada II. Title.
RC684.D5S7 2005   641.5'6311   C2005-903762-8

Project Editors: Tanya Trafford and Shelley Tanaka
Interior Photography: Robert Wigington
Food Styling: Olga Truchan

Design by CS Richardson

Printed and bound in Canada

10 9 8 7 6 5 4 3 2 1

FOR MY FAMILY,
WHO NOURISH ME

CONTENTS

HEART AND STROKE FOUNDATION OF CANADA ACKNOWLEDGEMENTS

The Heart and Stroke Foundation would like to thank the following people for their assistance in the development and review of the nutritional information for *HeartSmart™* by Bonnie Stern. Their expertise and advice have been invaluable in transforming the latest scientific information on healthy eating into practical consumer-friendly information.

Fran Berkoff, RD, for doing a wonderful job of presenting the science of healthy eating so that it is easy to understand and use.

A special thanks to Bonnie Stern for updating her terrific recipes and adding even more delicious recipes for you to enjoy.

Barb Selley from Food Intelligence for the nutritional analysis.

Christine LeGrand, Heather Rourke, Stephen Samis, Mary Elizabeth Harriman, Dominique Mongeon and Carol Dombrow for coordinating and reviewing the nutritional information.

Julie Desjardins and Chris Pon for their leadership in behind-the-scenes work on contracts and sponsorship.

All those people who worked so hard putting this beautiful book together, especially Tanya Trafford, Shelley Tanaka, Anne Collins and their teams of very talented people.

We would also like to thank everyone who worked on all the other books in the HeartSmart™ series. Their hard work helped to make this a terrific book.

The Beef Information Centre is committed to sharing with Canadians ways they can continue to make lean beef a part of a well-balanced, healthy diet. The Beef Information Centre is pleased to support the initiatives of the Heart and Stroke Foundation of Canada and their efforts to help people live healthier lives and reduce their risk of heart disease and stroke.

The Heart and Stroke Foundation gratefully acknowledges the generous support of the Beef Information Centre in helping to make this cookbook possible. The financial support received from our sponsor does not constitute an endorsement of the sponsor's products by the Heart and Stroke Foundation or the author.

AUTHOR ACKNOWLEDGEMENTS

When I went to university, I thought I was going to be a librarian. I loved books—choosing them, opening them, reading them. It never occurred to me how much work went into writing them, editing them, publishing them and selling them. It also never occurred to me then that I would write a book of my own.

It takes many people to put a cookbook together, and I've been very lucky to work with a core group of talented, dedicated individuals over the years:

All my colleagues, old and new, at my cooking school—Anne Apps, Dely Balagtas, Jenny Burke, Lorraine Butler, Rhonda Caplan, Leonie Eidinger, Lauren Gutter, Letty Lastima, Maureen Lollar, Jennifer Mahoney, Francine Menard and Linda Stephen.

My friend and lawyer, Marian Hebb.

The talented team that Random House puts together—Julie Chivers, Anne Collins, Marlene Fraser, Janine Laporte, Allyson Latta, Brad Martin, Teresa Napolitano, John Neale, Scott Richardson, Scott Sellers, Jennifer Shepherd, Shelley Tanaka, Susan Thomas, Tanya Trafford, Olga Truchan and Robert Wigington.

The committed individuals at the Heart and Stroke Foundation of Canada, and their expert professionals—Fran Berkoff, Julie Desjardins, Carol Dombrow, Dominique Mongeon, Chris Pon and Barbara Selley.

My friends and colleagues in the food community—the suppliers who produce great ingredients, the chefs who teach at my school, the media and buyers who support my books.

Finally, special thanks to all of you. It means a lot to me when you say I'm in your kitchens, nourishing your friends and family with my recipes.

PREFACE

The Heart and Stroke Foundation of Canada is pleased to bring you *HeartSmart™*, the latest great product of our long-standing relationship with best-selling author Bonnie Stern. This book combines all of the best recipes from classics like *Simply HeartSmart™ Cooking*, *More HeartSmart™ Cooking*, and *HeartSmart™ Cooking for Family and Friends*, and also brings you 100 new recipes.

The Heart and Stroke Foundation is always here to help you enjoy good nutrition and good health, with lots of information and delicious recipes. Maintaining a healthy weight is a challenge for many Canadians. Obesity is a health issue of increasing concern, and a risk factor for heart disease and stroke. That's why in addition to the great recipes, we've also included valuable nutritional information. It's all part of the Foundation's efforts to keep consumers informed with the latest knowledge about food choices that can help reduce the risk of heart disease and stroke.

We know healthy food choices are not always easy in a hectic world. That's why we also offer Health Check™, a food information program that makes it simple to identify healthy choices in the grocery store. Products that display the Health Check™ symbol have been reviewed by our nutrition experts and meet nutrition criteria based on *Canada's Food Guide to Healthy Eating*. Choosing these products is a great way to help you and your family enjoy healthy eating.

You can play a big role in lowering your risk and protecting your heart health. Nutritious, balanced eating is certainly a big part of it. An overall healthy lifestyle, including regular physical activity, staying smoke-free, limiting alcohol consumption and managing stress, will also help you enjoy life to the fullest. You can find more information on our web site at www.heartandstroke.ca.

This book is proof positive that the "right" choices aren't dull. There's plenty of delicious variety in the recipes that follow, and I hope you try them all!

Cleve Myers, CA
Chair
Heart and Stroke Foundation of Canada

INTRODUCTION

A lot has changed in the food world since I started working with the Heart and Stroke Foundation of Canada more than twelve years ago. That's one of the reasons I was so excited about this project. It is also wonderful to have a single volume containing our favourite 300 recipes from *Simply HeartSmart™ Cooking*, *More HeartSmart™ Cooking* and *HeartSmart™ Cooking for Family and Friends*, as well as 100 new recipes.

Many cooks now know what it takes to lower the fat and salt in their diets. We know which ingredients to avoid or use sparingly and which ingredients we can use freely. We are growing accustomed to reading nutrition labels on the products we buy.

Yet at the same time, more people are eating out and buying prepared meals from specialty stores, supermarkets, take-away places and restaurants—meals that come without ingredient lists and nutrition labels. People can fool themselves by eating a restaurant take-out stir-fry without realizing how much oil or sodium it contains, or by choosing a salad without knowing how much fat is in the dressing.

My goal is to get people back into the kitchen, with recipes that are delicious, easy to make and healthful. Not only will you know exactly what is in your food, but there is nothing more satisfying than having your friends and family love what you have cooked for them. I want people to feel the joy of nourishing their families with great-tasting, healthful food.

Years ago, when I did my chef's training, you wouldn't dream of cooking a special meal without using butter, cream, eggs, cheese and lots of salt, and topping it off with a rich dessert. Eventually, people wanted every meal to be special, which led to overindulgence.

But now, special no longer has to mean rich and high in calories. Today home cooks have a wide choice of ingredients from all over the world—culinary treats that are naturally low in fat but add huge amounts of flavour. Fresh herbs are available year round, not just in big cities but everywhere. Flavoured vinegars like balsamic are commonplace. A vast array of seasonings, chiles and spices are available. People are rediscovering wholesome staples like beans and grains. Whole-grain breads, pastas and rice are becoming more popular, and the quality is improving. Restaurants are serving bean and vegetable dips with bread instead of butter. Wild mushrooms and exotic fruits have become a regular part of our diets, and dried fruits like dates, apricots, figs and prunes (renamed dried plums by savvy marketers!) are appearing in appetizers, salads and baked goods of all kinds. Organic ingredients can be found in almost every grocery store, and markets highlight local, seasonal ingredients.

At the same time, kitchen gadgets like grill pans, yogurt cheese makers, food processors and non-stick skillets make healthy cooking easier than ever.

People who have been diagnosed with heart disease often fear that they will no longer be able to eat well. But they are so wrong. Heart-healthy food is not only better for you, it is really delicious. Fresh fruit and vegetables, grains, fish, chicken and lean meats, angel food cake, sorbets and meringues were not invented by HeartSmart™ cooks. They were always there, but they are attracting new attention from professional and home cooks alike.

I am lucky that I get lots of feedback from students and readers. They tell me what they need to succeed in the kitchen in order to provide their families with nourishing meals. They always say that if a dish isn't delicious, there's no point making it because no one will eat it. Then the words healthy and nutritious come to mean food to be avoided rather than food to be embraced. So my first rule is that food has to taste really good.

Today it is easier than ever to prepare wonderful, heart-healthy meals. So get into the kitchen. There's no better time to cook.

Bonnie Stern
Toronto, 2006

THE LATEST WORD ON HEALTHY EATING
BY FRAN BERKOFF, RD

The Heart and Stroke Foundation of Canada welcomes you to *HeartSmart™*, your guide to creating delicious meals, snacks and treats that support your heart health and well-being. More than just a cookbook, it's a guide to healthy, lifelong eating patterns, with explanations of the latest nutritional research.

Three of the most important principles of heart-healthy eating are balance, variety and moderation. There's increasing evidence that combining and varying healthful foods and ingredients in an inclusive diet can play a significant role in reducing the risk of heart disease, stroke and other diseases like cancer.

To support your healthy choices, the Heart and Stroke Foundation also provides the Health Check™ food information program. Over 500 food products carrying the Health Check symbol meet the Foundation's criteria for healthy food choices, based on Canada's food guide. For more information visit www.healthcheck.org.

HeartSmart™ is a collection of the best of the outstandingly creative recipes from the HeartSmart series that combine healthy, delicious ingredients in tempting dishes you'll love to make and serve to family and friends.

You'll also find useful information about which fats are good for you and which ones to avoid or eliminate, and about the amount of fat that should be part of your diet.

You'll read about carbohydrates that are part of healthy eating and those that bring little to the table and find out how dietary fibre can support heart health.

You can also find tips and tools for shopping, eating out and maintaining your optimal body weight, all with the goals of protecting your health and reducing your risk of heart disease.

The Heart and Stroke Foundation of Canada is pleased to bring you *HeartSmart™* and we wish you an enjoyable journey to better heart health.

FAT CHANCE

Don't think of all fat in the food you eat as something to avoid. Think of fat as an opportunity. Fats are sources of fatty acids that are essential for health.

Here's why. Fats
- are required for cell growth, development and maintenance
- produce important hormones
- help carry fat-soluble vitamins throughout the body
- help form cell membranes
- contribute to immunity

Fat—the right kind and the right amount—is actually good for you and an important part of a healthy diet. In fact, adults should get 20 to 35 percent of their calories from fat, children 4 to 18 years should get 25 to 35 percent of their calories from fat and children 1 to 3 years, 30 to 40 percent.

Consuming 20 to 35 percent of your calories from fat translates to about 45 to 75 grams/day for a woman and about 60 to 105 grams/day for a man.

But the wrong kind of fat? Not good. As much as possible, you should try to reduce your intake of saturated fats and minimize the trans fats found in so many processed and fast foods.

So how do you know which fat is friend and which is foe?

FIRST, A WORD ABOUT CHOLESTEROL

Cholesterol is produced by the body. It helps produce hormones, enables the brain to function properly and maintains the body's nerve structure. Cholesterol is transported to and from cells in the form of lipoproteins. The two main lipoproteins are HDL (high density lipoprotein) and LDL (low density lipoprotein). HDL-cholesterol is commonly called "good" cholesterol because it carries excess blood cholesterol back to the liver to be excreted from the body. LDL-cholesterol is called "bad" cholesterol because it is the kind that builds up on artery walls. A high level of LDL-cholesterol in the blood is associated with an increased risk of heart disease. Ideally, you should have high levels of HDL-cholesterol and low levels of LDL-cholesterol.

The body produces cholesterol regardless of what you eat, and the cholesterol in food has less impact on blood cholesterol than the saturated fat in food. So the best defence is a lower fat diet. However, for some people, eating too many cholesterol-containing foods can raise blood cholesterol. The foods that contain cholesterol are animal products such as egg yolks, liver, shrimp, squid and fatty meats. If your blood cholesterol is elevated, you should moderate your intake of these foods.

THE SKINNY ON FATS

There are several different kinds of fats, but they all fall into two categories: unsaturated fats that are good for you and saturated fats that are not.

Foods almost always contain both saturated and unsaturated fats but they are classified according to which fats are present in the greatest amount.

THE GOOD FATS

Unsaturated fats are liquid at room temperature. They can help lower your LDL-cholesterol level when they replace saturated fats in your diet. There are two types of unsaturated fats—monounsaturated and polyunsaturated.

Monounsaturated fats protect against heart disease by lowering LDL-cholesterol levels. They are found in olive, canola and peanut oils, non-hydrogenated margarines, nuts such as almonds and hazelnuts, and avocados.

Polyunsaturated fats are also liquid at room temperature and can lower LDL-cholesterol levels. There are two groups of polyunsaturated fats: omega-3 and omega-6 fats.

Omega-3 fats include EPA (eicosapentaenoic acid), DHA (docosahexaenoic acid) and ALA (alpha-linolenic acid). They are the stars of the fat world. For sources of EPA and DHA, go fishing. They're found primarily in oily cold-water fish such as salmon, mackerel, herring and sardines. ALA is found in flaxseed and flaxseed oils, canola oil, soy oil, omega-3 eggs, walnuts, soybeans and in smaller amounts in dark green leafy vegetables.

Here's why omega-3 fats in fish are so important: They help prevent stickiness and clotting of blood, reducing the risk of stroke. They also help lower triglycerides, the form in which your body stores fat, and can reduce abnormal heart rhythms (arrhythmias).

There are now a number of products on the market that contain omega-3 fats, including omega-3 eggs, milk and other dairy products, and bread. Eating a variety of these foods will help add the important omega-3 fats to your diet.

Omega-6 fats work together with omega-3 fats to promote good heart health by providing your body with linoleic acid, which helps lower LDL-cholesterol. But these are tricky ones and should be eaten in moderation, since there's some evidence that large amounts can lower your HDL-cholesterol as well. If omega-6 fats sound a little nutty, that may be because one of the best sources for them is nuts and seeds such as almonds, pecans, Brazil nuts, sunflower seeds and sesame seeds. They're also found in vegetable oils including safflower, sunflower, corn, soybean and sesame.

It's important to maintain a balance of omega-3 and omega-6 fats because, while omega-3 fatty acids help reduce inflammation, most omega-6 fatty acids tend to promote inflammation. An imbalance of these essential fatty acids can contribute to the development of disease. Typically, Canadian diets tend to include high amounts of omega-6 fat, so the best strategy is to concentrate on consuming sufficient omega-3 fats. You can do this by eating fish 2 times a week.

THE BAD FATS

Saturated fats are solid at room temperature. They're found in animal products including fatty meat, poultry with skin and full-fat dairy products and in certain tropical oils such as coconut and palm. A diet high in saturated fats can raise your LDL-cholesterol and increase your risk of heart disease.

To lower your intake of saturated fats, cook with lean meat, take the skin off poultry and use lower-fat dairy products.

Trans fats are created when a vegetable oil undergoes a process called hydrogenation, which makes liquids solid and helps to prolong shelf life. Like saturated fats, trans fats raise LDL-cholesterol and lower HDL-cholesterol. You'll find trans fats in partially hydrogenated vegetable oils and some margarines. They also lurk in many packaged foods such as crackers, cookies, snack foods and commercially baked products as well as commercial French fries and many other fast-food menu items. Health Canada's new food labels make it mandatory to state the amount of trans fats in packaged foods.

FISH FACTS

Fish is an excellent source of protein, niacin, vitamin B12, iron, selenium, zinc and more. Most fish contains fewer calories and less fat per serving than many cuts of meat. It is suggested that you eat fish 2 times a week.

The best sources of omega-3 fats are fish from deep, cold water. These include salmon, mackerel, herring, sardines, anchovies and trout. The second-best sources include halibut, bluefish, ocean perch, bass, red snapper and smelts.

Lean fish such as sole or flounder is low in fat and high in protein. Mixing fish high in omega-3 fats with leaner fish varieties lets you add the special oils to your diet while keeping your total fat intake low.

Shellfish is a rich source of protein as well as important vitamins and minerals. Shellfish is also low in fat—a 3-oz (90 g) serving of scallops, for example, has less than 1 g of fat. Shrimp and squid are higher in cholesterol, but research indicates that it is excess fat (especially saturated fat), not cholesterol, that has the biggest impact on your body's cholesterol levels. If your cholesterol is elevated, you should eat shrimp and squid in moderation. Lobster, crab and scallops are low in fat and calories as long as they are not dipped in butter or cooked in a rich, creamy sauce.

When you eat fast food, go easy on the fried fish and fried fish sandwiches. The breading and frying make them higher in fat than a burger. In fact, a fish sandwich contains about 400 calories and 19 g of fat, compared with a plain burger at 260 calories and 9 g of fat.

THE MEDITERRANEAN DIET

People of the Mediterranean have long been known for being robust. Research suggests that this may be partly due to diet. Thus, the Mediterranean diet is often looked to as a healthy way to eat. The diet contains lots of fruit, vegetables, legumes and grains, with olive oil and nuts as the main source of fat. Fish, poultry, eggs and dairy (mostly cheese and yogurt) are eaten a few times per week and lean red meat a few times per month.

Because this eating plan concentrates on more complex carbohydrates in the form of whole grains, pasta, legumes and beans, vegetables and fruit, it is high in fibre, low in fat and often low in calories, with lots of important vitamins and minerals. The healthy fats in the diet come from olive oil and nuts. The traditional diet consists of fresh, locally grown food. It contains almost no processed foods, making it low in trans fats. Most researchers believe that it is the total diet, not just one individual food or food group, that provides the health benefits of the Mediterranean diet.

The lifestyle and culture of the people of the Mediterranean also play a part in their good health. They take time to relax with meals—a

DIOXINS

Reports of high levels of dioxins in farmed salmon have raised some legitimate concerns. Canadian-farmed Atlantic salmon has considerably more dioxins than its wild Pacific relatives. The amount of dioxins in Atlantic salmon is still within government safety limits. However, you can lower the amount of dioxins in Atlantic salmon even more by removing the skin and cutting away the creamy white fat *before* the fish is cooked. Also, cook on a rack or grill so that fat drips away. Canned salmon is wild unless the label states "Atlantic salmon."

For more information on this or any other environmental concerns, visit Health Canada's web site at www.hc-sc.gc.ca

great stress reliever. And they tend to be more physically active than North Americans, another factor in lowering risk. Still to come is the verdict on red wine, but some research points to its benefits if consumed in moderation.

Too often you pick out one part of the diet and assume it to be the factor that gives you the health benefits. Most probably it is the combination of factors, both diet and lifestyle, that make Mediterraneans so heart healthy.

RED MEAT

There is no question that red meat is a highly nutritious food; not only is it a leading source of high quality protein, but a 4-oz (125 g) serving provides more than 100 percent of the Recommended Dietary Allowance (RDA) of vitamin B12, an essential nutrient found only in animal products. Beef is also an excellent source of vitamin B6, niacin and selenium, as well as the essential minerals iron and zinc.

If you are concerned about the fat in meat, choose the leanest cuts of beef, which include sirloin, sirloin tip, tenderloin, flank steak, inside round, eye of round and outside round. Then trim any visible fat from the edges of your meat. When choosing ground beef, look for lean or extra lean. Reduce the fat further by broiling, grilling or roasting on a rack, so that the fat can drip away.

NUTS AND SEEDS

Nuts and seeds are rich sources of vitamin E and potassium as well as good sources of fibre and other minerals including calcium, iron, magnesium and zinc. Many also contain folate, niacin and other B vitamins. Nuts are a good source of protein, especially when combined with legumes, and play an important role in the diets of vegetarians. And nuts are emerging as nutritional superstars as scientists continue to find positive health benefits from consuming them.

Most nuts, including almonds, walnuts, pecans, peanuts and macadamias, contain heart-healthy monounsaturated and polyunsaturated fats. And other research has shown that including some of this healthy fat in your diet can be a benefit to people trying to lose weight. Some, such as walnuts, contain heart-healthy omega-3 fats, and some also contain plant chemicals that offer protection against cancers. Walnuts, for example, are an especially rich source of ellagic acid, an antioxidant that may protect against both cancer and heart disease.

Most of the studies of the health benefits of nuts look at amounts of 1 to 2 oz (30 to 60 g). Eating large amounts can quickly start to add up in the calorie department. So go nuts . . . moderately, of course!

CARBOHYDRATES: HIGH-OCTANE FUEL

How do you keep your brain sharp, your muscles energized and your body in tip-top working order? In a word, carbohydrates. Even though they've received some bad press, carbohydrates, or "carbs," are the fuel that keeps your mind and body humming.

You'll find them in breads, grains, cereal, vegetables, fruit and sweets. When they're digested, they end up as glucose.

CARBS AND WEIGHT GAIN

Myth: Eating carbohydrates will make you gain weight.

Truth: Eating too many carbohydrates or loading your bread, potatoes or pasta with fatty sauces or toppings will contribute to weight gain.

Sad truth: Portions of carbohydrate-rich foods have grown not just huge, but monstrous in recent years. One regular bagel is now equivalent to 4 or 5 slices of bread. A serving of pasta can be 2 cups (500 mL) or more, far exceeding a standard 1/2 cup (125 mL) serving. Popcorn bags are giant-sized and muffins are the size of small cakes.

Most important truth: Not all carbohydrates are the same. You have to distinguish between the complex carbohydrates in whole-grain breads and cereals, lentils, legumes and other starchy vegetables and the over-processed carbohydrates in white bread, pastries, cookies, and desserts with high sugar content. Complex carbohydrates are digested gradually and serve as a steady fuel supply, providing important vitamins, minerals and plant chemicals to nourish your body and mind.

Truth to remember: Chosen well and eaten moderately, carbohydrates are important fuel for a high-energy lifestyle.

GLYCEMIC INDEX

The Glycemic Index (GI) is a ranking of carbohydrate-containing foods according to their effect on your blood sugar after they're digested. It can be a useful tool for choosing healthy carbohydrates.

Foods can have a low GI (<55), an intermediate GI (55–70) or a high GI

(>70). There are currently over 750 published GI values of various foods.

Low GI foods, including oatmeal, oat bran, brown rice, barley, lentils, whole-grain, high-fibre breads, pumpernickel bread, bulgur, sweet potatoes, apples, berries, peas and yogurt, take longer to digest. They're absorbed more slowly by the body and so release energy more slowly, bringing about a slower, more gradual rise in blood sugar and more consistent blood sugar levels. The low GI foods are generally higher in soluble fibre.

High GI foods, such as white bread, potatoes, cookies, rice cakes, parsnips and watermelon, are more quickly absorbed, causing blood sugar to rise quickly with a potential for an over-release of insulin. Higher GI foods should generally be eaten less often.

A CARBOHYDRATE THAT RATES

That would be whole grains—not just an excellent source of sustained energy and fibre but also of valuable vitamins, minerals, antioxidants and plant chemicals linked to lowered risk of disease. As with vegetables and fruit, it's probably the whole package of nutrients that provides the health benefits.

Several important studies have shown that eating whole grains protects you from diabetes and heart disease.

Eating foods made from whole grains means you are eating all parts of the grain. This includes the outer bran layer (where most of the fibre is), the nutrient-rich germ layer, and the endosperm where the starch is. When grains are processed, all that is usually left is the endosperm, making them much less nutritious than the whole grain. Besides taking out the fibre, the processing usually takes out important nutrients. While enriched grains will have some of the goodness added back, they will never be as nutritionally complete as the original whole grain.

When shopping for whole grain breads and cereals, read labels. Wheat bread can be 100 percent or 60 percent whole wheat—100 percent is your best choice.

When a bread is labelled "multigrain," check to see what appears first in the ingredient list. If it's "enriched wheat flour," you aren't getting as much of the whole grain as you want. Wheat flour does not mean whole wheat flour, and just because a bread is brown or dark in colour doesn't mean that it is whole wheat.

Other whole grains include barley, brown rice, buckwheat groats (kasha), bulgur, kamut, spelt, oatmeal, oat bran, whole wheat pasta and millet.

CHILDHOOD OBESITY

A lot has been written about the distressing problem of childhood obesity, and it is a complex issue. Putting kids on a low-carb diet is not the solution. Kids should not be starving and they should not be on a diet so restrictive that they are deprived of essential nutrients found in many carbohydrate-rich foods. Kids need carbs for their growth and also to keep their brain and muscles well stocked with energy. Without this fuel, their ability to learn could be compromised.

Kids are not getting fat simply from eating carbs. They may be putting on weight from large portions of overly processed carbohydrate- and fat-rich foods. It is best to cut back on processed snack foods that are heavy in both fats and carbs and skip the oversized portions.

HIGH FIVE, HIGH FIBRE

Hurray for fibre!

Let's hear it for the food component that contributes so much to good health while providing almost no calories. Here's what high-fibre diets can do:

- lower risk of heart disease and some cancers
- help control blood sugar in people with diabetes
- help prevent constipation
- provide a feeling of fullness and make weight control easier.

How can you take advantage of this plant food miracle? It's simple. Make sure your diet is a high-fibre one.

Eat 5 or more servings of vegetables and fruit and 5 or more servings of whole-grain products each day. Try to reach a total of 25 to 35 g of fibre daily—that's more than the average Canadian eats now.

SOME FIBRE IS ROUGH ON YOU

Fibre comes in two forms—soluble and insoluble. Both kinds are in most plants, but some foods are richer in one or the other.

Insoluble fibre is often called roughage. It's the kind that may lower the risk of some cancers, help in weight control and prevent constipation. Add these natural packages of roughage to your shopping list: wheat bran, whole wheat products, brown rice, vegetables including carrots, broccoli and peas, and fruit such as pears.

SOME FIBRE YOUR HEART WILL LOVE

Soluble fibre helps lower cholesterol (when eaten as part of a low-fat diet) and may also help control blood sugar in people with diabetes. Find soluble fibre in lentils, legumes, oat bran, oatmeal, flax, psyllium, barley and pectin-rich fruit such as apples, strawberries and citrus fruit.

TEN TIPS FOR A HIGH-FIBRE TARGET (AND ONE CAUTION)

1. Snack on high-fibre fruit such as apples, pears, raspberries or strawberries and dried fruit such as prunes, dried apricots or raisins. Leave the skins on when possible, but wash thoroughly.

2. Include higher fibre vegetables such as corn, peas, potatoes (with skin), sweet potatoes, broccoli, Brussels sprouts, carrots and turnip. Add fibre to a sandwich with tomatoes, cucumbers, peppers, shredded carrots or dark leafy greens.

3. Seek out products high in fibre and read labels. To be labelled a "source of fibre," a product must have 2 g of fibre per serving. Products labelled a "high source of fibre" contain 4 g and if they're marked "very high source of fibre," they must contain at least 6 g.

4. Eat more whole grains. Buy 100 percent whole wheat bread.

5. Make breakfast a high-fibre opportunity. Aim to get 5 to 10 g at breakfast by eating a fibre-rich cereal, whole-grain toast, pita or bagel and fresh or dried fruit. Eat breakfast cereals with at least 2 g of fibre per serving.

6. Up your fibre by adding 1 to 2 tbsp (15 to 25 mL) of wheat bran, oat bran or ground flax to cereals, yogurt, applesauce or casseroles.

7. Choose baked goods made with whole wheat flour, bran, oatmeal, raisins, poppy seeds or sesame seeds.

8. Try lentil soups, stews or casseroles. Substitute beans for meat in casseroles and soups. Add chickpeas to pasta or green salad or refried beans to tacos and burritos.

9. Add a handful of seeds or nuts to a salad or stir-fry.

10. Use whole-grain flour for pancakes, muffins or other baked goods.

As you start to increase your fibre intake, go easy. Too much, too quickly can make you pretty uncomfortable. Start slowly and spread your fibre throughout the day. Also, be sure to drink lots of water to help the fibre do its job.

WINNING TRIO: VEGETABLES AND FRUIT, SOY AND FLAX

Vegetables and fruit are delicious, versatile and brimming with top-quality nutrition. Most are excellent sources of vitamins C and A, fibre, folic acid and potassium. Plus, they're powerful little factories for phytochemicals, plant compounds that give colour and flavour to food. But phytochemicals do more than that. They may also help to protect you from disease. Many act as antioxidants, working hard to deactivate harmful free radicals, the highly reactive molecules released when your body uses oxygen. Free radicals make a two-pronged attack on your heart. They lead to cardiovascular disease by damaging cell structures. And they combine with oxygen to form compounds that build up LDL-cholesterol. Free radicals are even implicated in certain cancers and some of the processes of aging.

Isn't it great to know you can help fight free radicals and their threat to good health simply by eating luscious berries, sweet melons, leafy green salads and even pizza?

The army of antioxidants includes vitamins C and E, selenium, carotenoids including beta-carotene, lutein and lycopene and bioflavonoids including anthocyanins. Most vegetables and fruit have more than one antioxidant and phytochemical fighter. In fact, each apple and carrot is a whole army all by itself! Blueberries, for example, are an excellent source of disease-fighting anthocyanins and also contain many vitamins and minerals as well as fibre, and sweet potatoes are packed with beta-carotene, vitamin C, potassium, folate and fibre. It's a bonus that vegetables and fruit are low in fat and usually low in calories.

Altogether, it's not surprising that research shows that populations who eat more vegetables and fruit are generally healthier.

At present, there is no clear evidence to support the widespread use of antioxidant vitamin supplements to prevent heart disease and stroke. It is food's natural mix of vitamins, minerals, plant chemicals and fibre that creates the best disease-fighting team—and this complex interplay of nutrients is not yet available in pill form.

YOUR BEST FOOD SOURCES FOR ANTIOXIDANTS AND PHYTOCHEMICALS

Vitamin C: citrus fruit and juice, kiwi, strawberries, broccoli, Brussels sprouts, peppers, potatoes, cabbage

Beta-carotene: Deep yellow, orange or green vegetables and fruit including apricots, carrots, cantaloupe, sweet potatoes, pumpkin, broccoli, dark green leafy vegetables, mangoes, red peppers and squash

Lutein: Leafy greens, peas, corn, peppers

Lycopene: tomatoes, tomato sauce, tomato paste, red grapefruit

Anthocyanins: blueberries, cherries, cranberries, plums, red grapes, blackberries

Vitamin E: vegetable oils, wheat germ, nuts, seeds, avocados

Selenium: Brazil nuts, grain products, wheat germ, wheat bran, oat bran, fish, shellfish, meat, poultry, eggs, beans

GETTING YOUR FIVE OR MORE A DAY

"Get your 5 or more servings of vegetables and fruit" is advice heard these days from most health experts.

One serving is equal to:
- any medium-sized piece of vegetable or fruit (an apple, pear, carrot)
- $1/2$ cup (125 mL) vegetable or fruit juice
- $1/2$ cup (125 mL) fresh, frozen or canned vegetables or fruit
- 1 cup (250 mL) salad
- $1/4$ cup (50 mL) dried fruit

One serving could be the tomato sauce on your pizza, a bowl of vegetable soup, the extra veggies on your sub sandwich or the dried fruit in your trail mix.

TEN WAYS TO GET YOUR FIVE OR MORE

1. For convenience, shop for cut-up, cleaned and ready-to-eat fresh vegetables: a bag of peeled and cut carrots, lettuces ready-to-mix for a salad, cherry tomatoes, celery hearts, shredded cabbage, packages of broccoli, cauliflower and other veggies cut up for a stir-fry.

2. Top your breakfast cereal with sliced berries, bananas or kiwis or dried fruit such as raisins.

3. Keep single-serving cans of unsweetened fruit for snacks at work.

4. In restaurants, order fruit as a starter or dessert.

5. Start the day with a smoothie made with yogurt, milk and a variety of fresh or frozen fruits.

6. Top your sandwich or burger with tomatoes, shredded cabbage, peppers, onions and dark greens.

7. Add extra vegetables to pasta sauce, chili, soup or stew.

8. In restaurants, order extra vegetables as a side dish or grilled vegetables as an appetizer.

9. Snack on baby carrots, pepper slices, fresh broccoli or wedges of cabbage.

10. Try one new vegetable or fruit every week.

Soy is a favourite with vegetarians—and with scientists who are finding out more and more about its health effects. So far, soy foods seem to have a beneficial effect on a variety of conditions, especially heart disease.

Soybean protein contains all of the essential amino acids, making it the only plant protein that approaches or equals animal products in providing a complete source of protein. No wonder it's a smart choice for people who have given up or reduced their intake of animal products!

Soybeans are good sources of B vitamins and potassium, zinc and other minerals. Soy is also rich in phytochemicals, including isoflavones, lignans and phytosterols, all of which have positive effects on health.

Heart health is one area where soy's benefit is well known: replacing some animal products with soy protein can help reduce the risk of heart disease. That's because, according to evidence from several studies, soy helps lower levels of LDL-cholesterol without reducing levels of the beneficial HDL-cholesterol.

Soy's role in cancer prevention is less clear. Throughout Asia, where soy has long been a dietary staple, rates of breast and prostate cancer are much lower than in Western countries. This effect is attributed, in part, to the isoflavones. However, many researchers feel that it is soy intake early in life that is protective. The evidence regarding soy and its effect on cancer rates is still inconclusive, and much more research needs to be done. People who are being treated or have been treated for breast or prostate cancer should speak to their physician before adding soy to their diet.

The bottom line on soy? It's a great source of protein, especially as an alternative to animal foods. It can help lower cholesterol levels and may help with menopausal symptoms for some women. Research in other areas continues.

FIVE WAYS TO INCREASE YOUR INTAKE OF SOY

1. Drink a glass of soy beverage or use it in a smoothie, in your latte or on cereal. It's best to buy the soy beverages fortified with calcium and vitamin D.
2. Use firm tofu in a stir-fry, grilled on the barbecue or added to pasta sauce. Try soft tofu in a dip, creamy salad dressing, as a substitute for mayonnaise or in scrambled eggs.
3. Snack on soy nuts or add them to a green salad. Have a snack of edamame or soybeans in the shell.
4. Add soy protein powder to a breakfast shake.
5. Try a soy burger or other soy meats. You'll find them in the deli or produce section of grocery stores.

Flax, traditionally known as linseed, is a tiny seed packed with healthy components just bursting to bring good things to your life. Its star is quickly rising in the world of nutrition.

Here's a profile of this up-and-comer you should get to know:

- Flax is a great source of soluble fibre that can lower cholesterol levels and thus lower heart disease risk. Studies have shown that adding flax to your diet can lower cholesterol levels by more than 5 percent.
- Flax can add healthy bulk to your diet, helping prevent constipation.
- Flax is rich in omega-3 fatty acids, which can reduce heart disease risk.
- Flax also contains phytochemicals—naturally occurring plant chemicals called lignans. These compounds act as antioxidants and also appear to counter some of the harmful effects of estrogen. Studies are looking at the role flax may play in lowering the risk of breast and colon cancer.

You can buy whole flax seeds but there is some nutritional advantage to using it in ground form. Whole flax will give you more fibre, but grinding will release more of the other healthy ingredients.

To use flax:

- Add it to cereal, muffin batters, breads, pancake mixes and cookie mixes
- Mix it with yogurt, juice or applesauce
- Sprinkle it on salads or in soups
- Add it to casseroles or meatloaf

DASH FOR HIGH BLOOD PRESSURE

It's important to keep your blood pressure under control because high blood pressure, or hypertension, is a risk factor for heart disease and stroke. Weight management and increased physical activity can help. And so can sodium reduction.

The DASH (**D**ietary **A**pproaches to **S**top **H**ypertension) diet has been shown to be an effective tool in blood pressure management. The DASH diet is rich in fruit and vegetables (8+ servings/day) and low-fat dairy products (2+ servings per day), reduced in sodium and low in total and saturated fat.

Research studies show that people with mild hypertension who followed DASH were able to achieve a reduction in their blood pressure similar to that obtained by drug treatment. While this diet is particularly beneficial to people with high blood pressure, it is in line with Canada's food guide, and it is a heart-healthy diet that anyone can follow.

Here's what DASH is all about:

- Fruit, vegetables and low-fat dairy foods.
- Whole foods rather than single nutrients and whole grains rather than refined
- Foods rich in potassium, magnesium and calcium, all nutrients that have been shown to affect blood pressure
- High-fibre, low-saturated fat and total fats.

The DASH diet recommends the following per day:

- 8 to 10 servings of fruit and vegetables. (See Portion Sizes, page 34.) This may seem like a lot, but remember that it doesn't have to be 8 to 10 different foods, and 1 cup (250 mL) of juice, cooked fruit or vegetables (which is what many people eat as a serving at a meal) is 2 servings. Two per meal and a couple as snacks will get you to 8 easily. These are the foods that provide potassium, magnesium and fibre.
- 2 to 3 servings of low-fat dairy foods. One serving is a glass of milk, 1 cup (250 mL) of yogurt or 1½ oz (45 g) of low-fat cheese. These foods are major sources of calcium.
- 7 to 8 servings of whole grains. One serving is a slice of whole wheat bread, 1 oz (30 g) dry cereal, ½ cup (125 mL) of cooked rice, pasta or cereal. The emphasis here is on whole grains.
- Meat, fish and poultry should be lean, portions should be smaller and they should be cooked in ways that further reduce fat such as broiling, baking, roasting.
- Added fats should be used minimally and should include those that are heart friendly such as olive oil or canola oil.
- 4 to 5 servings per week of nuts, seeds and dry beans are also suggested. A serving is ⅓ cup (75 mL) or 1½ oz (45 g) nuts or 2 tbsp (25 mL) seeds or ½ cup (125 mL) cooked dry beans.

The DASH diet restricts:

- Sodium. The stuff in the salt shaker. We've known for a long time that reducing salt intake can be an effective way for some people to lower their blood pressure.

The sodium part of the salt is the culprit. Sodium is also found in MSG (monosodium glutamate), garlic salt or other seasoned salts, sea salt, meat tenderizers, commercially prepared sauces and condiments like ketchup, soy sauce, chili sauce and steak sauce, bouillon cubes, dried soup mixes, instant soups, cured or smoked foods, olives and pickles. In general, the more processed a food is, the higher the sodium content.

To reduce sodium:

- Use flavourings that don't contain sodium, such as fresh or dried herbs, garlic powder or fresh garlic, onion flakes (instead of onion salt), dry mustard, lemon, spices such as ground coriander, cumin, chili powder and curry powder, ginger, hot peppers and pepper.
- Make your own salad dressings rather than using the bottled ones, and try using flavoured vinegars instead of adding salt.
- Eat more fresh or frozen fruit and vegetables. If you use canned vegetables, buy sodium-reduced products. Use fresh potatoes rather than instant, fresh cucumbers instead of pickles. Omit

---

B VITAMINS

Folic acid, and vitamins B6 and B12 play a role in lowering heart disease risk by helping to regulate homocysteine levels in your body. Homocysteine is a protein substance found in your blood. Some evidence suggests that high levels damage the lining of the artery walls potentially leading to a build-up of plaque and increasing risk of heart attack or stroke.

- The best food sources of folic acid are dark green leafy vegetables (such as broccoli, spinach, romaine lettuce, peas and Brussels sprouts), orange juice, liver, dried peas and beans. White flour, enriched pasta and enriched cornmeal are now fortified with folic acid.
- Vitamin B6 is abundant in whole grains and cereals, bananas, lentils, beans, meat, fish, poultry, nuts and soybeans.
- Vitamin B12 is plentiful in all animal products—meat, fish, poultry, dairy and eggs. People who avoid all animal products or people who have a particular anaemia with an inability to absorb B12 from the intestinal tract may have concerns about a deficiency. Also, between 10 percent and 30 percent of older adults lose their ability to adequately absorb the naturally occurring form of B12 found in food. These people should meet most of their recommended intake with synthetic B12 from fortified foods or supplements. Some soy products are fortified with B12 but most aren't, so you have to read labels carefully. It is also found in some brands of nutritional yeast.

This doesn't mean that you should abandon your lower fat diet and substitute these vitamins as a way to lower heart disease risk. But there is evidence that the two dietary strategies—eating a lower fat, high-fibre diet with adequate intakes of the three B vitamins—work together as a healthy route to heart health.

salt from the cooking water when you are boiling pasta, rice or vegetables.

- Eat fresh or frozen fish instead of canned or dried varieties; choose sliced roast beef or chicken instead of bologna, salami or other processed meats.
- Retrain your taste buds. Taste food before adding salt. Cook from scratch instead of packages. Try using half the amount of salt specified in your favourite recipes.

VITAMIN E

Most people associate vitamin E with lowered risk of heart disease but this relationship may not be a strong one. The Heart Outcomes Prevention Evaluation study (HOPE) followed, for over 4 years, almost 10,000 people who were at high risk for heart attack or stroke. The people in the study who received a supplement of 400 IU of vitamin E daily (in comparison to those who received a placebo) did not seem to decrease their risk of heart disease. The study was extended for another 4 years as the HOPE-TOO (HOPE—The Ongoing Outcomes) study. Again they found that E had no impact on fatal and nonfatal cancers, major cardiovascular events or death.

An editorial in the Journal of the American Medical Association says that this closes the door on the prospect of a major protective effect of long-term exposure to this supplement, taken in moderately high doses, against complications of atherosclerosis and overall cancer.

While this research suggests there is no benefit in taking large amounts of E supplements, it does not negate the importance of including healthy amounts of vitamin E–rich foods in your diet. The best food sources of E are oils (especially safflower, sunflower, canola, olive, soybean), almonds, peanuts, sunflower seeds, avocado, wheat germ, wheat germ oil and peanut butter.

VEGETARIAN DIET

A study from the University of Toronto suggests that a low-fat vegetarian diet may be just as good as certain drugs at lowering high cholesterol levels. A group of adults with high cholesterol levels were put on either a low saturated fat diet, the same diet plus medication or a strict vegetarian diet that included soy proteins, high-fibre foods such as oats, barley and psyllium, fruit and vegetables such as eggplant and okra, nuts (especially almonds) and a special margarine containing plant sterols (also found in leafy green vegetables and vegetable oils). The researchers found that the people on the vegetarian diet lowered their cholesterol by almost 29 percent compared with a decrease of 30 percent in those who followed the low-fat diet with medication during that same time. The positive results of this study underline the importance of diet and exercise as an option for people working to lower cholesterol levels. There are a number of dietary factors in the vegetarian diet that help lower cholesterol: the soy protein, the plant sterols and the soluble fibre found in fruit, vegetables and grains such as oats and barley.

While this research is promising, it doesn't mean you should stop your medical therapy in favour of a vegetarian diet. Discuss this with your physician and dietitian to decide your best prescription for heart health.

WEIGHTY MATTER

Being overweight increases your risk of high cholesterol, high blood pressure and diabetes—all significant risk factors for heart disease. There's really no question about that.

The big question? How to lose weight.

Nobody says it's easy.

But first, let's establish what a healthy weight looks like and feels like—because weight is more than just a number. A healthy weight is the one you can maintain without starving, by eating foods that you enjoy and that are good for you.

To get there, to lose weight and to eat healthier meals, requires a commitment.

The right time to start is when you're ready to make changes that are healthier for you—and not because it's a new year or you think it will change other areas of your life.

Above all, be patient. Losing weight is a process, sometimes a long one. It took time to gain weight and it will take time to lose it.

A loss of 1 to 2 lb (5 to 1 kg) a week is healthy and realistic.

Start slowly:

Put margarine or butter on only one slice of bread in your sandwich. Use mustard instead of mayonnaise. Take the skin off your chicken. Buy 1 percent yogurt instead of 4 percent. Fry without oil or with less oil by using a non-stick pan. Use a sweet-flavoured vinegar instead of oil on your salad.

Small, realistic changes like these will add up and subtract pounds.

Think about why you're eating. If it's for reasons other than hunger, start to explore this.

Look for activities and strategies that help curb the urge to overeat. Learn your hunger patterns and emotional triggers (stress, boredom, a hard day at the office or a fight with your partner). Rearrange your eating schedule so that you eat often enough to avoid intense hunger, and find different ways to deal with other triggers.

Identify your good habits. Perhaps you already eat lots of vegetables and fruit, or you already eat a good breakfast every morning. Strengthen these habits and add new ones to the list.

Active living is an excellent partner in a weight-loss routine.

Find an activity you enjoy. It doesn't have to be aerobics or working out at the gym.

Consider walking the dog, dancing, cross-country skiing, skating, or even taking a break at the office and walking briskly around the building. You might enjoy using a pedometer to keep track of how much you move each day.

Try to increase the number of times or the length of time that you're physically active.

Exercise helps you feel better physically and mentally.

For more information on appropriate activities, refer to Canada's Guide to Physical Activity, available from your local Heart and Stroke Foundation office and www.paguide.com. Also visit http://www.heartandstroke.ca/healthyweight

MANAGING DIABETES

Beyond the Basics: Meal Planning for Healthy Eating, Diabetes Prevention and Management is the new meal-planning guide for healthy eating and diabetes prevention and management. *Beyond the Basics* is designed to make it easier for health professionals to assist consumers in including a variety of foods at mealtimes while keeping carbohydrate intake fairly consistent.

If you have diabetes or are at risk for diabetes, meet with a Registered Dietitian or Certified Diabetes Educator to develop your individual healthy eating plan.

Use food labels and the nutrient analysis provided for the recipes in this book to estimate the size of 1 carbohydrate choice.

You can obtain a copy of the *Beyond the Basics* meal-planning guide by visiting your local Diabetes Education Centre or health professional.

THE BEYOND THE BASICS CHART CAN HELP GUIDE YOUR MENU CHOICES

FOOD GROUPS	SERVING SIZE	NUTRIENTS	KCAL (APPROXIMATE)
Grains & Starches (includes corn, potatoes and yams)	1 slice of bread or 1/2 an English muffin or a portion up to the size of your fist	15 g carbohydrate 3 g protein 0 g fat	70
Fruit	1 fresh fruit or 1/2 cup (125 mL) of canned fruit up to the size of your fist	15 g carbohydrate 1 g protein 0 g fat	65
Milk & Alternatives (includes soy beverages)	Drink up to 1 cup (250 mL) of low-fat milk with a meal.	15 g carbohydrate 8 g protein variable fat	Skim—90 1%—110 2%—130 Whole—140
Other Choices (includes a variety of sweet and snack foods)	See Nutrition Facts Table (page 32)	15 g carbohydrate variable fat and protein	Variable
Vegetables (parsnips, peas & winter squash provide 15 g carbohydrate/cup)	Choose as much as you can hold in both hands	<5 g carbohydrate** 2 g protein 0 g fat	30
Meat & Alternatives	Choose an amount up to the size of the palm of your hand and the thickness of your little finger. (This would be a 3–4 oz/90–120 g serving.)	0 g carbohydrate 7 g protein 3–5 g fat	55–75
Fats	Limit fat to an amount the size of the tip of your thumb.	0 g carbohydrate 0 g protein 5 g fat	50
Extras (coffee, tea, diet soda, vinegar, mustard and other condiments)		< 5 g carbohydrate*	<20

* This chart has been adapted from information available on www.diabetes.ca

** Less than 5 g carbohydrate foods are considered carbohydrate free

LABELS AND TABLES

Canada has revised its food labels to help you make informed choices consistent with your personal health goals. The nutrition label on pre-packaged foods is now mandatory, has a consistent look, includes more detailed nutrient information and is on more foods.

WHAT'S ON A LABEL?

The Ingredient List: Items are listed in descending order by weight, with the ingredient present in the largest amount listed first. The list can alert you to ingredients to which you might be allergic as well as to indicate the presence of whole grains, the sources of salt/sodium, and the kinds of fat in the product.

The Nutrition Facts Table: The core label will provide information on serving size, calories, total fat, saturated fat, trans fat, cholesterol, sodium, carbohydrate, fibre, sugars, protein, vitamin A, vitamin C, calcium and iron. Nutrients will be described as % Daily Value. The Daily Values for vitamins and minerals are based on the Recommended Nutrient Intakes for Canadians and represent the highest recommendation for each age/sex group, not including needs for pregnancy and lactation.

The addition of trans fats to the labels will make it much easier to assess whether a food is heart healthy.

Nutrient Content Claims: Claims such as "low calorie" or "low in saturated fat" highlight a particular nutritional feature of the product. There are strict criteria that must be met for these claims to appear. For example "fat free" means that the product is free of fat (less than 0.5 g of fat per reference amount and per stated serving of food). The claim is optional.

Health Claims: In addition to the list of nutrients, manufacturers are now allowed to put certain health claims on food products. The claim can associate a nutrient in that food with a diet-related disease or health condition. The following diet-related claims are permitted:

- A healthy diet low in sodium and high in potassium may reduce the risk of high blood pressure.
- A healthy diet adequate in calcium and vitamin D may reduce the risk of osteoporosis.
- A healthy diet low in saturated fats and trans fats may reduce the risk of heart disease.

Nutrition Facts		
Per 125 mL (87 g)		
Amount		% Daily Value
Calories 80		
Fat 0.5 g		1 %
Saturated 0 g		
+ Trans 0 g		0 %
Cholesterol 0 mg		
Sodium 0 mg		0 %
Carbohydrate 18 g		6 %
Fibre 2 g		8 %
Sugars 2 g		
Protein 3 g		
Vitamin A 2 %	Vitamin C	10 %
Calcium 0 %	Iron	2 %

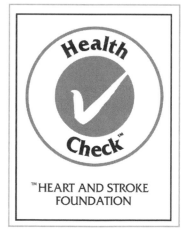

™HEART AND STROKE FOUNDATION

- A healthy diet rich in vegetables and fruit may reduce risk of certain cancers.

Health Check™: This is a food information program, brought to you by the Heart and Stroke Foundation, which will help you make wise food choices. The Health Check™ symbol on a food product means that the product's nutrition information has been reviewed and meets established nutrition criteria. Every food product involved in the program has an explanatory message describing how the food is part of a healthy diet, a Nutrition Facts table and the very recognizable Health Check™ symbol. There are different criteria for each food category, depending on the important nutrition components of that food. For example, the criteria for lean ground beef focuses on the amount of fat.

SOME SHOPPING TIPS

Here are a few tips to help ensure your cupboards are stocked with healthy foods:

- Plan ahead. Shop from a list that you made when you weren't hungry.
- Get the family involved in meal planning by having them contribute to your shopping list.
- Set a weekly routine time for shopping, with quick stops in between for perishables such as milk, fruit, vegetables, meat, fish and poultry.
- Buy seasonal, locally grown foods. They should be fresher and cheaper.
- Use the Nutrition Facts Table to help you select lower fat foods.
- Nutrition information is given per serving, so it is important to know exactly what the serving size is. If you eat more or less than the stated serving size, remember to reduce or increase the calories, fat, fibre and sodium you actually consume.
- Watch for store specials and plan meals around them.
- Think good nutritional thoughts when shopping. For example, buy whole-grain breads, brown rice, higher fibre breakfast cereals, lower fat muffin mixes, whole wheat flour for baking, lower fat crackers and cookies.
- Spend some time in the produce section. Select lots of dark green and orange vegetables and orange fruit.

- Buy the leanest meat products. These include:
  - Beef: Eye of round, inside and outside round; sirloin tip, sirloin roasts and steaks; rib eye steaks; stewing beef; tenderloin; flank steak; lean and extra-lean ground beef
  - Pork: ham; leg roasts and cutlets; tenderloin cuts; centre-cut chops and roasts; picnic shoulder; shoulder butt
  - Lamb: leg roast; loin chops
  - Veal: all cuts
  - Poultry: all cuts without skin
  - Deli meats: ham, turkey roll or pastrami, beef pastrami
- Visit the fish counter and try something new.
- When buying canned products, choose those that are labelled "low in sodium," "low in salt," "sodium free," or "salt free."

EATING OUT

Here are some tips on eating healthily when you're dining out:
- Ask questions. The restaurant staff should be able to answer questions about how the food is prepared and to make simple adjustments, such as leaving off sauces and dressings.
- Choose items that are baked, barbecued, stir-fried, broiled, grilled, poached or steamed.
- Order sauces and dressings on the side.
- Choose a restaurant where the style of food fits the diet that you're following. It's easier, for instance, to order a low-fat meal in a Japanese restaurant than it is in a steak house. The same Japanese meal, however, may supply much more sodium, making it an unwise choice for someone on a low-salt diet.
- Call ahead to ask about the day's specials so you can decide on your entrée in advance; you'll be less tempted to overindulge if you've already made up your mind about what you want. At the same time, if you are on a restricted diet, ask if there are menu items that are suitable. Most restaurants will accommodate such requests, especially if they have advance notice.
- To avoid overeating, pass up the fixed-price menu and select from the à la carte menu.
- Remember, you are the customer. Ask for what you want and don't be afraid to send it back if it's not just right. If you don't know what a menu item contains, ask.

- If the portion sizes are large, share a main course with a friend. Or order appetizer portions. Another option is to take the remainder home in a doggie bag.
- Check on the availability of foods that may not appear on the menu, like lower-fat milk, fresh fruit, lower-fat salad dressing.

PORTION SIZES

You may be constantly hearing that you should eat 1 or 2 servings of this or that, but if you're like most people, you have no idea what a serving actually is. So let's clear up the confusion with the help of a measuring cup, your hand and a few other props.

- A serving of vegetables and fruit is 1 piece of fresh fruit (about the size of a tennis ball) or vegetable—an orange, tomato, carrot, apple or pear.
- One serving is a small baked potato about the size of your fist, as is 1 cup (250 mL) of salad.
- One serving is also 1/2 cup (125 mL) of cooked vegetables or fruit (half of your fist) or 1/2 cup (125 mL) of juice.
- A 3 oz (90 g) serving of cooked meat, fish or chicken is about the size of your palm, a cassette tape or a deck of cards.
- One serving is also one egg, 1/2 can of fish, a small chicken leg and thigh or breast, 2 tbsp (25 mL) peanut butter (the size of a ping-pong ball), 1/3 cup (75 mL) of tofu or 1/2 cup (125 mL) of beans.
- A 1/2-cup (125 mL) serving of cereal, rice, noodles or pasta is about half a fistful. One cup (250 mL) of rice or pasta is about the size of a tennis ball or a whole fistful.

It's a good idea to actually measure out a cupful of some foods once or twice so you can see what a serving looks like. At the same time, you may want to measure how much your favourite soup bowl or dessert dish holds. For example, measure out the amount of cereal you put in your morning bowlful and then you will know if you are eating one, two or three portions. You may also discover that your pasta portion is the equivalent of 4 or 5 servings or that your regular drinking glass is 10 to 12 oz (300 to 350 mL) and your morning glass of juice is really 3 servings of fruit.

ALCOHOL

Chances are you have heard a lot about how alcohol may protect your heart. You also know of the many personal and social problems linked to alcohol and the dangers of excessive alcohol use.

Excessive alcohol is associated with elevated triglycerides (a type of fat in the blood) and high blood pressure, risk factors for heart disease and stroke.

However, there is some evidence that drinking moderate amounts of alcohol may lower the overall risk of heart disease and stroke. There are a number of theories as to why, including alcohol's ability to raise HDL-cholesterol and to reduce the formation of potentially harmful blood clots. It appears that any alcohol—red wine, white wine, spirits or beer—may have this effect, but some researchers believe it to be particularly true for red wine. They attribute this to polyphenols—compounds with antioxidant properties thought to prevent plaque build-up on artery walls.

Most experts suggest that 1 drink a day will do little harm even though the benefits may still be the subject of debate. For those healthy adults who drink alcohol, consumption should not exceed 2 drinks a day with a weekly limit of 14 drinks for men and 9 drinks for women. A standard drink is 12 oz (341 mL) of 5 percent beer, 5 oz (142 mL) of wine and 1¹/₂ oz (43 mL) of 40 percent spirits. More is definitely not better and if you don't drink now, this is no reason to start. The consensus is that the protective effects, if any, disappear with increased intake.

ABOUT THE NUTRIENT ANALYSIS

Computer-assisted calculation of the nutrient values was carried out by Food Intelligence (Toronto, Ontario) and Info Access (1988) Inc. (Don Mills, Ontario). The primary database was the Canadian Nutrient File, supplemented when necessary with information from other reliable sources. Values are rounded to whole numbers; amounts less than 0.5 appear as trace.

The calculations were based on
- imperial amounts unless a metric quantity would typically be purchased and used;
- smaller number of servings (larger portion) when there was a range;
- smaller ingredient quantity when there was a range; and
- first ingredient listed when there was a choice.

Canola vegetable oil, 1 percent milk and unsalted stocks were used. Optional ingredients and those in non-specific quantities were not included.

Nutritional labelling criteria (2003 Guide to Food Labelling and Advertising, Canadian Food Inspection Agency) were applied to recipe servings to identify excellent or good sources of vitamin A, thiamine, riboflavin, niacin, vitamin B6, vitamin B12, folate, vitamin C, calcium and iron. An excellent source provides 25 percent of the Daily Value for a nutrient (50 percent for vitamin C), and a good source provides 15 percent (30 percent for vitamin C).

Hummos with Sauteed Chickpeas and Zhoug
Black Bean and Corn Spread
Hummos with Butternut
Hummos with Sesame
Caramelized Onion Dip with Roasted Potatoes
Asian Eggplant Salsa
Guacamole
Tzatziki
Goat Cheese Dip with Potatoes
Creamy Salsa
White Bean and Roasted Garlic Spread
Roasted Butternut Spread
Smoked Trout Spread
Moroccan Cooked Tomato Salsa
Shrimp and Asparagus Sushi Rolls
Smoked Salmon Sushi Pizza
Roasted Tomato and Garlic Bruschetta
Bruschetta with Uncooked Tomato Salsa
Chickpea Bruschetta

Wild Mushroom Bruschetta with Goat Cheese
Ricotta Bruschetta
Asparagus Tarts with Goat Cheese
Smoked Salmon Tortilla Spirals
Grilled Tuna Satays with Sweet Mango Dipping Sauce
Corn Pancakes with Spicy Salsa
Grilled Shrimp Martinis
Grilled Tuna Tartare with Avocado
Grilled Shrimp Salad Rolls
Chicken Satays with Peanut Sauce
Naked Chicken Dumplings with Sweet and Sour Sauce
Asian Chicken Pot Stickers

HEART
SMART

APPETIZERS

HUMMOS WITH SAUTEED CHICKPEAS AND ZHOUG

My Israeli friend Hanoch Drori once described a hummos like this, and it sounded so good that I came up with this recipe. It is garnished with whole chickpeas and spicy zhoug (similar to a cilantro pesto), though you can omit the garnish if you prefer a classic hummos. Serve with whole wheat pita or pita chips (page 49).

Makes 1 1/2 cups (375 mL)

1 19-oz (540 mL) can chickpeas, rinsed and drained, or 2 cups
    (500 mL) cooked chickpeas
3 cloves garlic, coarsely chopped
1/4 cup (50 mL) lemon juice
2 tbsp (25 mL) tahina
1/2 tsp (2 mL) ground cumin
1/2 tsp (2 mL) salt
1/3 cup (75 mL) water, approx.
1/4 tsp (1 mL) hot red pepper sauce, optional

Sauteed Chickpeas

1 tsp (5 mL) olive oil
2 cloves garlic, finely chopped
1/4 cup (50 mL) cooked chickpeas from above
1/4 tsp (1 mL) ground cumin
1/4 tsp (1 mL) salt

Zhoug

1 clove garlic, coarsely chopped
1/2 jalapeño, seeded and coarsely chopped
1/2 cup (125 mL) packed fresh cilantro
1/2 tsp (2 mL) salt
1/4 tsp (1 mL) ground cardamom
1/4 tsp (1 mL) ground cumin
2 tbsp (25 mL) olive oil

1. Reserve about 1/4 cup (50 mL) chickpeas for garnish. In a food processor, combine remaining chickpeas, garlic, lemon juice, tahina, cumin and salt. Puree. Add water until mixture is creamy and smooth but still thick enough to spread. Season with hot pepper sauce. Taste and adjust seasonings.

TAHINA
Tahina is a paste made from ground sesame seeds. It has tremendous flavour but a high fat content. You can buy it in health food stores, Middle Eastern markets and many supermarkets. Use it in small quantities, and store it in the refrigerator.

PER TBSP (15 ML)	
Calories	28
Protein	1 g
Fat	1 g
Saturates	trace
Cholesterol	0 mg
Carbohydrate	3 g
Fibre	1 g
Sodium	69 mg
Potassium	38 mg

2. To prepare sauteed chickpeas, heat oil in a small skillet on medium heat. Add garlic, chickpeas, cumin and salt. Cook for 2 minutes.

3. To prepare zhoug, in a food processor, chop garlic and jalapeño. Add cilantro and puree. Add salt, cardamon and cumin. Blend in oil. Add a little water if mixture is too thick to drizzle.

4. Spread hummos on a serving plate. Spoon sauteed chickpeas on centre of hummos. Drizzle zhoug to taste around chickpeas.

BLACK BEAN AND CORN SPREAD

This makes a delicious dip or sandwich spread. Other beans such as red kidney beans or chickpeas could be used instead of the black beans. The tortillas can also be baked (page 49).

Makes about 2 to 2 ½ cups (500 to 625 mL)

1 19-oz (540 mL) can black beans, rinsed and drained, or 2 cups (500 mL) cooked beans
2 tbsp (25 mL) olive oil
2 tbsp (25 mL) lemon juice
2 tbsp (25 mL) yogurt cheese (page 391) or light mayonnaise
1 tbsp (15 mL) chipotle puree (page 183), or 1 jalapeño, seeded and finely chopped
2 tsp (10 mL) ground cumin
1 cup (250 mL) corn kernels
¼ cup (50 mL) chopped fresh cilantro, divided
Salt and pepper to taste
8 10-inch (25 cm) whole wheat or regular flour tortillas

1. In a food processor, combine beans, oil, lemon juice, yogurt cheese, chipotle and cumin. Blend until smooth or slightly chunky.

2. Partially blend or stir in corn and half the cilantro. Taste and add salt and pepper if necessary.

3. Grill tortillas on both sides until lightly browned. Cut into wedges.

4. Sprinkle dip with remaining cilantro and serve with grilled tortilla chips.

PER TBSP (15 ML) WITH 1/4 TORTILLA	
Calories	73
Protein	3 g
Fat	2 g
Saturates	trace
Cholesterol	0 mg
Carbohydrate	11 g
Fibre	2 g
Sodium	77 mg
Potassium	88 mg

HUMMOS WITH BUTTERNUT

Here's a delicious variation of hummos. Butternut squash is richly flavoured and has a drier texture than most squash, and as a bonus you can often find it peeled and precut. But if you are in a hurry, use 2 cups (500 mL) diced frozen squash and simmer for 5 minutes instead of roasting. You could also add 1 or 2 minced garlic cloves or 1 head roasted garlic (page 67). Serve this with pita or tortilla chips (page 49).

Makes about 3 cups (750 mL)

1 lb (500 g) peeled butternut or buttercup squash, cut in 2-inch
    (5 cm) chunks (about 4 cups/1 L)
1 tsp (5 mL) chopped fresh rosemary, or ¼ tsp (1 mL) dried
2 tbsp (25 mL) olive oil, divided
1 19-oz (540 mL) can chickpeas, rinsed and drained, or 2 cups
    (500 mL) cooked chickpeas
2 tbsp (25 mL) lemon juice
1 tsp (5 mL) ground cumin
¼ tsp (1 mL) hot red pepper sauce
Salt and pepper to taste

1. In a large bowl, toss squash with rosemary and 1 tbsp (15 mL) oil.
2. Spread squash on a baking sheet lined with parchment paper and roast in a preheated 400°F (200°C) oven for 40 minutes, or until tender and browned. Cool.
3. In a food processor, chop chickpeas finely. Add lemon juice, remaining 1 tbsp (15 mL) oil, cumin and hot pepper sauce. Combine well.
4. Add roasted squash and puree until smooth. Add salt and pepper if necessary. (If mixture is too thick, add a little yogurt or water to thin.)

Hummos with Roasted Red Peppers

Instead of squash, use 2 roasted, peeled, seeded and diced sweet red peppers (page 146).

Devilled Eggs with Hummos

Use hummos as a filling for devilled eggs. Shell hard-cooked eggs, cut in half and remove yolks. Pipe or spoon hummos into egg whites. Garnish with whole chickpeas and sprinkle with paprika.

CHICKPEAS

Chickpeas are delicious in dips, soups, salads and grain dishes.

I usually soak dried chickpeas in water overnight in the refrigerator and then cook them for 1½ hours, or until tender. But canned chickpeas are a good substitute; they retain more of their texture than other canned beans. I always keep a can of chickpeas on hand to make a last-minute appetizer like hummos, to add protein, fibre and flavour to a salad or soup, or just to eat as a snack.

PER TBSP (15 mL)	
Calories	20
Protein	1 g
Fat	1 g
Saturates	0 g
Cholesterol	0 mg
Carbohydrate	3 g
Fibre	0 g
Sodium	18 mg
Potassium	41 mg

HUMMOS WITH SESAME

I love this dip because it can be made in a minute with ingredients from the cupboard (it uses sesame oil instead of tahina). If you find it too thick, just thin with a little yogurt (or water). Serve it as a dip with pita bread or crackers or use it instead of mayonnaise in sandwiches.

Makes about 1½ cups (375 mL)

1 19-oz (540 mL) can chickpeas, rinsed and drained, or
      2 cups (500 mL) cooked chickpeas
2 cloves garlic, coarsely chopped
3 tbsp (45 mL) lemon juice
1 tbsp (15 mL) olive oil, optional
1 tbsp (15 mL) dark sesame oil
½ tsp (2 mL) ground cumin
½ tsp (2 mL) hot red pepper sauce
2 tbsp (25 mL) chopped fresh cilantro or parsley
Lemon slices

1. In a food processor, chop chickpeas coarsely.
2. Add garlic, lemon juice, olive oil, sesame oil, cumin and hot pepper sauce. Puree until smooth. Taste and adjust seasonings if necessary.
3. Garnish with cilantro and lemon slices.

PER TBSP (15 mL)	
Calories	27
Protein	1 g
Fat	1 g
Saturates	trace
Cholesterol	0 mg
Carbohydrate	4 g
Fibre	1 g
Sodium	18 mg
Potassium	41 mg

CARAMELIZED ONION DIP WITH ROASTED POTATOES

This is a fresher version of the old favourite, onion soup mix dip with potato chips. Place the dip in a bowl and surround with potatoes on a bed of parsley. Serve the potatoes with toothpicks or rosemary sprigs. (The potatoes can be prepared ahead; they taste great at room temperature.)

You can use sweet potato chunks in this recipe instead of regular potatoes. This would also make a great potato salad; use the dip as the dressing.

Makes 8 servings

2 lb (1 kg) Yukon Gold or baking potatoes, peeled
3 tbsp (45 mL) olive oil, divided
1 tbsp (15 mL) chopped fresh rosemary, or ½ tsp (2 mL) dried
½ tsp (2 mL) salt
¼ tsp (1 mL) pepper
2 large Spanish onions (about 12 oz/375 g each), chopped
1 cup (250 mL) yogurt cheese (page 391) or thick unflavoured
      low-fat yogurt

1. Cut potatoes into 1-inch (2.5 cm) chunks (or use whole or halved unpeeled baby potatoes). In a large bowl, toss potatoes with 2 tbsp (25 mL) oil, rosemary, salt and pepper.
2. Spread potatoes in a single layer on a large baking sheet lined with parchment paper. Roast in a preheated 400°F (200°C) oven for 45 to 50 minutes, or until brown and tender.
3. Meanwhile, in a large non-stick skillet, heat remaining 1 tbsp (15 mL) oil on medium-high heat. Add onions but do not stir until they begin to brown. Reduce heat to medium, stir and then leave onions alone again until they are brown on bottom. Then cook, stirring often, until onions are very brown, about 20 to 25 minutes. (If they begin to burn or stick, add a little water.) Cool completely.
4. Combine onions with yogurt cheese. Taste and adjust seasonings if necessary. Serve dip with roasted potatoes.

PER SERVING	
Calories	178
Protein	5 g
Fat	6 g
Saturates	1 g
Cholesterol	3 mg
Carbohydrate	27 g
Fibre	2 g
Sodium	176 mg
Potassium	486 mg
Good: Vitamin B6;	
Vitamin B12	

ASIAN EGGPLANT SALSA

People may think they don't like eggplant, but everyone seems to love this. The long skinny Asian eggplants are less bitter than the large ones.

Serve this with rice crackers or sesame crackers.

Makes about 2 cups (500 mL)
1 ½ lb (750 g) thin Asian eggplants (5 or 6)
2 tbsp (25 mL) soy sauce
2 tbsp (25 mL) brown sugar
2 tbsp (25 mL) water
1 tbsp (15 mL) rice vinegar
1 tsp (5 mL) dark sesame oil
½ tsp (2 mL) hot Asian chili paste
2 tsp (10 mL) olive oil
4 cloves garlic, finely chopped
1 tbsp (15 mL) finely chopped fresh ginger root
4 green onions, chopped
3 tbsp (45 mL) chopped fresh cilantro, divided

1. Trim eggplants and dice.
2. Combine soy sauce, sugar, water, vinegar, sesame oil and chili paste.
3. Heat olive oil in a large, deep non-stick skillet or wok on medium heat. Add garlic and ginger and cook for 30 seconds, or until fragrant. Add diced eggplant and cook for a few minutes.
4. Add soy sauce mixture and bring to a boil. Cover, reduce heat and simmer for 10 minutes, stirring every few minutes.
5. Uncover and continue to cook, stirring, until mixture is thick. Add green onions and 2 tbsp (25 mL) cilantro. Cook for another minute. Sprinkle remaining cilantro on top just before serving. Serve cold or at room temperature.

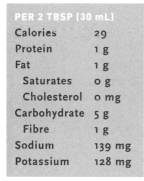

PER 2 TBSP (30 mL)	
Calories	29
Protein	1 g
Fat	1 g
Saturates	0 g
Cholesterol	0 mg
Carbohydrate	5 g
Fibre	1 g
Sodium	139 mg
Potassium	128 mg

GUACAMOLE

Many people have never tasted homemade guacamole, because most restaurants buy prepared mixtures from California. But the real thing is much better.

A few years ago people wouldn't touch avocados because they were high in fat. But now that they are recognized as being a source of "good" fat, they have become extremely popular again. Just don't eat too much—it's easy for a bowl of guacamole to disappear quickly.

Serve the guacamole as a dip with baked corn tortilla chips (page 49) or soft fresh flour or corn tortillas. Or use it as a topping for burgers, burritos, sandwiches, salads, grilled meats or fish.

Add the avocado just before serving to keep the colour bright. Or, if you want to make the guacamole an hour in advance, just add extra lime juice.

Makes about 1 cup (250 mL)

1 plum tomato, seeded and diced
1 small jalapeño, seeded and finely chopped
⅓ cup (75 mL) chopped fresh cilantro
1 tbsp (15 mL) lime juice, or more to taste
½ tsp (2 mL) salt
1 ripe avocado

1. Combine tomato, jalapeño, cilantro, lime juice and salt. (This can be done ahead.)
2. Just before serving, cut avocado in half, remove pit and dice. Add to tomato mixture and mash in with a potato masher. Mixture can be as smooth or as chunky as you wish. Taste and adjust seasonings, adding salt and/or lime juice if necessary. If not serving immediately, place plastic wrap directly on surface of guacamole to prevent discolouration.

Creamy Avocado Spread

Mash 1 cup (250 mL) light ricotta cheese into guacamole.

AVOCADOS

I try to buy the small, wrinkled, dark green Haas avocados. They are more dense and "buttery" than other varieties.

It is hard to find ripe avocados the day you need them, so buy them a few days ahead. Keep perfectly ripe avocados in the refrigerator.

Unripe ones can be left on the counter out of direct sunlight; they should ripen in two to three days. Dely Balagtas, who works with me at the cooking school, places them in a bag of rice, and they are usually ready in a day.

PER TBSP (15 mL)	
Calories	17
Protein	0 g
Fat	2 g
Saturates	trace
Cholesterol	0 mg
Carbohydrate	1 g
Fibre	1 g
Sodium	75 mg
Potassium	73 mg

CUTTING AN AVOCADO

Cut the avocado in half lengthwise. Gently rotate the two halves back and forth until you can separate them. To remove the pit, press the long side of a knife blade into the pit and gently wiggle the pit until it comes free.

To dice, hold a pitted avocado half in the palm of your hand skin side down and cut the avocado flesh in a cross-hatch pattern without cutting through the skin. Then scoop out the diced flesh.

To prevent a cut avocado from darkening, sprinkle the cut side with lemon juice or lime juice and cover tightly with plastic wrap.

PER TBSP (15 ML)	
Calories	13
Protein	1 g
Fat	trace
Saturates	trace
Cholesterol	1 mg
Carbohydrate	2 g
Fibre	trace
Sodium	82 mg
Potassium	54 mg

TZATZIKI

This is a popular concoction that can be used as a dip, spread or as a sauce for grilled chicken, lamb or fish (it is particularly good in pita sandwiches). Use less garlic if you are faint of heart, and peel and seed the cucumber if you wish. Salting the cucumber draws out excess liquid and prevents the dip from becoming watery.

If you like extra-thick tzatziki, drain your yogurt cheese overnight before serving.

Makes about 2 cups (500 mL)

1 English cucumber
1 tsp (5 mL) salt
1 1/2 cups (375 mL) yogurt cheese (page 391) or thick unflavoured
    low-fat yogurt
4 cloves garlic, minced
2 tbsp (25 mL) chopped fresh dill
1/4 tsp (1 mL) hot red pepper sauce, optional

1. Grate cucumber and combine with salt in a sieve. Set sieve over a bowl and allow to rest for 15 minutes. Rinse cucumber well, wrap in a tea towel and press out excess liquid.
2. Combine yogurt cheese, garlic, dill and hot pepper sauce.
3. Stir in cucumber. Taste and adjust seasonings if necessary.

Grilled Chicken in Pita with Tzatziki

In a large bowl, combine 1 tbsp (15 mL) olive oil, 2 minced cloves garlic, 1 tbsp (15 mL) chopped fresh oregano, 1 tbsp (15 mL) grated lemon peel, 3/4 tsp (4 mL) pepper, 1/2 tsp (2 mL) salt and pinch hot red pepper flakes. Add 6 boneless, skinless single chicken breasts that have been pounded thin (page 244). Coat chicken with marinade and refrigerate for up to 2 hours.

Grill chicken for 3 to 5 minutes per side, or until just cooked through.

Cut 3 pita breads in half. Place a chicken breast in each half and top with tzatziki, sliced tomatoes and lettuce.

Makes 6 servings.

GOAT CHEESE DIP WITH POTATOES

When creamy, fresh, unripened goat cheese is combined with other ingredients in a dip or spread, the flavour becomes milder, often appealing to people who may not like goat cheese.

Belgian endive, carrot sticks, cucumber rounds, green and yellow beans, broccoli and cauliflower florets can be used with or instead of the potatoes. You can also use roasted potatoes (page 44). For a great potato salad, just combine the potatoes with the dip.

Makes about 2 cups (500 mL)

2 lb (1 kg) baby new potatoes, unpeeled (about 32)
4 oz (125 g) soft unripened goat cheese
4 oz (125 g) light ricotta
1 cup (250 mL) yogurt cheese (page 391) or
        thick unflavoured low-fat yogurt
1 clove garlic, minced
2 tbsp (25 mL) chopped fresh parsley
2 tbsp (25 mL) chopped fresh basil or dill
2 tbsp (25 mL) chopped fresh chives or green onions
1 tsp (5 mL) chopped fresh thyme or rosemary, or pinch dried
$1/2$ tsp (2 mL) hot red pepper sauce
$1/4$ tsp (1 mL) pepper
Salt to taste

1. Boil potatoes in a large pot of water until tender. Drain and halve.
2. Meanwhile, blend goat cheese with ricotta and yogurt cheese. Mixture should be smooth.
3. Blend in garlic, parsley, basil, chives, thyme, hot pepper sauce, pepper and salt. Taste and adjust seasonings if necessary. Place dip in a bowl and surround with potatoes.

Blue Cheese Dip

Use mild Gorgonzola or Roquefort instead of goat cheese. Use 1 tbsp (15 mL) chopped fresh tarragon (or 1 tsp/5 mL dried) instead of basil. Omit thyme.

Tuna Dip

Omit goat cheese and ricotta. Blend yogurt cheese with a 7-oz (198 g) can white tuna (water-packed), drained and flaked.

PER SERVING (1/4 CUP/50 mL DIP WITH 4 POTATOES)	
Calories	177
Protein	10 g
Fat	5 g
Saturates	3 g
Cholesterol	14 mg
Carbohydrate	24 g
Fibre	2 g
Sodium	126 mg
Potassium	551 mg

Good: Riboflavin; Vitamin B6; Vitamin B12; Calcium

CREAMY SALSA

This is great served as a dip with baked tortilla chips. It also works well in burritos, fajitas and tacos. The salsa can be made without the yogurt cheese, but add 2 tbsp (25 mL) lime juice or lemon juice instead.

Makes about 2 cups (500 mL)

3 fresh plum tomatoes, seeded and diced
1 jalapeño, seeded and chopped
1 clove garlic, minced
3 green onions, chopped
¹/₂ cup (125 mL) chopped fresh cilantro or parsley
¹/₂ tsp (2 mL) ground cumin
³/₄ cup (175 mL) yogurt cheese (page 391) or
      thick unflavoured low-fat yogurt
Salt, pepper and hot red pepper sauce to taste

1. Combine tomatoes, jalapeño, garlic, green onions, cilantro and cumin.
2. Stir in yogurt cheese. Taste and adjust seasonings, adding salt, pepper and hot pepper sauce if necessary.

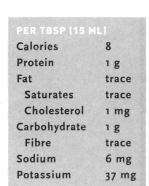

PER TBSP (15 ML)	
Calories	8
Protein	1 g
Fat	trace
Saturates	trace
Cholesterol	1 mg
Carbohydrate	1 g
Fibre	trace
Sodium	6 mg
Potassium	37 mg

HOMEMADE CHIPS

Make your own low-fat tortilla chips, corn chips, pita chips or bagel chips to serve with dips and spreads.

Cut pita breads or corn or flour tortillas into wedges (scissors work well) and arrange in a single layer on a baking sheet (cut bagels into thin slices). Bake in a preheated 400°F (200°C) oven for 8 to 10 minutes, or until lightly browned and crisp.

The chips can also be seasoned. Brush with lightly beaten egg white and sprinkle with chopped fresh or dried herbs, za'atar (page 140), sesame seeds or poppy seeds before cutting into wedges.

WHITE BEAN AND ROASTED GARLIC SPREAD

Use chickpeas or black beans instead of kidney beans if you wish. You can also serve this mixture hot as a side dish.

If the dip is too thick, thin it with a little yogurt or yogurt cheese (page 391). Serve with pita or grilled bread (page 58).

Makes about 1½ cups (375 mL)

1 19-oz (540 mL) can white kidney beans, rinsed and drained, or
    2 cups (500 mL) cooked beans
1 head roasted garlic (page 67), or 2 cloves raw garlic, chopped
2 tbsp (25 mL) lemon juice
1 tbsp (15 mL) olive oil
½ tsp (2 mL) hot red pepper sauce
½ tsp (2 mL) ground cumin
½ tsp (2 mL) pepper
Salt to taste

1. Place beans in a food processor. Squeeze garlic out of skins and add to beans. Blend.
2. Blend in lemon juice, oil, hot pepper sauce, cumin and pepper.
3. Taste and add salt or more lemon juice if necessary.

PER TBSP (15 mL)	
Calories	26
Protein	1 g
Fat	1 g
Saturates	trace
Cholesterol	0 mg
Carbohydrate	4 g
Fibre	1 g
Sodium	53 mg
Potassium	45 mg

ROASTED BUTTERNUT SPREAD

This is an unusual way to use up cooked squash. I discovered it by accident when I had leftover pureed vegetables and then, coincidentally, found the spread served with bread instead of butter on many fancy restaurant tables. I guess they had leftovers, too!

I like to use butternut squash because it is less watery than other winter squashes, and you can often find it already cut up.

Makes about 2 cups (500 mL)

2 lb (1 kg) butternut squash
10 sprigs fresh rosemary, or ½ tsp (2 mL) dried
1 head garlic
1 tbsp (15 mL) balsamic vinegar
1 tsp (5 mL) brown sugar
1 tsp (5 mL) ground cumin
½ tsp (2 mL) pepper
Salt to taste

PER TBSP (15 mL)	
Calories	13
Protein	trace
Fat	0 g
Saturates	0 g
Cholesterol	0 mg
Carbohydrate	3 g
Fibre	0 g
Sodium	1 mg
Potassium	81 mg
Good: Vitamin A	

1. Cut squash in half lengthwise and scoop out seeds. Place rosemary in hollow and place squash, cut side down, on a baking sheet lined with parchment paper.
2. Cut about ¼ inch (5 mm) off top of garlic. Wrap in foil and place on baking sheet beside squash.
3. Bake squash and garlic in a preheated 375°F (190°C) oven for 45 to 50 minutes, or until garlic and squash are tender. Cool. Discard rosemary.
4. Scoop squash out of peel into a food processor (you should have about 2 cups/500 mL). Squeeze roasted garlic out of skins into squash. Add vinegar, sugar, cumin and pepper and blend. Taste and season with salt if necessary.

SMOKED TROUT SPREAD

This is delicious spread on bagels for a weekend breakfast, or served in mini pitas or on rounds of baguette as an appetizer. Smoked salmon or whitefish can be used instead of the trout.

Makes about 2 cups (500 mL)

1/2 lb (250 g) filleted and boned smoked trout
        (1 1/2 or 2 small whole trout)
1 cup (250 mL) yogurt cheese (page 391) or light ricotta cheese
2 tbsp (25 mL) lemon juice
1 tbsp (15 mL) grated white horseradish
2 tbsp (25 mL) chopped fresh dill
2 tbsp (25 mL) chopped fresh chives or green onions
1/2 tsp (2 mL) pepper
Salt to taste

1. Break up trout and chop in a food processor or with a knife.
2. Blend in yogurt cheese, lemon juice and horseradish.
3. Stir in dill, chives and pepper. Taste and season with salt if necessary.

PER TBSP (15 ML)	
Calories	16
Protein	2 g
Fat	1 g
Saturates	trace
Cholesterol	2 mg
Carbohydrate	1 g
Fibre	0 g
Sodium	63 mg
Potassium	39 mg
Good: vitamin B12	

MOROCCAN COOKED TOMATO SALSA

Rhonda Caplan, who works with me at the cooking school, has an eye for a great recipe. She is from Montreal, where this cooked spread is very popular in Moroccan restaurants. You can serve it as a dip with pita chips (page 49) or vegetable sticks, but it also makes a terrific pasta sauce or spread for sandwiches. Or you can poach eggs in it for a wonderful breakfast dish.

If you are in a hurry, just dice the raw peppers and add them to the tomatoes. Although we usually make this with canned plum tomatoes, ripe fresh tomatoes taste sensational when they are in season.

I like this chunky, but it can also be pureed.

Makes about 5 cups (1.25 L)

4 sweet red peppers
2 tsp (10 mL) olive oil
12 cloves garlic, finely chopped
4 jalapeños, seeded and finely chopped
3 lb (1.5 kg) fresh plum tomatoes, peeled, seeded and chopped, or
    3 28-oz (796 mL) cans plum tomatoes, drained and chopped
Salt to taste

PER TBSP (15 ML)	
Calories	6
Protein	trace
Fat	trace
Saturates	0 g
Cholesterol	0 mg
Carbohydrate	1 g
Fibre	trace
Sodium	1 mg
Potassium	44 mg

1. Cut peppers in half and remove ribs and seeds. Arrange peppers, cut side down, on a baking sheet. Broil until skins turn black. Cool. Peel and dice peppers.
2. Heat oil in a large, deep non-stick skillet on medium heat. Add garlic and jalapeños and cook gently for a few minutes, or until soft and fragrant but not brown.
3. Add tomatoes and cook, stirring often, for about 20 minutes, or until mixture is very thick and sauce-like.
4. Add reserved peppers and salt. Continue to cook gently for 10 to 15 minutes, or until thick, stirring occasionally to prevent sticking. Taste and adjust seasonings if necessary.

SHRIMP AND ASPARAGUS SUSHI ROLLS

Some people hesitate to eat sushi because they think it always involves eating raw fish. But sushi refers to the vinegar flavouring of the rice (sushi actually means vinegared things), and it can be made with many ingredients, including raw or cooked seafood, tofu or vegetables.

This is a wonderful appetizer to serve at a party or special dinner. If you can't find extra-large shrimp, just use additional smaller ones. Leftover sushi can be broken up and served as a salad. For a vegetarian version, omit the shrimp, or use grilled tofu. The shrimp and asparagus could also be grilled.

Makes 4 rolls (about 24 pieces)
8 extra-large shrimp, cleaned (about 1 oz/30 g each)
8 spears asparagus, trimmed and peeled
1/4 cup (50 mL) honey-style mustard, or
    4 tsp (20 mL) prepared wasabi
1/4 cup (50 mL) yogurt cheese (page 391) or light mayonnaise
4 sheets toasted nori (about 8 x 7 inches/20 x 18 cm)
4 cups (1 L) cooked short-grain sushi rice
    seasoned with rice vinegar (page 56)
8 pieces lettuce, about 1 inch (2.5 cm) wide and
    4 inches (10 cm) long
8 fresh chives or strips green onion

1. Insert skewers lengthwise through shrimp to keep shrimp straight. Cook in a deep skillet of simmering water for 3 to 4 minutes, or until pink, opaque and cooked through. Cool and remove skewers.
2. Cook asparagus in a separate skillet of boiling water for 2 to 3 minutes, or until just cooked and bright green. Drain, rinse with very cold water and pat dry.
3. Cut asparagus spears to same length as nori; if shrimp are not long enough, cut them in half lengthwise.
4. In a small bowl, combine mustard and yogurt cheese. (Adjust amount of mustard or wasabi to taste.)
5. To roll sushi, arrange a sheet of nori on a bamboo mat (sudari), tea towel or zipper-style plastic bag, with longer side going east–west. Bumpy side of nori should be face up to help rice stick, and so shiny side of nori is on outside. Gently pat about 1 cup (250 mL) rice over nori, leaving about 1/2 inch (1 cm) space at top. (Dip your fingers in a

DIPPING SAUCE FOR SUSHI
Combine 1/2 tsp (2 mL) wasabi with 2 tbsp (25 mL) water. Stir in 1/4 cup (50 mL) soy sauce, 2 tbsp (25 mL) rice vinegar and 1 tbsp (15 mL) chopped fresh ginger root.

Makes about 1/2 cup (125 mL).

PER PIECE	
Calories	62
Protein	3 g
Fat	0 g
Saturates	0 g
Cholesterol	15 mg
Carbohydrate	12 g
Fibre	0 g
Sodium	67 mg
Potassium	54 mg

NORI

According to Japanese cooking expert Elizabeth Andoh, nori is made from laver, a type of sea vegetable that has been compressed and dried in thin sheets. Buy the pretoasted variety and store it in the freezer.

RICE VINEGAR

Rice vinegar is mild enough to be sprinkled on salads without any oil at all. If you don't have it, use cider vinegar, although the taste will be a little more acidic.

Seasoned rice vinegar (sushi vinegar) contains salt and sugar; it is used to flavour sushi rice but is also delicious sprinkled on regular salads and steamed rice. If you can't find it, use regular rice vinegar with or without a little salt and sugar added.

bit of cold water and shake off excess before working with sushi, as it is very sticky.)

6. Spread a bit of mustard mixture lengthwise along centre of rice. Line up 2 pieces of lettuce on mustard and arrange 2 shrimp, 2 asparagus spears and 2 chives on lettuce. Wet strip of nori at top and, using mat or towel to help you roll, roll up sushi. Do not roll mat into sushi! (It gets easier after the first roll.) Repeat until you have four rolls. If you are not serving immediately, wrap each roll in plastic wrap.

7. Just before serving, using a knife dipped in cold water, trim off ends of each roll (chef's treat). Cut each roll in half and then cut each half in thirds. Wipe knife with a wet cloth before each cut.

Southwest Sushi Rolls

Combine 1 tsp (5 mL) chipotle puree (page 183) with 1/3 cup (75 mL) yogurt cheese (page 391) or mayonnaise and 2 tbsp (25 mL) chopped fresh cilantro. Spread on rice instead of mustard/yogurt mixture.

Smoked Salmon Sushi Rolls

Use 3 oz (90 g) smoked salmon, cut in strips, instead of shrimp. Use 1/4 English cucumber, unpeeled and cut in strips 8 inches (20 cm) long, instead of asparagus. Use 8 long sprigs fresh dill in addition to fresh chives.

SMOKED SALMON SUSHI PIZZA

This healthful moulded version of deep-fried restaurant-style sushi pizza is quick and easy. You can also make individual moulds using small ring moulds or washed tuna or salmon cans with the tops and bottoms removed.

For a spectacular garnish, use flying fish roe or green wasabi caviar.

Makes 36 to 64 pieces

2 cups (500 mL) short-grain sushi rice
2 1/4 cups (550 mL) cold water
1/4 cup (50 mL) seasoned rice vinegar
36 thin slices English cucumber
1/4 lb (125 g) smoked salmon, thinly sliced
2 tbsp (25 mL) honey-style mustard, or 1 tbsp (15 mL)
      prepared wasabi
1/4 cup (50 mL) light mayonnaise or yogurt cheese (page 391)
1 sheet toasted nori (about 8 x 7 inches/20 x 18 cm)
1/4 cup (50 mL) chopped fresh chives or green onions
1 tbsp (15 mL) toasted sesame seeds

1. Rinse rice in several changes of cold water until water runs clear. Drain rice well. In a medium heavy pot, combine rice and cold water. Allow to rest for 15 to 30 minutes.
2. Bring rice to a boil, covered, on medium-high heat. Boil for 1 minute. Reduce heat to low and cook for 10 minutes. Remove from heat and allow to rest for 10 minutes. Do not lift lid at any time during cooking and resting.
3. Transfer rice to a large bowl and gently toss with vinegar. If rice tastes perfect, add a bit more vinegar (vinegar taste will dissipate as rice cools). Cover rice with a damp towel if not using right away.
4. Line an 8-inch (1.5 L) square baking dish with plastic wrap. Arrange cucumber slices, overlapping slightly, on bottom. Arrange smoked salmon slices on top of cucumber. Combine mustard and mayonnaise and spread over salmon.
5. Gently and carefully spread half the sushi rice on top of salmon. Dip your fingers into a bowl of cold water and gently pat down rice. Place nori on top of rice. Pat on remaining rice. Cover with plastic wrap and weigh down with cans of food or bricks covered with foil. Allow to rest at room temperature for 15 to 30 minutes, or refrigerate.
6. To serve, unwrap and invert onto a serving platter. Sprinkle with chives and sesame seeds. Cut into squares.

WASABI

Wasabi is the green horseradish used in Japanese cooking. It is typically used to put the "kick" in sushi. You can buy it in paste form in a tube, or in powdered form in a small can. Use the dry version in rubs, or turn it into a paste by combining it with a little water. Cover and let rest for 2 to 3 minutes.

PER PIECE

Calories	187
Protein	5 g
Fat	5 g
Saturates	1 g
Cholesterol	5 mg
Carbohydrate	29 g
Fibre	1 g
Sodium	207 mg
Potassium	90 mg

Excellent: Folate
Good: Vitamin B12

ROASTED TOMATO AND GARLIC BRUSCHETTA

Even winter tomatoes become intense and flavourful when they are roasted. Combined with garlic and herbs, they make a great bruschetta topping. Serve the bruschetta on its own or on top of a salad or soup. The roasted tomato mixture can also be used as a crêpe or omelette filling, sandwich topping, pasta sauce or pizza topping, and it is delicious served over grilled or roasted fish.

Makes 20 pieces
Roasted Tomato Topping
8 plum tomatoes, cut in quarters lengthwise (about 1 1/2 lb/750 g)
1 tbsp (15 mL) olive oil
1/2 tsp (2 mL) salt
1/4 tsp (1 mL) pepper
2 heads garlic
2 tbsp (25 mL) chopped fresh basil
2 tbsp (25 mL) chopped fresh mint or parsley
2 tbsp (25 mL) balsamic vinegar

Grilled Bread
20 slices whole wheat or regular baguette
1 tbsp (15 mL) olive oil
1 tbsp (15 mL) chopped fresh rosemary, or 1/2 tsp (2 mL) dried
1/4 tsp (1 mL) salt
1/4 tsp (1 mL) pepper

1. Place tomato wedges, cut side up, on a baking sheet lined with parchment paper. Spray or drizzle with oil. Sprinkle with salt and pepper.
2. Cut top quarter off heads of garlic. Wrap heads in foil.
3. Roast tomatoes and garlic in a preheated 400°F (200°C) oven for 40 to 45 minutes, or until garlic is squeezable and tomatoes have dried a bit and are slightly brown on bottom. Cool.
4. Chop tomatoes coarsely and place in a bowl. Squeeze garlic from cloves and add to tomatoes. Add basil, mint and vinegar and combine well. Taste and adjust seasonings if necessary.
5. Brush bread with oil. Sprinkle with rosemary, salt and pepper. Grill for 1 minute on each side, or until outside is crusty but inside is still chewy.
6. Top each slice with a spoonful of tomatoes just before serving.

PER PIECE	
Calories	69
Protein	2 g
Fat	2 g
Saturates	0 g
Cholesterol	0 mg
Carbohydrate	11 g
Fibre	1 g
Sodium	172 mg
Potassium	148 mg

BRUSCHETTA WITH UNCOOKED TOMATO SALSA

Although there are many commercial salsas on the market, I prefer to make my own using fresh, unprocessed ingredients. This easy homemade version is my idea of what a salsa should be.

Makes 16 servings

Tomato Salsa

1 sweet red pepper, raw or roasted (page 146), peeled,
      seeded and diced
1 tomato, seeded and diced
$^1/_2$ cup (125 mL) chopped fresh basil
2 tbsp (25 mL) chopped black olives
1 tbsp (15 mL) olive oil
1 tbsp (15 mL) balsamic vinegar
1 clove garlic, minced
$^1/_4$ tsp (1 mL) pepper
Salt to taste

Grilled Bread

1 tbsp (15 mL) olive oil
1 tsp (5 mL) chopped fresh rosemary, or $^1/_4$ tsp (1 mL) dried
$^1/_4$ tsp (1 mL) pepper
Pinch salt
16 slices whole wheat or regular baguette

PER 1/2 PIECE	
Calories	57
Protein	2 g
Fat	2 g
Saturates	trace
Cholesterol	0 mg
Carbohydrate	9 g
Fibre	1 g
Sodium	92 mg
Potassium	47 mg

1. To prepare salsa, combine red pepper and tomato. Stir in basil, olives, oil, vinegar, garlic and pepper. Allow to marinate for at least 10 minutes while preparing grilled bread. Taste and adjust seasonings, adding salt if necessary.
2. To prepare bread, in a small bowl, combine oil, rosemary, pepper and salt. Brush on one side of bread slices.
3. Grill bread slices for 1 minute per side, or until outside is crusty but inside is still chewy.
4. Serve bread, herb side up, topped with salsa.

CHICKPEA BRUSCHETTA

Bruschetta is so popular that there are restaurants in Italy that specialize in it. This is an easy and delicious version. Use any leftover topping in sandwiches, or add more stock or yogurt and serve as a dip.

Makes 26 pieces

2 tbsp (25 mL) olive oil, divided
1 small onion, chopped
3 cloves garlic, finely chopped
Pinch hot red pepper flakes
1 19-oz (540 mL) can chickpeas, rinsed and drained, or
      2 cups (500 mL) cooked chickpeas
1 tbsp (15 mL) lemon juice
2 tbsp (25 mL) chopped fresh parsley
1 tsp (5 mL) chopped fresh rosemary, or $1/4$ tsp (1 mL) dried
1 tsp (5 mL) chopped fresh thyme, or $1/4$ tsp (1 mL) dried
$1/2$ tsp (2 mL) pepper
$1/2$ cup (125 mL) homemade vegetable stock (page 109) or water
26 slices whole wheat or regular baguette

PER PIECE	
Calories	58
Protein	3 g
Fat	2 g
Saturates	trace
Cholesterol	0 mg
Carbohydrate	9 g
Fibre	2 g
Sodium	96 mg
Potassium	155 mg

1. Heat 1 tbsp (15 mL) oil in a large, deep non-stick skillet on medium-high heat. Add onion, garlic and hot pepper flakes. Cook for a few minutes until tender.

2. Add chickpeas, lemon juice, parsley, rosemary, thyme and pepper. Cook for a few minutes. Add stock and bring to a boil.

3. Mash chickpea mixture with a potato masher until spreadable but not pureed. Taste and adjust seasonings if necessary.

4. Brush one side of bread slices with remaining 1 tbsp (15 mL) oil. Grill bread for 1 minute per side, or until outside is crusty but inside is still chewy. Spread oiled side of bread with about 1 tbsp (15 mL) chickpea mixture.

WILD MUSHROOM BRUSCHETTA WITH GOAT CHEESE

If you cannot find wild mushrooms (page 289) or if they are too expensive, simply use regular mushrooms (preferably brown), or top goat cheese with caramelized onions (page 329) or salsa. You could also use Gorgonzola or Cambozola instead of goat cheese.

Makes 20 pieces

2 tsp (10 mL) olive oil
2 shallots or 1 small onion, finely chopped
2 cloves garlic, finely chopped
1 lb (500 g) portobello or other wild mushrooms, trimmed and sliced
2 tsp (10 mL) chopped fresh thyme, or ½ tsp (2 mL) dried
1 tsp (5 mL) pepper, divided
Salt to taste
2 tbsp (25 mL) chopped fresh parsley
3 oz (90 g) soft unripened goat cheese
2 tbsp (25 mL) yogurt cheese (page 391) or light ricotta cheese
1 clove garlic, minced
20 slices whole wheat or regular baguette
20 small sprigs fresh basil or parsley

1. Heat oil in large, deep non-stick skillet on medium heat. Add shallots and chopped garlic and cook gently for 2 minutes.

2. Add mushrooms, thyme and ½ tsp (2 mL) pepper. When mushrooms begin to render liquid, increase heat and cook for 5 to 10 minutes, or until liquid evaporates and mushrooms are cooked. Add salt. Stir in parsley.

3. In a bowl or food processor, blend goat cheese, yogurt cheese, minced garlic and remaining ½ tsp (2 mL) pepper. Add a little more yogurt if necessary to make mixture spreadable (you should have about ½ cup/125 mL).

4. Grill bread for about 1 minute per side, or until crusty on outside but still chewy inside. Spread with cheese mixture (about 1 tsp/5 mL per slice). Top with mushrooms and garnish with basil.

PER PIECE	
Calories	49
Protein	2 g
Fat	2 g
Saturates	1 g
Cholesterol	3 mg
Carbohydrate	6 g
Fibre	2 g
Sodium	77 mg
Potassium	100 mg

RICOTTA BRUSCHETTA

You can also use this spread on crackers, as a sandwich filling or stuffed into vegetables or small pita breads. Or try serving it on slices of cucumber, zucchini, apples, pears, radishes or sweet peppers. For a smoky flavour, barbecue the toasts instead of broiling them.

I always try to buy the driest ricotta cheese available, but if your brand is very moist, drain the cheese first—cut it in quarters, place in a strainer and let drain for a few hours or overnight in the refrigerator.

My husband hates mint in savoury dishes. I love it, but you decide.

Makes about 24 pieces

24 slices whole wheat or regular baguette
1 lb (500 g) light ricotta
2 tbsp (25 mL) chopped fresh parsley
2 tbsp (25 mL) chopped fresh chives or green onions
2 tbsp (25 mL) chopped fresh basil or dill
1 tbsp (15 mL) chopped fresh mint, or 1/4 tsp (1 mL) dried
1/2 tsp (2 mL) pepper
2 cloves garlic, minced
1/4 tsp (1 mL) hot red pepper flakes
2 tbsp (25 mL) olive oil, optional
Salt to taste

1. Grill bread slices for about 1 minute per side, or until crusty on outside but still chewy inside.
2. Combine ricotta, parsley, chives, basil, mint and pepper. Stir in garlic, hot pepper flakes and oil. Taste and adjust seasonings, adding salt if necessary.
3. Spread each piece of bread with about 4 tsp (20 mL) ricotta mixture.

PER PIECE	
Calories	57
Protein	3 g
Fat	2 g
Saturates	1 g
Cholesterol	6 mg
Carbohydrate	8 g
Fibre	trace
Sodium	96 mg
Potassium	40 mg

ASPARAGUS TARTS WITH GOAT CHEESE

The idea for these fanciful spring tarts came from Buffalo Mountain Lodge in Banff. You can also fill the phyllo cups with caramelized onions (page 44) and Gorgonzola, or sauteed wild mushrooms and mashed potatoes.

I like to use panko breadcrumbs (page 204) in phyllo recipes, because they keep the pastry crisp.

Makes 8 servings

Phyllo Cups

3 tbsp (45 mL) unsalted butter, melted, or olive oil
3 tbsp (45 mL) water
8 sheets phyllo pastry
1/2 cup (125 mL) dry breadcrumbs

Filling

1 lb (500 g) asparagus
2 tsp (10 mL) olive oil
2 leeks, trimmed and sliced
3 shallots or 1 small onion, finely chopped
2 cloves garlic, finely chopped
1 tbsp (15 mL) chopped fresh thyme, or 1/2 tsp (2 mL) dried
1 tsp (5 mL) chopped fresh rosemary, or pinch dried
Salt and pepper to taste
3 oz (90 g) soft unripened goat cheese, crumbled
1 bunch fresh chives or slivered green onions,
        cut in 4-inch (10 cm) lengths

1. To prepare phyllo cups, in a small bowl, combine melted butter and water.
2. Working with one sheet of phyllo at a time (cover remaining sheets with plastic wrap and a damp tea towel), brush phyllo with butter mixture and sprinkle with breadcrumbs. Cut into 6 squares. Place squares on top of each other at irregular angles and press into bottom of a muffin cup so edges stick up. Repeat with remaining phyllo to make eight cups.
3. To prepare filling, trim asparagus and peel about 2 inches (5 cm) from bottom of stalks. Bring a large skillet of water to a boil. Add asparagus and cook for 3 minutes. Trim off 2-inch (5 cm) tips and reserve. Cut stalks into 1/2-inch (1 cm) slices.

PER SERVING	
Calories	197
Protein	6 g
Fat	9 g
Saturates	4 g
Cholesterol	19 mg
Carbohydrate	24 g
Fibre	2 g
Sodium	253 mg
Potassium	154 mg
Excellent: Folate	

4. Heat oil in a large, deep non-stick skillet on medium heat. Add leeks, shallots and garlic and cook gently for 5 minutes, or until vegetables are very tender (add a few spoonfuls of water if they start to stick). Add chopped asparagus, thyme and rosemary. Taste and adjust seasonings, adding salt and pepper if necessary.

5. Divide mixture among phyllo shells. Top with crumbled cheese. Arrange asparagus tips on top so they stick out of filling.

6. Bake in a preheated 375°F (190°C) oven for 20 minutes, or until golden brown. Garnish with chives inserted into filling.

Dessert Phyllo Cups

Use melted butter or unflavoured vegetable oil for brushing. Dust the phyllo with a combination of granulated sugar and ground nuts instead of breadcrumbs. Bake the unfilled cups for 15 to 18 minutes, or until crisp. Cool and remove from pans. Fill with fruit sorbet and top with fresh berries. You can also fill the cups with caramelized fruit or compotes. Sprinkle with icing sugar before serving.

PHYLLO

- If your phyllo pastry is frozen, defrost it overnight in the refrigerator and allow the package to stand at room temperature for about an hour before using.
- Be organized. Have your fillings ready and all your equipment close at hand. Give yourself as much counter space as possible.
- Once you open the package, cover the phyllo that you are not using with a large piece of plastic wrap and a slightly dampened tea towel (to hold the plastic in place).
- If you are using melted butter, mix some water with the butter so it will go farther.
- Use a large pastry brush to brush on the butter or oil. I like the silicone pastry brushes; the bristles don't fall off into the pastry.
- Sprinkle breadcrumbs, sugar, ground nuts, etc., between the layers of phyllo for added texture and flavour.
- Extra pastry will keep in the refrigerator for a few weeks, or you can refreeze it if you wrap it well.
- Phyllo pastries freeze beautifully, either baked or unbaked. Freeze small pastries in a single layer on a baking sheet lined with plastic wrap and then pack the frozen pastries in bags.

SMOKED SALMON TORTILLA SPIRALS

These are an all-time favourite and make a perfect appetizer for an outdoor dinner. You can also serve them as a sandwich for a light lunch. For people who are lactose intolerant, use soy cream cheese.

Make the rolls ahead but slice them just before serving.

Whole wheat tortillas with flax taste great in this recipe.

Makes 32 pieces

8 oz (250 g) light cream cheese or ricotta
2 tbsp (25 mL) honey-style mustard
4 10-inch (25 cm) whole wheat or regular flour tortillas
½ lb (250 g) thinly sliced smoked salmon
2 tbsp (25 mL) chopped fresh dill
2 tbsp (25 mL) chopped fresh chives or green onions
¼ tsp (1 mL) pepper
4 leaves soft Boston lettuce

1. In a food processor, blend cheese and mustard until smooth and spreadable.
2. Arrange tortillas on work surface in a single layer. Spread with cheese as evenly as possible.
3. Arrange smoked salmon in a single layer on top of cheese, leaving a 1-inch (2.5 cm) border at top of each tortilla. Sprinkle with dill, chives and pepper. Place a lettuce leaf across middle.
4. Roll tortillas up tightly, pressing firmly to seal. Wrap well in plastic wrap and refrigerate until ready to serve.
5. To slice, unwrap, trim ends and cut each roll slightly on diagonal into 8 pieces. Arrange cut side up on a serving platter.

PER PIECE	
Calories	61
Protein	3 g
Fat	3 g
Saturates	1 g
Cholesterol	7 mg
Carbohydrate	6 g
Fibre	1 g
Sodium	157 mg
Potassium	50 mg

GRILLED TUNA SATAYS WITH SWEET MANGO DIPPING SAUCE

These beautiful appetizers are spicy and delicious. I prefer the tuna very rare, but you can cook it for the extra two minutes if you wish. The dipping sauce is also great with dumplings (page 72) and salad rolls (page 70).

Makes 32 skewers

1 lb (500 g) fresh tuna steak, about 1 inch (2.5 cm) thick
1 tsp (5 mL) dark sesame oil
1 tbsp (15 mL) wasabi powder (page 56)
1 tsp (5 mL) coarsely ground black pepper
1/2 tsp (2 mL) coarse salt
1/4 cup (50 mL) thinly sliced pickled ginger
2 cups (500 mL) watercress sprigs or other greens

Sweet Mango Dipping Sauce

1/2 ripe mango, peeled
2 tbsp (25 mL) sweet Thai chili sauce (page 183) or red pepper jelly

1. Pat tuna dry and cut into 4 "sticks" about 5 to 6 inches (12 to 15 cm) long. Rub with sesame oil.
2. In a small bowl, combine wasabi powder, pepper and salt. Pat into tuna on all sides.
3. Grill tuna on a very hot grill or grill pan, rotating until cooked on all sides but still very rare inside (2 to 4 minutes in total).
4. To prepare dipping sauce, cut up mango. In a food processor, puree mango and sweet Thai chili sauce until smooth. Taste and adjust seasonings, adding more sweet sauce if necessary. Place in a dipping bowl. You should have about 1/2 cup (125 mL).
5. Just before serving, slice each tuna stick into 8 pieces lengthwise. Skewer them (with sturdy toothpicks or small skewers) with a piece of pickled ginger and watercress leaf. Arrange remaining watercress on a serving platter and place tuna skewers on top. Serve with dipping sauce.

PER SKEWER	
Calories	27
Protein	3 g
Fat	1 g
Saturates	trace
Cholesterol	5 mg
Carbohydrate	1 g
Fibre	trace
Sodium	77 mg
Potassium	64 mg
Excellent: Vitamin B12	

CORN PANCAKES WITH SPICY SALSA

These pancakes are very tender, with a sweetness that is the perfect foil for a spicy topping. Other spreads and dips such as guacamole (page 46) also make good toppings. Leftover pancakes can be sliced and sprinkled on salads or soups.

On their own, these pancakes make a great side dish. You can also make mini pancakes using 1 tsp (5 mL) batter for each one, or you can make bigger pancakes and serve them for brunch with smoked salmon, drizzled with yogurt cheese (page 391).

Makes about 24 pancakes

Corn Pancakes

3 eggs
1 cup (250 mL) buttermilk or sour milk (page 407)
1 cup (250 mL) all-purpose flour
1/2 cup (125 mL) cornmeal
2 tbsp (25 mL) granulated sugar
1 tsp (5 mL) baking soda
1/2 tsp (2 mL) ground cumin
1/2 tsp (2 mL) salt
1/2 tsp (2 mL) pepper
1 tbsp (15 mL) vegetable oil
3/4 cup (175 mL) corn kernels
1/4 cup (50 mL) diced roasted sweet red pepper (page 146)

Spicy Salsa

3 plum tomatoes, seeded and chopped
1 jalapeño, seeded and finely chopped, or
        1 tbsp (15 mL) chipotle puree (page 183)
1 clove garlic, minced
1 tbsp (15 mL) olive oil
1 tbsp (15 mL) lime juice
1/4 cup (50 mL) chopped fresh cilantro
2 tbsp (25 mL) chopped fresh chives
Salt and pepper to taste

PER PANCAKE AND 1 TBSP (15 ML) SALSA	
Calories	64
Protein	2 g
Fat	2 g
Saturates	0 g
Cholesterol	27 mg
Carbohydrate	9 g
Fibre	1 g
Sodium	116 mg
Potassium	63 mg

1. To prepare pancakes, in a large bowl, combine eggs and buttermilk.
2. In a separate bowl, combine flour, cornmeal, sugar, baking soda, cumin, salt and pepper. Mix together well.
3. Whisk dry ingredients into egg mixture. Stir in oil, corn and red pepper.
4. Heat a large lightly oiled non-stick skillet on medium heat. Add batter,

using about 2 tbsp (25 mL) per pancake; they should be about 2 inches (5 cm) in diameter. Cook for a few minutes, or just until surface loses its sheen. Turn and cook second side. Continue until all pancakes are cooked (arrange pancakes in a single layer on a serving platter).

5. To prepare salsa, combine tomatoes, jalapeño, garlic, oil, lime juice, cilantro and chives. Taste and adjust seasonings, adding salt and pepper as necessary. Spoon some salsa on each pancake.

Breakfast Corn Pancakes

Omit red pepper and cumin. Serve pancakes with maple syrup instead of salsa.

GARLIC

When I use raw garlic in a salad dressing, spread or dip, I like to mince it or put it through a garlic press, so there are not actual pieces of raw garlic in the mixture. But when I cook garlic, I chop it finely with a knife, as minced garlic tends to burn and stick when it is sauteed.

When you are cooking garlic, do not let it brown too much, or it will become bitter. If you are sauteing chopped garlic with other ingredients (e.g., onions), add the other ingredients to the hot skillet first to soften the heat and help prevent the garlic from burning. If you are sauteing in a very small amount of oil, reduce the heat and try covering the skillet. If the garlic still browns too quickly, simply add a few spoonfuls of water to cool the pan and slow down the cooking, and then keep cooking, uncovered, until the water evaporates.

Be cautious with quantity when you use raw garlic, as it is very strong. If the garlic is to be cooked, you can be more generous, as it becomes sweeter and more gentle in flavour the longer it cooks. You can also add chopped raw garlic to stews or sauces towards the end of the cooking time to add a stronger garlic taste to a dish.

ROASTED GARLIC

Roasted garlic adds a wonderful flavour to dishes, and it thickens sauces, dips, salad dressings and soups without adding fat. Use it in soups, salads, salad dressings, pasta sauces, mashed potatoes, rice and vegetable dishes. Or spread it on grilled bread with some goat cheese (which is the way roasted garlic became so popular in the first place).

To roast garlic, cut the top quarter off the heads and remove any parchment-like skin that comes away easily. Wrap the garlic heads in foil in a single layer and place on a baking sheet. Bake at 400°F (200°C) for 40 to 45 minutes, or until tender. When cool, turn the head upside down and gently squeeze the garlic flesh out of the cloves into a bowl.

Roasted garlic lasts for a few weeks in the refrigerator, so make lots.

GRILLED SHRIMP MARTINIS

Chopped-up shrimp cocktail served in a martini glass is a sensational presentation, and the taste and textures are fabulous, too. In this recipe a few shrimp go a long way.

This would also make a great brunch or lunch salad served on Boston lettuce.

Makes 6 to 8 servings

1 lb (500 g) shrimp, cleaned
1 tbsp (15 mL) olive oil
1 tsp (5 mL) salt, divided
2 ears corn, husked
1 small red onion, sliced in rounds ¼ inch (5 mm) thick
1 sweet red pepper, halved and seeded
1 jalapeño, seeded and diced
⅓ cup (75 mL) chopped fresh cilantro
½ small ripe avocado, diced (page 47)
3 tbsp (45 mL) lime juice
1 clove garlic, minced
½ tsp (2 mL) ground cumin
1½ tsp (7 mL) chipotle puree (page 183)
2 tbsp (25 mL) tequila, optional
1 cup (250 mL) coarsely crushed baked whole wheat or regular
        tortilla chips (page 49)

1. Pat shrimp dry and toss with oil and ½ tsp (2 mL) salt. Grill for a few minutes per side, or until shrimp are pink, opaque and starting to curl. Cut into ½-inch (1 cm) chunks and place in a large bowl.
2. Grill corn on all sides until lightly browned. Cut corn from cobs (page 333) and add to shrimp.
3. Grill onion slices for a few minutes per side until browned. Grill red pepper, skin side down, until blackened. Peel. Dice onion and pepper and add to shrimp along with jalapeño, cilantro and avocado.
4. In a small bowl, combine lime juice, garlic, cumin, chipotle and remaining ½ tsp (2 mL) salt. Taste and adjust seasonings if necessary.
5. Toss shrimp and vegetables with dressing and tequila. Spoon into martini glasses and top with chips.

PER SERVING	
Calories	204
Protein	15 g
Fat	7 g
Saturates	1 g
Cholesterol	112 mg
Carbohydrate	21 g
Fibre	4 g
Sodium	371 mg
Potassium	434 mg

Excellent: Niacin; Vitamin B12; Vitamin C
Good: Vitamin B6; Folate; Iron

GRILLED TUNA TARTARE WITH AVOCADO

Sometimes referred to as a Japanese pub or tapas bar, Hapa Izakaya is a happening place in Vancouver. The restaurant serves a wide range of Asian appetizers, and their chopped tuna and avocado salad inspired this concoction. Although most things called "tartare" are served raw, I like to grill fish and meat briefly first.

You can also serve the tuna with rice crackers instead of the cucumber rounds.

Makes about 48 pieces

1/2 lb (250 g) fresh tuna steak, about 1 inch (2.5 cm) thick
1 tsp (5 mL) dark sesame oil
1/2 tsp (2 mL) coarse salt
1/2 tsp (2 mL) coarsely ground black pepper
1 tbsp (15 mL) seasoned rice vinegar or lime juice
1 tbsp (15 mL) soy sauce
2 tbsp (25 mL) chopped fresh chives or green onions
2 tbsp (25 mL) finely chopped fresh cilantro
1/2 ripe avocado
48 thin (about 1/4 inch/5 mm thick) slices cucumber, patted dry

PER PIECE	
Calories	12
Protein	1 g
Fat	trace
Saturates	0 g
Cholesterol	2 mg
Carbohydrate	trace
Fibre	trace
Sodium	37 mg
Potassium	36 mg
Good: Vitamin B12	

1. Pat tuna dry and brush with sesame oil. Combine salt and pepper and press into both sides of tuna.

2. Grill tuna on a very hot grill or barbecue for 1 minute per side. Cool. Dice tuna into tiny pieces and place in a large bowl.

3. Add vinegar, soy sauce, chives and cilantro and toss gently.

4. Just before serving, peel avocado, cut it in half, remove pit and coarsely mash one half (page 47). (Wrap other half tightly and use another time.) Gently combine with tuna. Taste and adjust seasonings if necessary.

5. Line a 2-cup (500 mL) bowl or mould with plastic wrap and pack in tuna mixture firmly. Unmould onto a serving platter. Serve with cucumber rounds.

GRILLED SHRIMP SALAD ROLLS

If you are making these ahead, wrap each roll in waxed paper to prevent them from drying out. This is also a great way to use up left-over Asian salads or stir-fries.

These rolls can also be served with Ponzu Dipping Sauce (page 71).

Makes about 20 rolls
Thai Dipping Sauce
¼ cup (50 mL) rice vinegar
2 tbsp (25 mL) Thai fish sauce
2 tbsp (25 mL) lime juice
2 tbsp (25 mL) granulated sugar
½ tsp (2 mL) hot Asian chili paste

Salad Rolls
20 extra-large shrimp, cleaned
2 oz (60 g) rice vermicelli noodles
20 rice paper wrappers (or more if necessary)
1 carrot, cut in thin strips
1 sweet red pepper, seeded and cut in thin strips
½ ripe mango, peeled and cut in thin strips
20 large leaves fresh cilantro
20 leaves fresh mint
20 pieces soft Boston lettuce

1. To prepare sauce, in a small bowl, combine vinegar, fish sauce, lime juice, sugar and chili paste.
2. Insert skewers into shrimp from head to tail to straighten them. Grill for a few minutes on each side (or cook in a deep skillet of boiling water) until barely cooked. Cool and remove shrimp from skewers.
3. Soak noodles in warm water for 15 minutes. Drain well. Toss with 1 tbsp (15 mL) dipping sauce.
4. Working with 2 or 3 wrappers at a time, soften rice paper wrappers for 20 to 30 seconds in a shallow bowl of very warm water. Arrange on damp tea towels in a single layer.
5. Lay a shrimp on middle bottom third of each wrapper. Arrange a piece or two of carrot, pepper, mango, noodles and herbs on shrimp and top with a piece of lettuce. Fold up bottom third, fold in one end and roll up snugly. Repeat with remaining ingredients. Serve rolls with dipping sauce.

RICE PAPER WRAPPERS

Rice paper wrappers come in different shapes and sizes. They are used in Asian dishes and can be used raw, steamed, baked or fried. Soak two or three at a time in a large bowl of warm water for about 20 to 30 seconds, or until they are pliable.

Arrange the wrappers in a single layer on a damp tea towel. Place the filling down the middle of the wrapper, fold in the ends and roll up. The moist wrappers should stick together well.

Rice paper wrappers can be found in Asian food stores. In some recipes you can substitute lettuce leaves (if the recipe calls for the wrappers to be used raw or steamed) or spring roll wrappers (if the wrappers are to be fried or baked).

PER ROLL

Calories	95
Protein	8 g
Fat	1 g
Saturates	0 g
Cholesterol	67 mg
Carbohydrate	14 g
Fibre	1 g
Sodium	221 mg
Potassium	135 mg

Excellent: Vitamin B12
Good: Vitamin A; Vitamin C

PONZU DIPPING SAUCE

This is a great dipping sauce for satays and salad rolls.

Combine 2 tbsp (25 mL) soy sauce, 2 tbsp (25 mL) rice wine and 2 tbsp (25 mL) lime juice. Makes about 1/3 cup (75 mL).

CHICKEN SATAYS WITH PEANUT SAUCE

This recipe is also good made with pork, lamb or extra-firm tofu strips. Serve it as an appetizer or as a main course with stir-fried vegetables and rice. It is delicious with or without the sauce.

Using chickpeas in the peanut sauce is a great way to adapt a normally high-fat sauce. The sauce also makes a good vegetable dip, or you can toss it with linguine.

To avoid the problem of burning wooden skewers, skewer food after grilling. For chicken satays, for example, grill the whole chicken breast, cut it into strips and thread onto skewers before serving.

Makes 16 skewers

1 tsp (5 mL) curry powder or paste
1 clove garlic, minced
1 tbsp (15 mL) soy sauce
1 tbsp (15 mL) lemon juice
1 tbsp (15 mL) honey
1 tbsp (15 mL) water
1 lb (500 g) boneless, skinless chicken breasts

Peanut Sauce

1/2 cup (125 mL) cooked chickpeas
1 tbsp (15 mL) smooth peanut butter
2 tbsp (25 mL) rice wine
2 tbsp (25 mL) honey
2 tbsp (25 mL) soy sauce
2 tbsp (25 mL) water
Dash hot red pepper sauce

1. In a large bowl, combine curry powder, garlic, soy sauce, lemon juice, honey and water. Add chicken and combine. Refrigerate for 10 to 60 minutes.
2. To prepare sauce, in a food processor, combine chickpeas, peanut butter, rice wine, honey, soy sauce, water and hot pepper sauce and puree. Taste and adjust seasonings if necessary.
3. Grill chicken breasts for 4 to 5 minutes per side, or until cooked through. Cut chicken into 16 strips and thread onto skewers. Serve with peanut sauce drizzled on top or as a dip.

PER SKEWER

Calories	60
Protein	7 g
Fat	1 g
Saturates	trace
Cholesterol	18 mg
Carbohydrate	5 g
Fibre	trace
Sodium	164 mg
Potassium	86 mg
Good: Niacin	

NAKED CHICKEN DUMPLINGS WITH SWEET AND SOUR SAUCE

Asian-style dumplings are usually wrapped in thin wheat or rice flour wrappers, but it is much faster to make the dumplings "naked" and serve them as meatballs. These can be served with toothpicks or cocktail forks as an appetizer, or you can spoon them over noodles or rice for a main course. For a great variation, use half chicken and half shrimp or pork.

Sweet and sour sauce has a reputation for being sugary and sticky, but this recipe is based on an authentic version I learned at the Wei-Chuan School of Cooking in Taiwan. You can also toss the sauce with pieces of grilled or broiled chicken or cooked shrimp, or you can use it in meat and vegetable stir-fries.

Makes about 32 meatballs

1 lb (500 g) lean ground chicken breast
1 egg white
1 tbsp (15 mL) cornstarch
1/2 tsp (2 mL) salt
1/4 tsp (1 mL) hot Asian chili paste

Sweet and Sour Sauce

1/3 cup (75 mL) ketchup
3 tbsp (45 mL) rice vinegar or cider vinegar
2 tbsp (25 mL) granulated sugar
1/2 cup (125 mL) water
1 tbsp (15 mL) soy sauce
1 tsp (5 mL) dark sesame oil
2 tsp (10 mL) cornstarch
2 tsp (10 mL) olive oil

Garnish

1 1/2 tbsp (20 mL) sesame seeds, toasted (page 384)
2 tbsp (25 mL) chopped fresh cilantro or parsley

1. In a large bowl, combine ground chicken, egg white, cornstarch, salt and chili paste.
2. Line a baking sheet with waxed paper. With wet hands, shape mixture into 1-inch (2.5 cm) balls and flatten slightly. Place on baking sheet. Refrigerate or freeze until ready to cook.

PER DUMPLING	
Calories	31
Protein	4 g
Fat	1 g
Saturates	0 g
Cholesterol	9 mg
Carbohydrate	2 g
Fibre	0 g
Sodium	109 mg
Potassium	60 mg

3. To prepare sauce, in a small bowl, combine ketchup, vinegar, sugar, water, soy sauce, sesame oil and cornstarch.

4. Heat olive oil in a large non-stick skillet over medium-high heat. Add chicken balls in a single layer. Cook for 2 to 3 minutes, or until lightly browned on bottom. Loosen meatballs and turn. Add sauce and cover pan. Cook gently for 3 to 5 minutes, or until chicken feels firm. Stir to combine well. Sauce should thicken.

5. Turn chicken balls out onto a serving platter and sprinkle with sesame seeds and cilantro.

ASIAN SEASONINGS

Black Bean Sauce

The black beans used in Asian recipes are fermented and salted, and they are commonly used in small amounts as a seasoning. Do not confuse them with the dried or canned black turtle beans used in Southwestern chilis and soups.

If they are old and dried out, fermented beans can be soaked in boiling water for about 10 minutes before being drained and chopped. You can also buy black bean sauce—fermented beans combined with ingredients like garlic, oil, sugar and rice wine. My favourite brand is Lee Kum Kee black bean and garlic sauce. Once the jar has been opened, store it in the refrigerator.

To make your own black bean sauce, heat 1 tsp (5 mL) dark sesame oil in a skillet. Add 2 finely chopped cloves garlic, 1 tsp (5 mL) finely chopped fresh ginger root and 2 tbsp (25 mL) minced fermented black beans. Cook for about 1 minute, or until fragrant. Add 1 to 2 tbsp (15 to 25 mL) water.

Hoisin Sauce

Hoisin sauce is a sweet bean paste that is readily available in most supermarkets. It is great used as a glaze or in barbecue sauces and is traditionally used on the Mandarin pancakes served with Chinese roast duck. I like the Koon Chun brand the best. Keep opened jars in the refrigerator.

Oyster Sauce

Oyster sauce adds richness without a fishy taste, and it can be used in place of salt (you can also buy a vegetarian version). It keeps indefinitely in the refrigerator. My favourite brand is Lee Kum Kee.

ASIAN CHICKEN POT STICKERS

Whenever Hugh Carpenter teaches at my school, everyone who attends his classes (including me and my staff) rushes home afterwards to cook. Hugh makes great dumplings, and these are Hugh-inspired. (Instead of chicken, you can use shrimp finely chopped in a food processor.) I prefer them lightly glazed, but you can double the sauce recipe if you wish.

Serve these in individual bowls as a first course, or place in a large serving bowl and serve with toothpicks as an hors d'oeuvre with drinks.

You can also turn the dumplings into wontons by folding the dough into triangles and sealing closed. Cook them in a large pot of boiling water for about 5 minutes, or until they are cooked through, and add them to soups.

These can be made ahead and frozen uncooked. Cook from the frozen state but for twice the cooking time. They can also be cooked ahead and reheated, but you will have to add a bit of water or stock to the skillet.

Makes about 35 dumplings

1 lb (500 g) lean ground chicken breast
1 egg white
1 tbsp (15 mL) cornstarch
1 tbsp (15 mL) soy sauce
1 tsp (5 mL) dark sesame oil
1/4 tsp (1 mL) salt
1/2 cup (125 mL) chopped cooked spinach, squeezed very dry
1 small carrot, finely chopped or grated
2 green onions, chopped
1 tsp (5 mL) chopped fresh ginger root
1/4 tsp (1 mL) hot Asian chili paste
35 Chinese dumpling wrappers, approx.
1 tbsp (15 mL) vegetable oil, divided

Curried Tomato Sauce
1/3 cup (75 mL) pureed tomatoes, tomato sauce or
        light coconut milk
1/3 cup (75 mL) water
1 tbsp (15 mL) dry sherry
1 tbsp (15 mL) oyster sauce or hoisin sauce

PER DUMPLING	
Calories	42
Protein	4 g
Fat	1 g
Saturates	0 g
Cholesterol	8 mg
Carbohydrate	5 g
Fibre	0 g
Sodium	71 mg
Potassium	75 mg

1 tbsp (15 mL) curry powder or paste
1 tsp (5 mL) granulated sugar

Garnish
1 tsp (5 mL) sesame seeds, toasted (page 384)
¼ cup (50 mL) chopped fresh cilantro or chives

1. In a large bowl, combine ground chicken, egg white, cornstarch, soy sauce, sesame oil and salt. Stir in spinach, carrot, green onions, ginger and chili paste. Mix well.
2. Place a few dumpling wrappers on work surface in a single layer. Place a teaspoon of filling in centre of each wrapper. Place one dumpling in palm of your hand and bring up sides of wrappers to cover filling, leaving top slightly open. Squeeze slightly around middle to give each dumpling a "waist." Flatten filling that is exposed on top. Place dumplings, open side up, on a baking sheet lined with waxed paper and brushed with a little vegetable oil. Continue until all filling is used.
3. To prepare sauce, combine pureed tomatoes, water, sherry, oyster sauce, curry powder and sugar.
4. Heat remaining vegetable oil in a large, deep non-stick skillet on medium-high heat. Arrange dumplings, open side up, in skillet. Cook for 2 to 3 minutes, or until lightly browned on bottom.
5. Spoon sauce over and between dumplings, and cover pan. Cook for 3 to 5 minutes, or until tops feel firm and cooked through. Shake pan gently to prevent sticking.
6. Toss dumplings gently and sprinkle with sesame seeds and cilantro.

Carrot Soup with Cumin
Roasted Cauliflower Shooters
Jerusalem Artichoke Soup
Grilled Corn Chowder with Cilantro and Chipotles
French Onion Soup
Leek and Potato Soup
Celeriac and Potato Soup
Swiss Chard and Pine Nut Soup
Thai Chicken Noodle Soup
Japanese-style Chicken Noodle Soup
Chicken Soup with Matzo Balls
Roasted Tomato Soup
Curried Butternut Soup
Barbecued Tomato and Corn Soup
Hot and Sour Soup
Spicy Gazpacho
Pasta e Fagioli
Mexican Green Lentil Soup
Israeli Red Lentil Soup
White Bean Soup with Salad Salsa
Mushroom, Bean and Barley Soup
Moroccan Mixed Bean Soup with Pasta
Black Bean Soup with Yogurt and Spicy Salsa

Split Pea Soup with Dill
Green Minestrone with Parmesan Cheese Crisps
Chickpea and Spinach Soup
Seafood Soup with Ginger Broth
Malka's Bouillabaisse
Quick Miso Soup
Fast Pho

HEART
SMART

SOUPS

CARROT SOUP WITH CUMIN

When I am entertaining, I make soups with vegetable stock whenever possible, in case guests have not mentioned that they are vegetarian (it happens all the time).

Makes 8 to 10 servings
2 tsp (10 mL) olive oil
1 onion, chopped
2 cloves garlic, chopped
1 tsp (5 mL) ground cumin
2 lb (1 kg) carrots (about 12), chopped (about 5 cups/1.25 L)
6 cups (1.5 L) homemade vegetable stock (page 109), chicken
        stock or water
Salt and pepper to taste
2 tbsp (25 mL) chopped fresh cilantro, mint or parsley

1. Heat oil in a large saucepan over medium heat. Add onion and garlic and cook gently for about 5 minutes, or until very fragrant. (If mixture starts to stick or brown too much, add a few spoonfuls of water.)
2. Add cumin and cook for 30 to 60 seconds, or until fragrant, stirring constantly.
3. Add carrots and stock. Bring to a boil. Reduce heat and simmer gently until vegetables are very tender, about 30 minutes.
4. Puree soup and return to heat. Add water if soup is too thick. Taste and season with salt and pepper. Sprinkle with cilantro before serving.

PER SERVING	
Calories	79
Protein	2 g
Fat	2 g
Saturates	trace
Cholesterol	0 mg
Carbohydrate	16 g
Fibre	3 g
Sodium	618 mg
Potassium	225 mg
Excellent: Vitamin A	

There are many ways to puree soups. Immersion blenders puree the soup right in the pot; the strong, high-powered ones work the best. Counter-top blenders tend to give you a very smooth texture, though you may have to puree the soup in several batches. Food processors also work well. The old-fashioned food mill (page 450) strains and purees at the same time, which means you can leave the skins on tomatoes, asparagus, apples, etc., during cooking.

PER SERVING

Calories	29
Protein	1 g
Fat	1 g
Saturates	trace
Cholesterol	0 mg
Carbohydrate	4 g
Fibre	1 g
Sodium	343 mg
Potassium	79 mg
Good: **Vitamin C**	

ROASTED CAULIFLOWER SHOOTERS

My staff and I went to The Beard House in New York to cook a brunch to celebrate the publication of my cookbook, *Essentials of Home Cooking*. After shopping for the event all day in the pouring November rain, we decided to go to Hearth, a tiny but popular Italian restaurant in the Village. We were soaked, but as soon as we sat down, the server handed us warm shooters of roasted cauliflower soup. It took the chill right out of us, as well as being a delicious treat.

You can warm your guests on frosty nights, too, with soup shooters. They are also a fabulous way to use up that cup or two of leftover soup that you've hidden away in the freezer. If you don't have shooter glasses, espresso cups or small coffee cups work well.

Roasting cauliflower intensifies the flavour and gives the soup a rich taste. If you serve this in a bowl as a first course, garnish it with toasted walnuts, thinly sliced green onions and a little crumbled Gorgonzola.

Makes 12 to 16 shooters or 8 regular servings

1 cauliflower (about 1 1/2 lb/750 g after trimming), broken in florets (about 4 cups/1 L)
1 tbsp (15 mL) olive oil
1 tsp (5 mL) salt
1 tsp (5 mL) chopped fresh thyme, or pinch dried
1/4 tsp (1 mL) pepper
3 cups (750 mL) homemade vegetable stock (page 109), chicken stock or water

1. Toss cauliflower with oil, salt, thyme and pepper. Spread cauliflower on a baking sheet lined with parchment paper and roast in a preheated 350°F (180°C) oven for 30 to 40 minutes, or until very tender.
2. Puree cauliflower and stock. Transfer to a saucepan and bring to a boil. Reduce heat and simmer for a few minutes. Soup should be thin enough to drink (or serve with little demi-tasse spoons). Taste and adjust seasonings if necessary. Serve in shooter glasses or espresso cups.

JERUSALEM ARTICHOKE SOUP

Jerusalem artichokes are not really artichokes, and they do not come from Jerusalem. They don't look like regular artichokes, either, but are knobby little roots. They are actually a type of sunflower (*girisole* in Italian), and some believe "Jerusalem" came from a misinterpretation of the Italian. In California they are called sunchokes, which makes more sense. They have a unique delicious flavour and can be added to mashed potatoes or roasted root vegetable mixtures. Some people like them raw in salads, but I prefer them cooked.

People with sensitive stomachs sometimes have trouble digesting Jerusalem artichokes. I usually serve them in small quantities, but they are so good that everyone always wants more!

Oddly enough, I first had this soup in Jerusalem (where chefs there love them, too). Making a "cream" with nuts and adding it to enrich the soup is a trick I learned from Jerusalem star chef Moshe Basson.

Makes 8 to 10 servings

2 tsp (10 mL) olive oil
2 onions, chopped
2 cloves garlic, finely chopped
2 lb (1 kg) Jerusalem artichokes, scrubbed or peeled and sliced
6 cups (1.5 L) homemade vegetable stock (page 109),
    chicken stock or water
Pinch crushed saffron threads
1 tsp (5 mL) salt
1/4 tsp (1 mL) pepper
1 tbsp (15 mL) lemon juice
1/4 cup (50 mL) almonds, optional
1/4 cup (50 mL) water, optional

1. Heat oil in a large saucepan on medium heat. Add onions and garlic and cook gently for 5 minutes, or until tender and fragrant but not brown. Add about 1/4 cup (50 mL) water if onions start to stick.
2. Add Jerusalem artichokes and cook for a few minutes longer. Add stock and bring to a boil.
3. Add saffron, salt and pepper. Reduce heat, cover and simmer for 30 minutes.
4. Puree soup and return to heat. Stir in lemon juice. Taste and adjust seasonings if necessary. If soup is too thick, add water.
5. Puree almonds with water until very smooth and stir into soup.

COMMERCIAL SOUP STOCKS

Salt-free, fat-free homemade stocks (page 109) are the best, but if you do not have homemade stocks, there are substitutes.

- I like to use the stocks sold in Tetra Paks. They can be resealed and stored in the refrigerator. Taste different brands to see which ones you like the best.
- Frozen stock is usually salt free, with the fat removed, but it can be quite expensive, so dilute it with water.
- Canned broth, bouillon cubes and powdered soup bases usually contain a lot of salt; they can also

PER SERVING

Calories	81
Protein	2 g
Fat	1 g
Saturates	trace
Cholesterol	0 mg
Carbohydrate	16 g
Fibre	2 g
Sodium	302 mg
Potassium	381 mg

Good: Thiamine; Iron

contain MSG, fat and food colouring. Buy lower-salt, lower-fat products if possible and refrigerate canned broth before opening. The fat will solidify on the surface, and you can remove it before using. I then dilute the canned broth more than the directions recommend, and freeze any extra.

- If you use bouillon cubes or powdered soup bases, dilute them with lots of water, and look for lower-salt, lower-fat brands.
- Water can be a good substitute for stock when there are many other flavourful ingredients in the recipe.

GRILLED CORN CHOWDER WITH CILANTRO AND CHIPOTLES

This smoky-tasting chowder is especially delicious in the fall when local corn is at its sweetest. You can grill the corn on a barbecue or in a grill pan, or use the corn without grilling it at all. For extra flavour and colour, add about 1 cup (250 mL) diced butternut squash when you add the potatoes.

Makes 6 to 8 servings

6 ears corn, husked
2 tsp (10 mL) olive oil
1 onion, diced
1 tsp (5 mL) chipotle puree, or 1 jalapeño, seeded and diced
1 large Yukon Gold or baking potato, peeled and diced
3 cups (750 mL) homemade vegetable stock (page 109), chicken stock or water
1 tsp (5 mL) salt
1 cup (250 mL) milk or water
1 tomato, seeded and diced
2 tbsp (25 mL) chopped fresh cilantro
2 tbsp (25 mL) pine nuts, toasted

1. Remove kernels from 4 ears of corn (page 92) and reserve. You should have about 3 cups (750 mL).
2. Grill remaining 2 ears of corn directly on a hot grill, turning frequently, until some kernels are tinged with brown. This will take about 5 minutes. Cool, remove corn from cobs and reserve separately.
3. In a large saucepan, heat oil on medium heat. Add onion and cook gently for 5 to 8 minutes, or until tender but not brown. Add chipotle and potato. Cook for about 2 minutes.
4. Add stock and salt. Bring to a boil. Add reserved ungrilled corn kernels. Reduce heat and cook gently for 15 minutes, or until potatoes are tender.
5. Partially puree soup and return to heat. Soup should be creamy with chunks of corn and vegetables. Return soup to saucepan.
6. Add milk and bring to a boil. Taste and adjust seasonings if necessary.
7. Sprinkle with grilled corn, tomato, cilantro and pine nuts just before serving.

FRENCH ONION SOUP

This is delicious with or without the croutons and cheese. It will look as though you have a truckload of sliced onions, but don't worry; they cook down to less than half. If you have leftovers, transfer everything (croutons and soup) to a baking dish. Bake at 350°F (180°C) until the bread absorbs the liquid and serve as a casserole.

If you like your cheese topping gooey, use half mozzarella cheese. For a vegetarian version, use roasted vegetable stock (page 109) instead of chicken or beef stock.

If you don't have ovenproof soup bowls, sprinkle the baked croutons with the Parmesan and bake for about 15 minutes, or until the cheese melts. Place croutons on soup just before serving.

Makes 8 servings

2 tsp (10 mL) olive oil
3 lb (1.5 kg) onions, thinly sliced (about 9)
1 cup (250 mL) dry white wine or stock
1 tbsp (15 mL) red wine vinegar or sherry vinegar
8 cups (2 L) homemade chicken or beef stock (page 109) or
        low-sodium commercial broth
Salt and pepper to taste

Croutons

8 3-inch (7.5 cm) rounds whole wheat or regular French or
        Italian bread (about 1/2 inch/1 cm thick)
1 tbsp (15 mL) olive oil
1 clove garlic, minced
1 tsp (5 mL) chopped fresh thyme, or pinch dried
1/4 tsp (1 mL) salt
1/4 tsp (1 mL) pepper
1/2 cup (125 mL) grated Parmesan, Swiss or Fontina cheese

1. Heat oil in a Dutch oven on medium-high heat. Add onions but do not stir. When onions begin to brown, stir, reduce heat to medium and cook for 15 to 20 minutes, or until onions are tender and evenly browned.

2. Add wine and bring to a boil. Reduce heat again and cook gently until wine has evaporated, about 15 minutes. Add vinegar and cook for a few minutes longer.

3. Add stock, bring to a boil, reduce heat and simmer for 20 minutes. Season with salt and pepper.

PER SERVING	
Calories	181
Protein	6 g
Fat	6 g
Saturates	2 g
Cholesterol	6 mg
Carbohydrate	27 g
Fibre	3 g
Sodium	311 mg
Potassium	494 mg
Excellent: **Niacin**	
Good: **Vitamin B12**	

LEEKS

I use only the white and light-green portions of leeks (unless the leeks are very young, in which case the whole thing is tender). Cut off the root ends and dark-green tops; then peel off the dark-green outside layers until you reach the light-green part.

Leeks collect sand between their layers as they grow, so they must be cleaned thoroughly. Slice the leeks and place them in a large bowl of cold water. Swish the pieces around until the grit sinks to the bottom of the bowl and the leeks float to the top. Lift out the leeks gently and dry them.

PER SERVING	
Calories	101
Protein	2 g
Fat	2 g
Saturates	1 g
Cholesterol	1 mg
Carbohydrate	20 g
Fibre	1 g
Sodium	28 mg
Potassium	253 mg

4. Meanwhile, to prepare croutons, arrange bread in a single layer on a baking sheet. In a small bowl, combine oil, garlic, thyme, salt and pepper. Brush on top of bread. Bake in a preheated 400°F (200°C) oven for 10 minutes, or until lightly browned.

5. To serve, ladle soup into 8 ovenproof onion soup bowls. Place a crouton on each. Sprinkle evenly with cheese. Return to oven and bake for 10 minutes. Allow to rest for 5 minutes before serving.

LEEK AND POTATO SOUP

When I first opened my cooking school, this soup was "hot." Now, twenty years later, it is hot again. (When it is served cold, it becomes the classic Vichyssoise.)

The soup can be served pureed or chunky style, and sometimes it is cooked with half milk and half stock. For a really trendy presentation, drizzle it with a little balsamic vinegar before serving.

Makes 8 servings

1 tbsp (15 mL) olive oil
3 large leeks, trimmed and chopped
1 clove garlic, finely chopped
3 large Yukon Gold or baking potatoes, peeled and diced
5 cups (1.25 L) homemade vegetable stock (page 109), chicken
    stock or water
1 tsp (5 mL) chopped fresh thyme, or pinch dried
1/2 tsp (2 mL) pepper
Salt to taste
1/4 cup (50 mL) chopped fresh chives or green onions

1. Heat oil in a large saucepan on medium heat. Add leeks and garlic and cook gently for 5 to 7 minutes, or until leeks wilt. Add potatoes and combine well.

2. Add stock and bring to a boil. Add thyme and pepper. Reduce heat and simmer gently for 20 minutes, or until potatoes are tender.

3. Puree soup and return to heat. Heat thoroughly. Taste and adjust seasonings, adding salt if necessary. Sprinkle with chives before serving.

Potato and Roasted Garlic Soup

Use 1 chopped onion instead of leeks. Use 3 heads roasted garlic (page 67) instead of raw garlic. Squeeze garlic out of skins before pureeing.

CELERIAC AND POTATO SOUP

Celeriac is available in nearly all supermarkets and many specialty markets. My kids think it looks like a knobby, hairy brain, but it has a wonderfully intense celery-like flavour. I use it in roasted vegetable mixtures, in mashed potatoes, in mixed vegetable soups and in potato soups like this one. See if your guests can guess the secret ingredient.

To peel celeriac, cut a flat piece off the top and bottom. Place a flat side on a cutting board and cut off the peel from top to bottom with a sharp knife.

Makes 6 to 8 servings

1 tbsp (15 mL) olive oil
1 onion, chopped
1 clove garlic, finely chopped
1 lb (500 g) celeriac, peeled and diced
1 lb (500 g) Yukon Gold or baking potatoes, peeled and diced
6 cups (1.5 L) homemade vegetable stock (page 109),
        chicken stock (page 00) or water
1 tbsp (15 mL) chopped fresh thyme, or ½ tsp (2 mL) dried
Salt and pepper to taste

1. Heat oil in a large saucepan on medium-high heat. Add onion and garlic. Cook for a few minutes until tender.

2. Add celeriac and potatoes. Cook for a few minutes. Add stock and thyme. Bring to a boil, reduce heat and simmer gently, uncovered, for 20 to 25 minutes, or until very tender.

3. Remove about ½ cup (125 mL) diced vegetables and reserve for garnish.

4. Puree soup, adding liquid if soup is too thick. Taste and season with salt and pepper. Garnish soup with reserved vegetables.

Celery and Potato Soup

Use celery instead of celeriac. The flavour will be less intense and the texture less creamy, but it will still be delicious. You can also use turnip or rutabaga instead of celeriac.

PER SERVING	
Calories	130
Protein	2 g
Fat	3 g
Saturates	1 g
Cholesterol	1 mg
Carbohydrate	24 g
Fibre	2 g
Sodium	97 mg
Potassium	585 mg
Good: **Vitamin B6**	

SWISS CHARD AND PINE NUT SOUP

This soup was inspired by Israeli chef Moshe Basson, who made it with nettles that he picked in the hills around Jerusalem. He enriched the soup with ground pine nuts, which adds a creamy texture without using dairy products.

Basson is a world-famous chef who owned Eucalyptus, one of the best restaurants in Jerusalem. After the intifada he closed the restaurant, as did many other chefs, because of the decline in tourism. When I met him he had decided to help the community by opening a soup kitchen in the city, where people pay what they can afford. At night he cooks special biblical banquets (using foods mentioned in the Bible) for visiting groups to help pay for the food he serves at the soup kitchen.

Makes 8 servings

2 tsp (10 mL) olive oil
1 onion, chopped
2 cloves garlic, chopped
1 large bunch Swiss chard (about 1 1/2 lb/750 g), stalks and leaves
      chopped separately
4 cups (1 L) homemade vegetable stock (page 109), chicken stock
      or water
1/4 lb (125 g) fresh baby spinach
1/4 cup (50 mL) pine nuts, preferably toasted (page 219)
1/4 cup (50 mL) water
Salt and pepper to taste

1. Heat oil in a large saucepan on medium heat. Add onion and garlic and cook for 5 to 8 minutes, or until tender but not brown. Add Swiss chard stalks. Cook for 5 minutes.
2. Add stock and bring to a boil. Cook for 10 minutes.
3. Add Swiss chard leaves and spinach and cook for 5 minutes.
4. Meanwhile, in a food processor or blender, puree pine nuts with water until very smooth. Add soup and puree. Return to saucepan and heat thoroughly. Season with salt and pepper.

PER SERVING	
Calories	69
Protein	3 g
Fat	3 g
Saturates	1 g
Cholesterol	0 mg
Carbohydrate	8 g
Fibre	2 g
Sodium	165 mg
Potassium	500 mg
Excellent: Vitamin A	
Good: Iron	

THAI CHICKEN NOODLE SOUP

This soup has a bright, fresh flavour. If you want to serve it as a main course, double the amount of chicken. You can also marinate the chicken in 2 tbsp (25 mL) oyster sauce and grill it for 5 minutes per side before slicing and adding it to the soup.

Makes 6 servings

¼ lb (125 g) thin rice vermicelli or angelhair pasta
1 tsp (5 mL) vegetable oil
1 tbsp (15 mL) finely chopped lemongrass
1 tsp (5 mL) finely grated lime peel
1 tsp (5 mL) finely chopped fresh ginger root
Pinch hot red pepper flakes
6 cups (1.5 L) homemade chicken stock (page 109) or
    low-sodium commercial broth
½ lb (250 g) boneless, skinless chicken breasts, thinly sliced
1 carrot, grated
1 sweet red pepper, seeded and diced
1 tbsp (15 mL) Thai fish sauce or soy sauce
½ tsp (2 mL) hot Asian chili paste
¼ cup (50 mL) lime juice
¼ cup (50 mL) coarsely chopped fresh cilantro or parsley
Salt to taste

1. Cover rice vermicelli with warm water and let sit for 15 minutes. Drain well and reserve. (If you are using angelhair pasta, cook in boiling water until tender.)
2. Heat oil in a large saucepan on low heat. Add lemongrass, lime peel, ginger and hot pepper flakes and cook for about 30 seconds, or until fragrant.
3. Add stock and bring to a boil.
4. Add chicken, carrot, red pepper, fish sauce and chili paste. Reduce heat and simmer for 5 minutes. Add drained noodles and cook for 2 minutes longer, or until heated through.
5. Stir in lime juice and cilantro. Taste and adjust seasonings, adding salt if necessary.

LEMONGRASS

Lemongrass has an aromatic lemony flavour. The centre of the stalk should be moist and easy to chop. If it is dry and coarse, add it to the soup in large pieces and remove them before serving. If you cannot find lemongrass, use 1 tsp (5 mL) grated lemon peel.

PER SERVING

Calories	172
Protein	16 g
Fat	3 g
Saturates	1 g
Cholesterol	23 mg
Carbohydrate	19 g
Fibre	1 g
Sodium	326 mg
Potassium	395 mg

Excellent: Vitamin A; Vitamin C; Niacin
Good: Vitamin B6; Vitamin B12

JAPANESE-STYLE CHICKEN NOODLE SOUP

A big bowl of this soup makes a great main course, or you can serve it in smaller portions as a starter. Use chopsticks for the noodles, chicken and vegetables and drink the rest right out of the bowl, or provide spoons if you think your guests would not be comfortable slurping!

When I serve a clear soup with pasta in it, I like to cook the pasta separately so the broth stays clear.

For a vegetarian version, use vegetable stock (page 109) and more tofu instead of adding chicken.

Makes 6 to 8 servings

8 cups (2 L) homemade chicken stock (page 109) or
    low-sodium commercial broth
2 1-inch (2.5 cm) pieces fresh ginger root, smashed
1/4 cup (50 mL) rice wine
2 tbsp (25 mL) soy sauce
3/4 lb (375 g) udon noodles, soba (buckwheat) noodles or
    whole wheat spaghetti
1/2 lb (250 g) boneless, skinless chicken breasts,
    cut in 1/2-inch (1 cm) chunks
8 fresh shiitake mushrooms, stemmed and sliced
6 oz (175 g) fresh baby spinach
1 cup (250 mL) peas
2 carrots, grated
1/4 lb (125 g) firm or Japanese-style silken tofu (page 189),
    cut in 1/2-inch (1 cm) cubes
8 green onions, sliced on diagonal
1/4 cup (50 mL) coarsely chopped fresh cilantro

PER SERVING	
Calories	350
Protein	31 g
Fat	5 g
Saturates	1 g
Cholesterol	24 mg
Carbohydrate	50 g
Fibre	4 g
Sodium	798 mg
Potassium	828 mg

Excellent: Vitamin A; Niacin; Folate; Iron
Good: Riboflavin; Vitamin B6; Vitamin B12

1. In a large saucepan, combine stock, ginger, rice wine and soy sauce. Bring to a boil, reduce heat and simmer gently for 10 minutes. Discard ginger.
2. Meanwhile, cook noodles in a separate saucepan of boiling water for 5 to 6 minutes, or until almost tender. Rinse with cold water to help prevent sticking. Drain well.
3. Add chicken and mushrooms to stock and cook for 2 minutes. Add spinach, peas, carrots, tofu, green onions and noodles. Heat thoroughly for about 5 minutes. Taste and adjust seasonings if necessary. Sprinkle with cilantro.

CHICKEN SOUP WITH MATZO BALLS

Chicken soup with matzo balls has almost become a Jewish cliché. But matzo balls break down all ethnic barriers, because everyone seems to love them.

Texturally, there are two kinds of matzo balls—hard ones and soft fluffy ones. I have always preferred the latter, but I never seemed to be able to have any control over whether they turned out hard or fluffy. Then Rhonda Caplan, who works with me at the cooking school, told me about her mother's recipe. So I started making Sally Caplan's matzo balls, and my problem was solved. They are not only fluffy, but also lighter than most in calories and fat.

When it comes to the soup, use the best chicken you can. If it is not a kosher chicken, it should be organic or naturally raised.

Leftover soup makes a great homemade chicken stock; I usually dilute it a bit before using.

I like to make chicken soup a day ahead so I can refrigerate it overnight; the fat rises to the surface and solidifies, making it easy to remove.

Makes 8 to 10 servings

1 4-lb (2 kg) chicken
12 cups (3 L) cold water (approx.)
2 onions, quartered
2 stalks celery with leaves, sliced
2 carrots, sliced
2 parsnips, peeled and sliced
1 bay leaf
1 bunch fresh parsley
1 tsp (5 mL) salt
¼ tsp (1 mL) pepper

Matzo Balls

1 egg
2 egg whites
½ cup (125 mL) matzo meal
1 ½ tsp (7 mL) salt
2 tbsp (25 mL) chicken soup
2 tbsp (25 mL) chopped fresh parsley

MATZO
Matzo is an unleavened flatbread traditionally served at Passover. Matzo meal is ground matzo. Both can be purchased at Jewish delicatessens and many supermarkets.

PER SERVING	
Calories	104
Protein	10 g
Fat	3 g
Saturates	1 g
Cholesterol	29 mg
Carbohydrate	8 g
Fibre	0 g
Sodium	715 mg
Potassium	338 mg
Excellent: Niacin	
Good: Vitamin B12	

1. Cut chicken into 8 pieces. Remove and discard any visible fat. Place chicken in a large pot and add cold water just to cover. Bring to a boil and skim off scum that rises to surface.

2. Add onions, celery, carrots, parsnips, bay leaf, parsley, salt and pepper. Bring to a boil again, reduce heat and simmer very gently, uncovered, for 2 hours. Keep chicken covered with water.

3. Strain soup into another pot. Remove chicken from bones and use in the soup or in sandwiches if you wish. If you are serving soup right away, skim off fat.

4. Meanwhile, to prepare matzo balls, beat egg with egg whites. Add matzo meal, salt, 2 tbsp (25 mL) chicken soup and chopped parsley. Cover and refrigerate for 30 minutes.

5. With wet hands, shape mixture into 10 to 12 balls.

6. Bring a large pot of water to a boil. Add matzo balls gently and simmer, covered, for 40 minutes. Remove from water and serve in strained chicken soup.

Vegetarian Matzo Ball Soup

Use homemade roasted vegetable stock (page 109) in the soup and matzo balls, but season well. You can also use vegetable stock in the matzo balls and add them to another soup such as carrot (page 78) or Israeli lentil (page 97).

STOCK POTS

You need a big pot to make stock. A pasta pot, if you happen to have one, works well. It comes with a built-in colander that allows you to lift the pasta out of the cooking water to drain it. The pots are also great for making stock. Just pull out the bones, meat and vegetables, and you won't even have to strain the stock.

FREEZING STOCK

If you don't have a lot of freezer space, make your own condensed frozen homemade bouillon cubes. Boil down stock to one-eighth the original amount. Freeze in ice cube trays and pack in bags (label them clearly). Or freeze stock flat in small zipper-style plastic freezer bags (page 300).

Before using, reconstitute condensed stock by diluting it with boiling water.

ROASTED TOMATO SOUP

Roasting the tomatoes transforms a traditional tomato soup into something spectacular. I like to use a food mill (page 450) to puree the soup, because it removes the skins and seeds of the peppers and tomatoes, but you can also use a food processor or blender.

You can use two 28-oz (796 mL) cans of plum tomatoes (I like San Marzano the best) instead of the roasted tomatoes. Simply drain and add them to the saucepan with the roasted onions and peppers. Cook the soup for 15 minutes after adding the stock.

Use leftover soup as a sauce on pasta, or combine with vinegar and olive oil to make a salad dressing.

You can omit the chive/goat cheese garnish and simply swirl a spoonful of unflavoured yogurt in the centre of each serving. You can also top the soup with chopped toasted pine nuts or a little fresh tomato salsa.

Makes 6 to 8 servings

3 lb (1.5 kg) plum tomatoes (12 to 15), quartered lengthwise
3 sweet red peppers, halved and seeded
1 jalapeño, halved and seeded, or 1 tbsp (15 mL) chipotle puree
       (page 183)
1 onion, cut in chunks
1 tbsp (15 mL) olive oil
1 tbsp (15 mL) chopped fresh thyme, or 1/2 tsp (2 mL) dried
1 tbsp (15 mL) chopped fresh rosemary, or 1/2 tsp (2 mL) dried
1/2 tsp (2 mL) salt
1/4 tsp (1 mL) pepper
4 heads garlic
2 1/2 cups (625 mL) homemade vegetable stock (page 109),
       chicken stock or water
2 tbsp (25 mL) balsamic vinegar
1/4 cup (50 mL) crumbled soft unripened goat cheese
1 bunch fresh chives

1. Arrange tomatoes cut side up on baking sheets lined with parchment paper. Arrange red peppers and jalapeño skin side up alongside tomatoes (if you are using chipotle puree, add to soup in Step 3). Break up onion and scatter over vegetables. Drizzle vegetables with oil and sprinkle with thyme, rosemary, salt and pepper.
2. Cut top quarter off each head of garlic and wrap heads in foil in a single layer. Place vegetables and garlic in a preheated 400°F (200°C) oven and roast for 30 to 45 minutes, or until vegetables are brown

10 QUICK SOUP GARNISHES

- chopped fresh herbs
- swirl of plain or seasoned yogurt cheese (page 391)
- crushed baked corn chips (page 49)
- croutons (page 121)
- sprinkling of seeds (sesame, poppy, cumin, caraway)
- light sprinkling of grated low-fat cheese
- light dusting of finely chopped toasted nuts
- finely chopped salad or salsa
- thinly sliced baked potato skins (page 344)
- chopped or whole cooked chickpeas

PER SERVING	
Calories	151
Protein	6 g
Fat	5 g
Saturates	1 g
Cholesterol	3 mg
Carbohydrate	26 g
Fibre	5 g
Sodium	253 mg
Potassium	719 mg
Excellent: Vitamin A; Vitamin C; Vitamin B6	
Good: Thiamine; Iron	

and garlic is very squeezable. Peel peppers if skin comes off easily; otherwise don't worry.

3. Combine tomatoes, peppers and onion in a large saucepan. Squeeze in roasted garlic. Add stock and bring to a boil. Cook, uncovered, for 5 minutes.

4. Puree soup and return to heat. If soup is too thick, add stock; if it is too thin, cook, uncovered, until reduced.

5. Add vinegar and simmer for a few minutes. Taste and adjust seasonings if necessary.

6. Spoon soup into shallow bowls. Spoon a little crumbled goat cheese on each serving. Chop chives or hold bunch of chives over each serving and cut into 2-inch (5 cm) lengths so they fall like pick-up sticks.

CURRIED BUTTERNUT SOUP

My editor Shelley Tanaka and I have worked on my cookbooks for more than twenty years. One of the biggest compliments she pays me is that she often cooks my recipes as she edits them, saying she just can't resist. She gave me the inspiration for this yummy soup. My students say that when they're cooking my recipes at home they can hear me saying "delicious," but I hear Shelley saying "yummy."

Makes 6 to 8 servings

2 tsp (10 mL) olive oil
1 onion, chopped
3 cloves garlic, finely chopped
1 tbsp (15 mL) curry paste or powder
4 cups (1 L) diced peeled butternut squash (1 1/2 lb/750 g)
4 cups (1 L) homemade vegetable stock (page 109),
        chicken stock or water
Salt to taste
2 tbsp (25 mL) toasted sliced almonds, optional

1. Heat oil in a large saucepan on medium heat. Add onion and garlic and cook gently for 5 to 8 minutes, or until tender and fragrant. If mixture starts to burn or pan becomes dry, add a little water.

2. Stir in curry paste and cook for about 30 seconds.

3. Add squash and cook for a few minutes. Add stock and bring to a boil. Reduce heat and cook gently for 30 minutes.

4. Puree soup until smooth. Return to heat. Thin with some water if necessary. Add salt if necessary. Serve with toasted almonds sprinkled on top.

PER SERVING	
Calories	95
Protein	2 g
Fat	3 g
Saturates	trace
Cholesterol	0 mg
Carbohydrate	17 g
Fibre	2 g
Sodium	461 mg
Potassium	334 mg
Excellent: Vitamin A	
Good: Vitamin C	

BARBECUED TOMATO AND CORN SOUP

I like to make this recipe in barbecue classes so people will know that they can add wonderful smoky flavours to soups as well as salads, pasta dishes and sandwiches.

Leftovers can be used as a pasta sauce or made into a stew by adding cooked chicken, shrimp, meat or chickpeas.

Makes 8 servings

3 lb (1.5 kg) plum tomatoes, halved and seeded (12 to 15)
2 onions, cut in ½-inch (1 cm) slices
3 ears corn, husked
1 tbsp (15 mL) olive oil
4 cloves garlic, finely chopped
1 tbsp (15 mL) chipotle puree (page 183) or 1 jalapeño,
      seeded and finely chopped
4 cups (1 L) homemade vegetable stock (page 109),
      chicken stock or water
1 tbsp (15 mL) balsamic vinegar
Salt and pepper to taste
¼ cup (50 mL) shredded fresh basil

1. Grill tomatoes for a few minutes on each side until soft and brown.
2. Grill onion slices for a few minutes on each side until tender and brown. Dice.
3. Cook corn for a few minutes directly on grill until browned, turning to cook all sides. Cut or break cobs in half and stand upright, cut side down, on a cutting board. Cut kernels off cob from top to bottom.
4. Heat oil in a large saucepan on medium heat. Add garlic and cook gently for few minutes, or until tender and fragrant. Add chipotle and tomatoes. Stir and cook until hot.
5. Add stock and bring to a boil. Reduce heat and simmer for about 15 minutes.
6. Puree soup and return to heat. Add grilled onions and corn and cook for 5 minutes.
7. Add vinegar and season with salt and pepper. Serve garnished with shredded basil.

HOT ASIAN CHILI PASTE
Made with garlic and hot peppers, this is hot and delicious. Although it is traditionally an Asian ingredient, I use it in sauces, dips and spreads. I like the Vietnamese brand with the rooster on it.

PER SERVING

Calories	122
Protein	4 g
Fat	2 g
Saturates	1 g
Cholesterol	1 mg
Carbohydrate	25 g
Fibre	4 g
Sodium	38 mg
Potassium	611 mg

Excellent: Vitamin C
Good: Vitamin A;
Thiamine; Folate

HOT AND SOUR SOUP

Black Chinese vinegar is made from a variety of grains and adds a smoky, complex flavour to this popular soup that is easy to make at home.

Makes 6 to 8 servings

10 dried or fresh shiitake mushrooms
2 tbsp (25 mL) cornstarch
1/4 cup (50 mL) water
6 cups (1.5 L) homemade vegetable stock (page 109), chicken stock or water
3 leeks, trimmed and shredded, or 1 onion, very thinly sliced
1 cup (250 mL) thinly sliced bamboo shoots
1/2 lb (250 g) extra-firm tofu, cut in thin strips
3 tbsp (45 mL) black Chinese vinegar, balsamic vinegar or Worcestershire sauce
2 tbsp (25 mL) soy sauce
2 tbsp (25 mL) finely chopped fresh ginger root
1 tsp (5 mL) dark sesame oil
1/2 tsp (2 mL) pepper
1/2 tsp (2 mL) hot Asian chili paste
2 egg whites or 1 egg, beaten
3 green onions, thinly sliced

1. If you are using dried mushrooms, cover with hot water and let soften for 20 minutes. Drain and rinse. Discard shiitake stems and slice caps.
2. In a small bowl, blend cornstarch and water.
3. In a large saucepan, combine stock, mushrooms, leeks, bamboo shoots and tofu. Bring to a boil. Skim if necessary and cook for about 3 minutes.
4. Add vinegar, soy sauce, ginger, sesame oil, pepper and chili paste. Taste and adjust seasonings if necessary.
5. Stir cornstarch mixture and add to soup. Cook for a few minutes until slightly thickened, stirring to prevent lumps.
6. Remove soup from heat and slowly add beaten egg whites, stirring constantly so egg forms strands and cooks thoroughly. Add green onions.

PER SERVING	
Calories	139
Protein	10 g
Fat	2 g
Saturates	trace
Cholesterol	1 mg
Carbohydrate	23 g
Fibre	3 g
Sodium	428 mg
Potassium	384 mg

SPICY GAZPACHO

Gazpacho is really a salad in a bowl. It should be cool and refreshing. I like it spicy, but it's up to you. You can also add ½ cup (125 mL) corn kernels or chopped cooked shrimp, crab or lobster to the topping.

Makes 6 servings

3 large ripe tomatoes, seeded and coarsely chopped
1 sweet green pepper, seeded and coarsely chopped
1 sweet red pepper, seeded and coarsely chopped
1 stalk celery, coarsely chopped
1 English cucumber, coarsely chopped
3 green onions, coarsely chopped
2 cloves garlic, coarsely chopped
1 ½ cups (375 mL) V-8 or tomato juice
1 cup (250 mL) water
1 tbsp (15 mL) olive oil
1 tbsp (15 mL) Worcestershire sauce
1 tbsp (15 mL) sherry vinegar or balsamic vinegar
½ tsp (2 mL) hot red pepper sauce
Salt and pepper to taste

Garnish

1 tomato, seeded and diced
1 cup (250 mL) diced English cucumber
2 tbsp (25 mL) chopped fresh chives or green onions
2 tbsp (25 mL) chopped fresh parsley
2 tbsp (25 mL) shredded fresh basil or chopped parsley
1 ½ cups (375 mL) croutons (page 121)

1. In a food processor, combine tomatoes, peppers, celery, cucumber, green onions and garlic. Chop finely.
2. Add V-8, water, oil, Worcestershire, vinegar and hot pepper sauce. Puree until smooth. Taste and adjust seasonings with salt and pepper, vinegar and hot sauce.
3. To prepare garnish, combine tomato, cucumber, chives, parsley and basil. Sprinkle on soup. Add croutons and serve.

PER SERVING	
Calories	133
Protein	4 g
Fat	3 g
Saturates	1 g
Cholesterol	0 mg
Carbohydrate	24 g
Fibre	4 g
Sodium	368 mg
Potassium	627 mg

Excellent: Vitamin A; Vitamin C; Folate
Good: Thiamine; Vitamin B6

PASTA E FAGIOLI

This soup is delicious and heart-warming. Serve it in large bowls with crusty bread and a salad for a main course or in smaller portions as an appetizer. For a vegetarian version, omit the ham and use vegetable stock or water instead of chicken stock.

Any leftover soup will be very thick. You can reheat the soup and thin it with extra liquid, or add cubes of bread and more cheese and bake it in a casserole at 350°F (180°C) for about 30 minutes. It will be like a ribollita (page 196)—a casserole made with leftover minestrone.

Makes 8 servings

1 tbsp (15 mL) olive oil
2 onions, chopped
3 cloves garlic, finely chopped
1 carrot, chopped
1/4 tsp (1 mL) hot red pepper flakes, optional
1 28-oz (796 mL) can plum tomatoes, with juices
4 cups (1 L) homemade chicken stock (page 109) or low-sodium
      commercial broth
2 oz (60 g) smoked ham, in one piece, trimmed of any fat,
      optional
1 19-oz (540 g) can white kidney beans, rinsed and drained, or
      2 cups (500 mL) cooked beans
1 cup (250 mL) small wholewheat macaroni or soup pasta
Salt and pepper to taste
2 tbsp (25 mL) grated Parmesan cheese

PER SERVING	
Calories	181
Protein	10 g
Fat	4 g
Saturates	1 g
Cholesterol	2 mg
Carbohydrate	29 g
Fibre	7 g
Sodium	371 mg
Potassium	516 mg
Excellent: Vitamin A	
Good: Niacin; Folate	

1. Heat oil in a large saucepan on medium-high heat. Add onions, garlic and carrot and cook for 5 to 7 minutes, or until tender. Add hot pepper flakes.

2. Add tomatoes with their juices and break up tomatoes with a spoon. Add stock and bring to a boil. Add ham, reduce heat and simmer gently for about 30 minutes.

3. Add beans and cook for 10 minutes. Remove ham (dice and use as a garnish if you wish).

4. Puree half of soup and return all soup to saucepan. Bring to a boil.

5. Add pasta and cook for about 10 minutes, or until pasta is very tender. Stir often, as pasta easily sticks to bottom of pan. If soup is too thick, add some water. Taste and add salt and pepper if necessary. Serve sprinkled with Parmesan.

MEXICAN GREEN LENTIL SOUP

There are many types of lentil soups. I love this one, modelled after a version I tasted at a Banff restaurant called Coyotes Deli and Grill. Green lentils are used in this soup so they retain their shape and texture. I like the tiny French ones the best.

Makes 8 to 10 servings

1 tbsp (15 mL) olive oil
2 onions, chopped
2 cloves garlic, finely chopped
1 tbsp (15 mL) ground cumin
1 tbsp (15 mL) chipotle puree (page 183), or
    1 jalapeño, seeded and finely chopped
2 carrots, diced
2 stalks celery, diced
2 parsnips, peeled and diced
1 potato, peeled and diced
2 cups (500 mL) dried green lentils, rinsed and picked over
8 cups (2 L) homemade vegetable stock (page 109),
    chicken stock or water
1 1/2 cups (375 mL) corn kernels
2 tbsp (25 mL) lemon juice
Salt and pepper to taste
3 oz (90 g) soft unripened goat cheese
3 tbsp (45 mL) milk
1/4 cup (50 mL) chopped fresh cilantro or basil

1. Heat oil in a large saucepan on medium-high heat. Add onions and garlic and cook for 5 to 8 minutes, or until tender. Add cumin and chipotle and cook for 30 seconds.
2. Add carrots, celery, parsnips and potato. Cook for about 5 minutes. Stir in lentils and stock and bring to a boil. Reduce heat and simmer gently, uncovered, for about 30 minutes, or until lentils are very tender.
3. Add corn. Cook for 3 minutes. Add lemon juice. Taste and season with salt and pepper if necessary.
4. In a small bowl, combine goat cheese and milk until smooth. Serve soup drizzled with goat cheese mixture and sprinkled with cilantro.

LENTILS

Small red (pink or orange) lentils are commonly used in soups because they cook quickly, lose their shape and act as a thickener. The large green or brown lentils are usually used when you want the lentils to keep their shape (e.g., in salads and side dishes). I especially like the tiny green French Puy lentils for their clean taste and texture.

Lentils do not need to be soaked, and they are easy and quick to cook. I am not fond of canned green lentils, as they have a mushy texture.

PER SERVING

Calories	323
Protein	17 g
Fat	5 g
Saturates	2 g
Cholesterol	5 mg
Carbohydrate	55 g
Fibre	9 g
Sodium	127 mg
Potassium	889 mg

Excellent: Vitamin A; Thiamine; Vitamin B6; Folate; Iron
Good: Niacin

ISRAELI RED LENTIL SOUP

Every Middle Eastern cook has a favourite lentil soup. This easy, lemony version is thinner than most lentil soups. Use red lentils, as they dissolve and thicken when cooked, unlike green lentils, which hold their shape.

This is a good family soup, but if you are cooking it for children, reduce or omit the jalapeño and/or the cilantro.

Makes 6 to 8 servings

1 cup (250 mL) dried red lentils
2 tsp (10 mL) vegetable oil
1 large onion, chopped
3 cloves garlic, finely chopped
1 jalapeño, seeded and chopped
1 tsp (5 mL) ground cumin
8 cups (2 L) homemade vegetable stock (page 109),
      chicken stock or water
1 tsp (5 mL) salt
$^{1}/_{4}$ tsp (1 mL) pepper
2 tbsp (25 mL) lemon juice
$^{1}/_{3}$ cup (75 mL) chopped fresh cilantro

PER SERVING	
Calories	167
Protein	9 g
Fat	2 g
Saturates	trace
Cholesterol	0 mg
Carbohydrate	29 g
Fibre	5 g
Sodium	468 mg
Potassium	414 mg
Excellent: Folate; Iron	
Good: Vitamin A; Thiamine	

1. Place lentils in a sieve and rinse well. Spread out on a baking sheet and pick over to discard any stones.
2. Heat oil in a large saucepan on medium heat. Add onion, garlic and jalapeño and cook gently for 5 to 10 minutes, or until tender and fragrant. Add cumin and cook for about 30 seconds, or until fragrant.
3. Add rinsed lentils and stock and bring to a boil. Reduce heat and simmer gently, uncovered, for about 30 minutes, or until lentils are very tender and mixture is thick. (If soup is too thick, add stock or water.)
4. Add salt, pepper and lemon juice. Taste and adjust seasonings if necessary. Add cilantro before serving.

WHITE BEAN SOUP WITH SALAD SALSA

For a quick version of this soup, use canned beans (two 19-oz/ 540 mL cans) and cook the beans with the potatoes until the potatoes are tender, about 15 to 20 minutes.

Makes 8 to 10 servings

1 1/2 cups (375 mL) dried white kidney beans or navy beans
2 tsp (10 mL) olive oil
1 onion, finely chopped
3 cloves garlic, finely chopped
1/4 tsp (1 mL) hot red pepper flakes
8 cups (2 L) homemade vegetable stock (page 109),
    chicken stock or water
1/2 cup (125 mL) whole wheat or regular macaroni or soup pasta
1/2 tsp (2 mL) pepper
Salt to taste

Salad Salsa

2 large tomatoes, seeded and chopped
1/2 cup (125 mL) chopped arugula or watercress
2 tbsp (25 mL) chopped fresh chives or green onions
2 tbsp (25 mL) shredded fresh basil
2 tbsp (25 mL) chopped fresh parsley
1 small clove garlic, minced
1/2 tsp (2 mL) pepper
Salt to taste

1. Cover beans with plenty of water and soak for 3 hours at room temperature or overnight in refrigerator. Rinse and drain well.
2. Heat oil in a large saucepan on medium heat. Add onion, garlic and hot pepper flakes and cook gently for a few minutes without browning.
3. Add beans and stock. Bring to a boil, reduce heat and simmer gently, covered, for 1 hour, or until beans are tender.
4. Puree all or half of soup. Return to heat and thin with additional stock or water until soup reaches desired consistency.
5. Add pasta and cook for 10 minutes. Pasta will thicken soup slightly, so thin soup again if necessary. Add pepper. Taste and adjust seasonings, adding salt if necessary.
6. Meanwhile, to prepare salsa, combine tomatoes, arugula, chives, basil, parsley, garlic and pepper. Taste and adjust seasonings, adding salt if necessary. Serve soup with spoonful of salsa.

PER SERVING	
Calories	191
Protein	10 g
Fat	2 g
Saturates	trace
Cholesterol	0 mg
Carbohydrate	35 g
Fibre	10 g
Sodium	65 mg
Potassium	547 mg

Excellent: Folate; Iron
Good: Vitamin A; Thiamine

MUSHROOM, BEAN AND BARLEY SOUP

A chapter on soups would not be complete without a version of this hearty classic. I always make lots so that I have it for a few days. Thin leftover soup with water if necessary, as it thickens when it sits in the refrigerator. One 19-oz (540 mL) can white kidney beans, rinsed and drained, can be used instead of the dried beans; add them in Step 4 after the soup has cooked for 30 minutes.

Makes 12 to 14 servings

1 cup (250 mL) dried white kidney beans or navy beans
1/2 oz (15 g) dried wild mushrooms
2/3 cup (150 mL) pearl barley, rinsed
10 cups (2.5 L) homemade vegetable stock (page 109),
    chicken stock or water
1 onion, chopped
2 carrots, diced
2 stalks celery, diced
3 cloves garlic, finely chopped
1/2 lb (250 g) fresh mushrooms, sliced (about 3 cups/750 mL)
1/2 tsp (2 mL) pepper
Salt to taste
1/4 cup (50 mL) chopped fresh parsley

PER SERVING	
Calories	140
Protein	6 g
Fat	1 g
Saturates	trace
Cholesterol	0 mg
Carbohydrate	30 g
Fibre	8 g
Sodium	43 mg
Potassium	338 mg

Excellent: Vitamin A; Folate
Good: Niacin; Iron

1. Cover beans generously with water and soak for a few hours at room temperature or overnight in refrigerator. Rinse and drain.
2. Cover dried wild mushrooms with 1 cup (250 mL) warm water and allow to rest for 30 minutes. Strain liquid through a sieve lined with paper towel and reserve liquid. Rinse each mushroom to remove any sand or grit. Chop dried mushrooms and reserve.
3. Place barley, beans, reserved mushroom juice and stock in a large saucepan. Bring to a boil. Remove any scum that rises to surface.
4. Add onion, carrots, celery, garlic, fresh mushrooms and dried mushrooms. Cook for 1 hour, or until beans are tender and soup thickens. Stir occasionally. If soup is too thick, add water. Add pepper. Taste and adjust seasonings, adding salt if necessary. Serve sprinkled with parsley.

MOROCCAN MIXED BEAN SOUP WITH PASTA

This soup has an exotic flavour, but it is easy to make. Garam masala is a blend of spices. It is commercially available at specialty stores or East Indian markets, but if you cannot find it, make your own or just use cumin.

Makes 8 to 10 servings

1 tbsp (15 mL) olive oil
2 onions, chopped
2 cloves garlic, finely chopped
1 tbsp (15 mL) finely chopped fresh ginger root
1 tsp (5 mL) garam masala
1/2 tsp (2 mL) ground turmeric
1/4 tsp (1 mL) cayenne
3/4 cup (175 mL) dried red lentils, rinsed
1 28-oz (796 mL) can plum tomatoes, with juices
8 cups (2 L) homemade vegetable stock (page 109),
      chicken stock or water
1 19-oz (540 mL) can chickpeas, rinsed and drained, or 2 cups
      (500 mL) cooked chickpeas
1 19-oz (540 mL) can white kidney beans, rinsed and drained, or
      2 cups (500 mL) cooked kidney beans
1/2 cup (125 mL) broken whole wheat or regular spaghettini
3 tbsp (45 mL) lemon juice
1/4 tsp (1 mL) pepper
Salt to taste
1/3 cup (75 mL) chopped fresh cilantro or parsley

1. Heat oil in a large saucepan on medium heat. Add onions, garlic and ginger and cook gently for a few minutes, or just until onions wilt.
2. Add garam masala, turmeric and cayenne. Cook for 3 minutes. If mixture begins to stick or burn, add 1/2 cup (125 mL) water.
3. Stir in lentils, tomatoes and stock. Bring to a boil, reduce heat and simmer gently for 20 minutes.
4. Add chickpeas and beans and simmer for 20 minutes.
5. Puree about one-third of soup and return to saucepan. If soup is too thick, add some water.
6. Add spaghettini and cook for 15 minutes, or until pasta is very tender. Stir in lemon juice and pepper. Taste and adjust seasonings, adding salt if necessary. Serve sprinkled with cilantro.

GARAM MASALA
Combine 1 tbsp (15 mL) each ground cardamom, ground cinnamon and ground coriander, and 1 tsp (5 mL) each ground cloves, black pepper and ground nutmeg.
    Makes about 1/4 cup (50 mL).

PER SERVING

Calories	284
Protein	14 g
Fat	4 g
Saturates	1 g
Cholesterol	1 mg
Carbohydrate	51 g
Fibre	10 g
Sodium	407 mg
Potassium	725 mg

Excellent: Vitamin B6; Folate; Iron
Good: Thiamine; Niacin

BLACK BEAN SOUP WITH YOGURT AND SPICY SALSA

Black bean soup can be served as a starter or main course. Be sure to use dried black turtle beans and not the fermented black beans used in Asian cooking. You could also use canned black beans in this soup; use two 19-oz (540 mL) cans, rinsed and drained, and cook the soup for only 30 minutes after adding the beans.

Makes 8 to 10 servings

1 lb (500 g) dried black beans (about 2 cups/500 mL)
2 tsp (10 mL) olive oil
1 onion, chopped
6 cloves garlic, finely chopped
1 tbsp (15 mL) ground cumin
1 tbsp (15 mL) paprika
1/2 tsp (2 mL) cayenne
8 cups (2 L) homemade vegetable stock (page 109),
     chicken stock or water
1 tbsp (15 mL) chipotle puree (page 183) or 1 jalapeño, seeded and
     chopped, optional
Salt to taste

Spicy Salsa
2 tbsp (25 mL) chopped onion, preferably red
1 tomato, seeded and diced
1 jalapeño, seeded and chopped
1 small clove garlic, minced
1/4 cup (50 mL) chopped fresh cilantro or parsley

1/2 cup (125 mL) unflavoured low-fat yogurt

PER SERVING	
Calories	257
Protein	15 g
Fat	3 g
Saturates	1 g
Cholesterol	2 mg
Carbohydrate	45 g
Fibre	10 g
Sodium	48 mg
Potassium	665 mg

Excellent: Thiamine; Folate; Iron
Good: Niacin; Vitamin B12

1. Cover beans with water and soak for a few hours at room temperature or overnight in refrigerator. Rinse and drain.
2. Heat oil in a large saucepan on medium heat. Add onion and garlic and cook gently for a few minutes, or until fragrant. Add cumin, paprika and cayenne. Cook for about 30 seconds.
3. Add stock, chipotle and beans and bring to a boil. Cover, reduce heat and simmer for 1 1/2 hours, or until beans are very tender.
4. Puree soup until smooth. Taste and adjust seasonings, adding salt if necessary.
5. To prepare salsa, combine onion, tomato, jalapeño, garlic and cilantro.
6. To serve, ladle soup into shallow bowls. Spoon a little yogurt on each serving and top with salsa.

SPLIT PEA SOUP WITH DILL

This is one of our favourite family soups. Split peas do not need soaking, so this can be prepared more quickly than most soups based on dried legumes. I usually buy green split peas, but the yellow ones are also delicious and are traditionally used in French-Canadian pea soup and in East Indian and Scandinavian recipes.

 If you make the soup a day ahead, it will thicken even more. If necessary, thin it with water and adjust the seasonings when you reheat it.

Makes 8 to 10 servings

1 tbsp (15 mL) vegetable oil
2 onions, diced
2 cloves garlic, finely chopped
2 carrots, diced
2 parsnips, peeled and diced
1 large potato, peeled and diced
1 cup (250 mL) dried split green peas, rinsed
8 cups (2 L) homemade vegetable stock (page 109),
       chicken stock or water
1 cup (250 mL) broken whole wheat or regular spaghetti
2 tbsp (25 mL) chopped fresh dill
¼ tsp (1 mL) pepper
Salt to taste

1. Heat oil in a large saucepan on medium heat. Add onions and garlic and cook for 5 minutes, or until fragrant and tender. Do not brown.
2. Add carrots, parsnips and potato and combine well. Cook for 5 minutes.
3. Add peas and stock. Bring to a boil, reduce heat and simmer gently, covered, for 1 hour, or until peas are tender and soup is very thick. (Soup will probably not need pureeing.) Thin with water if necessary.
4. Add spaghetti and cook for 10 to 15 minutes, or until pasta is very tender. Thin soup again if necessary.
5. Stir in dill and pepper. Taste and adjust seasonings, adding salt if necessary.

PER SERVING	
Calories	252
Protein	10 g
Fat	3 g
Saturates	1 g
Cholesterol	1 mg
Carbohydrate	46 g
Fibre	7 g
Sodium	51 mg
Potassium	554 mg
Excellent: Vitamin A; Folate	
Good: Thiamine; Niacin; Iron	

GREEN MINESTRONE WITH PARMESAN CHEESE CRISPS

This is a tomato-free minestrone that is bright in colour and fresh in flavour. The cheese crisps (sometimes called frico) can be made ahead; they are an amazing garnish for many soups and salads. For a tomato-based minestrone, see the ribollita (page 196).

Makes 8 to 10 servings

2 tsp (10 mL) olive oil
1 onion, chopped
2 leeks, trimmed and chopped
3 cloves garlic, finely chopped
1 bunch Swiss chard, rapini or broccoli, trimmed and chopped
2 zucchini, sliced
8 cups (2 L) homemade vegetable stock (page 109), chicken stock
    or water
$1/2$ cup (125 mL) whole wheat macaroni or soup pasta
$1/2$ lb (250 g) green beans, cut in $1/2$-inch (1 cm) pieces
2 cups (500 mL) peas
$1/4$ cup (50 mL) chopped fresh parsley
2 tbsp (25 mL) chopped fresh basil
$1/4$ tsp (1 mL) pepper
Salt to taste
$3/4$ cup (175 mL) grated Parmesan cheese
$1/4$ cup (50 mL) pesto (page 166), optional

PER SERVING	
Calories	166
Protein	9 g
Fat	5 g
Saturates	2 g
Cholesterol	9 mg
Carbohydrate	25 g
Fibre	5 g
Sodium	325 mg
Potassium	568 mg

Excellent: Folate
Good: Vitamin A;
Riboflavin; Vitamin B12;
Vitamin C; Calcium;
Iron

1. Heat oil in a large saucepan on medium heat. Add onion, leeks and garlic and cook gently for 5 minutes without browning.
2. Add Swiss chard, zucchini and stock. Bring to a boil. Add pasta and cook for 5 minutes.
3. Add beans and peas and cook for 3 minutes longer. Add parsley, basil and pepper. Taste and adjust seasonings, adding salt if necessary.
4. Meanwhile, to prepare cheese croutons, spread Parmesan in a thin layer on a non-stick baking sheet. Bake in a preheated 350°F (180°C) oven for 2 to 5 minutes, or until cheese is melted and browned. Cool until crisp. Remove from baking sheet and break into chunks.
5. Stir pesto into each serving and top with croutons.

CHICKPEA AND SPINACH SOUP

This high-fibre soup is always a hit with my students. If you are making it ahead, add the spinach just before serving to retain the bright green colour.

Makes 8 servings

2 tsp (10 mL) olive oil
1 onion, chopped
2 cloves garlic, finely chopped
1 tsp (5 mL) ground cumin or curry powder
Pinch hot red pepper flakes
1 19-oz (540 mL) can chickpeas, rinsed and drained, or
      2 cups (500 mL) cooked chickpeas
4 cups (1 L) homemade vegetable stock (page 109),
      chicken stock or water
1/2 cup (125 mL) whole wheat macaroni or small soup pasta
10 oz (300 g) fresh baby spinach, chopped
1/4 tsp (1 mL) pepper
Salt to taste
2 tbsp (25 mL) chopped fresh parsley

1. Heat oil in a large saucepan on medium heat. Add onion, garlic, cumin and hot pepper flakes and cook gently for 5 minutes, or until onion is tender.

2. Add chickpeas and stock and bring to a boil. Reduce heat and simmer gently for 10 minutes. Puree half of soup and return to saucepan.

3. Add pasta and cook for 8 to 10 minutes, or until pasta is almost tender.

4. Add spinach and pepper and cook for 2 to 3 minutes, or just until spinach wilts (do not overcook or spinach will discolour). Taste and adjust seasonings, adding salt if necessary. Sprinkle with parsley.

PER SERVING	
Calories	220
Protein	10 g
Fat	3 g
Saturates	1 g
Cholesterol	1 mg
Carbohydrate	39 g
Fibre	5 g
Sodium	191 mg
Potassium	378 mg

Excellent: Vitamin A; Folate
Good: Vitamin B6; Iron

SEAFOOD SOUP WITH GINGER BROTH

This fresh, light-tasting soup is gentle and soothing. Diced chicken breasts can be used instead of the seafood.

Makes 8 servings

1 tsp (5 mL) vegetable oil
2 cloves garlic, finely chopped
1 tbsp (15 mL) finely chopped fresh ginger root
1 tsp (5 mL) grated lemon peel
1/4 tsp (1 mL) hot red pepper flakes
4 cups (1 L) homemade chicken or fish stock (page 109) or
      low-sodium commercial broth
2 tbsp (25 mL) Thai fish sauce or soy sauce
1 tbsp (15 mL) lemon juice
3 carrots, sliced
1/4 lb (125 g) scallops, diced
1/4 lb (125 g) cleaned shrimp, diced
1 tsp (5 mL) dark sesame oil
4 green onions, finely chopped
2 tbsp (25 mL) chopped fresh cilantro or parsley

1. Heat oil in a large saucepan on medium heat. Add garlic, ginger, lemon peel and hot pepper flakes and cook gently for a few minutes, or until very fragrant.
2. Add stock, fish sauce and lemon juice and bring to a boil.
3. Add carrots. Reduce heat and simmer gently for 15 minutes.
4. Add scallops, shrimp, sesame oil and green onions. Cook for just a few minutes, or until seafood is barely cooked. Taste and adjust seasonings if necessary. Serve sprinkled with cilantro.

PER SERVING	
Calories	73
Protein	8 g
Fat	2 g
Saturates	trace
Cholesterol	21 mg
Carbohydrate	5 g
Fibre	1 g
Sodium	282 mg
Potassium	267 mg

Excellent: Vitamin A
Good: Niacin;
Vitamin B12

MALKA'S BOUILLABAISSE

My friend Malka Marom is a talented singer, broadcaster and author. When I had this dish at her home, she told me that the secret to great food is good ingredients, good friends, good wine, good love and all sorts of other wonderful things!

Makes 8 large servings

2 cups (500 mL) dry white wine or water, divided
1 lb (500 g) clams, cleaned (about 16)
1 lb (500 g) mussels, cleaned (about 16)
1 tbsp (15 mL) olive oil
3 leeks, trimmed and thinly sliced
1 onion, chopped
2 tbsp (25 mL) all-purpose flour
1 28-oz (796 mL) can plum tomatoes, with juices,
      pureed or broken up
3 fresh tomatoes, chopped
1/4 cup (50 mL) chopped fresh thyme, or 1 tsp (5 mL) dried
2 bay leaves
3 cups (750 mL) homemade fish stock (page 109) or water
1/4 cup (50 mL) chopped fresh parsley, divided
Salt and pepper to taste
1 tbsp (15 mL) saffron threads
3/4 lb (375 g) cleaned shrimp
2 lb (1 kg) firm-fleshed white fish fillets, skin removed (e.g., halibut
      or cod), cut in 3-inch (7.5 cm) chunks
1 whole wheat or regular baguette, cut in chunks

1. In a large saucepan, bring 1 cup (250 mL) wine to a boil. Add clams. Cover and cook for 3 minutes. Add mussels and cover. Continue to cook for 3 to 5 minutes, or until mussels open. Strain and reserve juices, mussels and clams in shells (discard any clams or mussels that do not open).

2. Heat oil in a large saucepan on medium heat. Add leeks and onion. Cook gently, covered, until very tender, about 10 minutes. Stir in flour and cook for a few minutes, stirring.

3. Add canned tomatoes, fresh tomatoes, thyme, bay leaves, stock, remaining 1 cup (250 mL) wine and half the parsley. Bring to a boil and cook for 25 minutes. Taste and season with salt and pepper.

SAFFRON

Saffron is the most expensive spice, but it adds a wonderful colour and flavour to foods (usually rice, breads, curries, sauces and soups). Use it in small quantities, as it tends to taste medicinal if it is used to excess.

Try to buy saffron threads, as ground saffron is sometimes blended with the less expensive turmeric. The threads can be used whole or crushed with a mortar and pestle. They can also be toasted (but be careful not to burn).

PER SERVING

Calories	360
Protein	42 g
Fat	6 g
Saturates	1 g
Cholesterol	129 mg
Carbohydrate	31 g
Fibre	3 g
Sodium	520 mg
Potassium	1230 mg

Excellent: Thiamine; Niacin; Vitamin B6; Vitamin B12; Iron
Good: Vitamin A; Riboflavin; Vitamin C; Folate

MISO

Miso is a fermented soybean paste that has become very popular with the increased interest in Japanese food and soy products. It is available in different strengths, but the light/yellow version is the mildest and most popular.

To add miso to a soup or sauce, place it in a strainer and immerse the strainer in the hot liquid. You can also combine the miso with a little hot liquid before incorporating it into the dish.

PER SERVING

Calories	179
Protein	14 g
Fat	6 g
Saturates	1 g
Cholesterol	0 mg
Carbohydrate	19 g
Fibre	5 g
Sodium	407 mg
Potassium	586 mg

Excellent: Vitamin A; Folate; Iron
Good: Thiamine

4. Crush saffron with a mortar and pestle or back of a spoon. Add to soup and cook for about 5 minutes.

5. Add shrimp and fish. Cook for 5 minutes. Add reserved clams, mussels and juices and cook for another 5 minutes, but do not overcook.

6. Ladle soup into large bowl. Sprinkle with remaining parsley and serve with bread.

QUICK MISO SOUP

Here is a fast, easy miso soup that is totally vegetarian. Edamame are fresh soybeans, and they are growing in popularity. You can buy them frozen in the shell (just cook them in boiling water for 5 minutes, drain and salt, and serve as an appetizer) or shelled (add them frozen to soups, stir-fries and casseroles, or cook them for 3 to 4 minutes, drain and use in salads).

Makes 4 to 6 servings

4 cups (1 L) homemade vegetable stock (page 109)
4 fresh shiitake mushrooms, stemmed, thinly sliced
1/4 lb (125 g) fresh baby spinach
1 cup (250 mL) shelled edamame
1 cup (250 mL) diced tofu
2 tbsp (25 mL) light miso
2 green onions, thinly sliced on diagonal

1. Combine stock and mushrooms in a saucepan and bring to a boil. Cook for 5 minutes.

2. Add spinach, edamame and tofu. Cook for 2 minutes.

3. Place miso in a strainer and mash slightly. Lower strainer into broth and stir soup with miso (in strainer) to dissolve it.

4. Add green onions and cook for 1 minute.

FAST PHO

On a trip to Vietnam we had many versions of pho, the delicious national soup that is full of noodles, meat, vegetables, herbs and seasonings. You can add all the ingredients at the end or arrange them on the table Vietnamese style and let guests add their own seasonings. This is a very quick version but comforting and homey nevertheless. It is Vietnamese comfort food.

Instead of filet, very thinly sliced cooked brisket (page 286) can be cooked in the soup for about 5 minutes at the end of Step 1.

Makes 6 to 8 servings

8 cups (2 L) homemade chicken or beef stock (page 109) or
    low-sodium commercial broth
4 thin slices fresh ginger root, unpeeled
1 cinnamon stick, broken in half
4 star anise
1 stalk lemongrass, cut in 2-inch (5 cm) lengths
4 shallots, thinly sliced
6 oz (175 g) rice vermicelli (about ¼ inch/5 mm wide)
2 cups (500 mL) very fresh bean sprouts
3 tbsp (45 mL) Thai fish sauce or soy sauce
½ lb (250 g) beef filet, sirloin or flank steak, partially frozen and
    shaved in very thin slices
1 jalapeño, seeded and cut in thin slivers
8 lime wedges
16 fresh Thai basil leaves, coarsely chopped
16 fresh cilantro leaves, coarsely chopped
16 fresh mint leaves, coarsely chopped

1. In a large saucepan, combine stock, ginger, cinnamon stick, star anise, lemongrass and shallots. Bring to a boil, reduce heat and simmer gently for 15 minutes. Strain.

2. Meanwhile, soak noodles in warm water for 15 minutes.

3. Add noodles, bean sprouts and fish sauce to soup and heat for a couple of minutes.

4. Place slices of beef in each bowl. Ladle in hot noodles and broth. The Vietnamese custom is to allow guests to add their own hot pepper, lime juice and herbs, but I often add beef, pepper, lime juice and herbs to the saucepan and cook for just a minute before serving.

PER SERVING	
Calories	213
Protein	13 g
Fat	3 g
Saturates	1 g
Cholesterol	18 mg
Carbohydrate	32 g
Fibre	3 g
Sodium	768 mg
Potassium	468 mg

Excellent: Vitamin B12;
Vitamin C
Good: Folate; Iron

STOCKS

Homemade Chicken Stock

I always remove any visible fat from the chicken before making stock, but I do use the skin, because it has a lot of flavour. (Even though the skin contains fat, when the stock cools, any fat will rise to the surface to be skimmed off and discarded.)

Place 4 lb (2 kg) chicken pieces in a large pot. Add enough cold water to cover by about 2 inches (5 cm). Bring to a boil and skim off any scum.

Add 2 onions, 2 carrots, 2 stalks celery and 2 leeks (all cut in chunks). Bring to a boil and skim again if necessary. Add 1 bay leaf, ¹/₂ tsp (2 mL) dried thyme, 6 peppercorns and a small handful of fresh parsley. Reduce heat and cook gently, uncovered, for 1¹/₂ hours. If necessary, add water to keep chicken covered.

Strain stock. Even though most of the flavour will be cooked out of the chicken, it can be used in sandwiches, quesadillas and salads. Makes about 3 qt (3 L).

Homemade Beef Stock

Place 3 lb (1.5 kg) beef bones, 3 lb (1.5 kg) veal bones and 3 lb (1.5 kg) chicken pieces in a large roasting pan. Roast in a preheated 425°F (220°C) oven for 1¹/₂ hours, or until browned. Add 4 large onions, 4 large carrots, 3 stalks celery and 2 leeks (all cut in chunks) and brown for 30 minutes longer.

Transfer bones and vegetables to a large pot. Add a little boiling water to roasting pan, scrape off any browned bits and add to stock pot.

Cover bones and vegetables with cold water, bring to a boil and skim off scum. Add 2 bay leaves, ¹/₂ tsp (2 mL) dried thyme and 6 whole peppercorns. Simmer for 8 to 10 hours or overnight. Add water if necessary during cooking.

Strain and place stock in a clean pot. Cook until reduced to 4 qt (4 L). Refrigerate and remove fat. Makes about 4 qt (4 L).

Homemade Vegetable Stock

In a large pot, combine 2 onions, 2 carrots, 2 stalks celery, 2 leeks and ¹/₄ lb (125 g) mushrooms (all cut in chunks). Add 3 qt (3 L) cold water, 1 bay leaf, ¹/₂ tsp (2 mL) dried thyme, 4 peeled cloves garlic, 6 peppercorns and a handful of fresh parsley. Bring to a boil and remove any scum. Cover and simmer gently for 1¹/₂ hours. Strain stock.

For a more strongly flavoured vegetable stock, place vegetables in an oiled roasting pan and sprinkle with 1 tbsp (15 mL) granulated sugar. Roast in a preheated 425°F (220°C) oven for 30 to 45 minutes, or until well browned but not burnt. Add roasted vegetables and browned scrapings from pan to stock pot. Makes about 3 qt (3 L).

Homemade Fish Stock

Good fish stock is hard to find, so it is worth making your own. Use only lean, white-fleshed fish.

Place 3 lb (1.5 kg) fish bones, tails and heads in a large pot with 2 onions, 2 carrots, 2 stalks celery and 1 leek (all cut in chunks). Add a small handful of fresh parsley, 1 bay leaf, ¹/₂ tsp (2 mL) dried thyme, 6 peppercorns and 1 cup (250 mL) dry white wine or water. Cover with about 3 qt (3 L) cold water, bring to a boil and skim off any scum. Reduce heat and cook gently for 30 minutes. Strain.

Makes about 3 qt (3 L).

Roasted Squash, Baby Spinach and Bocconcini Salad
Middle Eastern Roasted Cauliflower Salad
Roasted Cherry Tomato Salad
Asian Coleslaw with Sweet Sushi Ginger
Grilled Tomato Salad
Grilled Vegetable Salad with Grilled Lemon Vinaigrette
Raita with Tomatoes and Cucumber
Roasted Vegetable Pasta Salad
Grilled Corn Salad
Caesar Salad with Creamy Roasted Garlic Dressing
Carrot Salad with Moroccan Dressing
Asian Chopped Salad
Grilled Chicken Salad with Peanut Sauce
Wheat Berry and Feta Salad with Dill
Wheat Berry and Grilled Corn Salad
Tabbouleh Salad with Fresh Herbs
Black Bean, Corn and Rice Salad
Chopped Grilled Chicken Salad
Sushi Salad
Spaghetti Salad with Tuna
Spaghetti Salad with Roasted Garlic and Tomato Salsa
Thai Chicken and Noodle Salad
Spaghettini with Salad Greens

Roasted Salmon Salad Niçoise
Arugula Salad with Grilled Shrimp, Asparagus and Fennel
Asian Grilled Steak Salad
Chopped Tuna Salad
Greek Salad with Grilled Chicken
Balsamic Spa Dressing
Mustard Pepper Dressing
Creamy Garlic Dressing
Citrus Vinaigrette
Sesame Ginger Dressing
Roasted Red Pepper Dressing
Honey Lime Vinaigrette

HEART

SMART

SALADS
AND SALAD
DRESSINGS

ROASTED SQUASH, BABY SPINACH AND BOCCONCINI SALAD

I interviewed Jamie Oliver for my column in the *National Post* a few years ago and I loved the casual style of his cooking. When I saw that he does not peel butternut squash before he roasts it, I decided to do the same. And it's true, it is delicious, skin and all.

This colourful salad tastes as good as it looks.

Makes 6 servings

2 lb (1 kg) butternut squash, halved lengthwise, seeded and cut in
    8 to 12 wedges
2 cups (500 mL) cherry tomatoes
1 tbsp (15 mL) chopped fresh thyme, or ½ tsp (2 mL) dried
1 tsp (5 mL) salt, divided
½ tsp (2 mL) pepper, divided
5 oz (150 g) fresh baby spinach
3 oz (90 g) bocconcini (fresh mozzarella), diced
2 tbsp (25 mL) balsamic vinegar
2 tbsp (25 mL) olive oil

1. Arrange squash skin side down on a baking sheet lined with parchment paper. Place cherry tomatoes on another baking sheet lined with parchment. Sprinkle squash and tomatoes with thyme, ½ tsp (2 mL) salt and ¼ tsp (1 mL) pepper.

2. Roast squash in a preheated 400°F (200°C) oven for 45 to 55 minutes, or until tender and browned. Roast cherry tomatoes for 12 to 15 minutes, or until skins are just starting to split.

3. Line salad plates with spinach. Place wedges of squash and a spoonful of cherry tomatoes on each plate. Top with cheese.

4. Combine vinegar, oil and remaining ½ tsp (2 mL) salt and ¼ tsp (1 mL) pepper. Drizzle over salad.

PER SERVING	
Calories	163
Protein	5 g
Fat	8 g
Saturates	2 g
Cholesterol	9 mg
Carbohydrate	23 g
Fibre	4 g
Sodium	439 mg
Potassium	739 mg

Excellent: Vitamin A; Vitamin C; Folate
Good: Thiamine; Vitamin B6; Calcium; Iron

MIDDLE EASTERN ROASTED CAULIFLOWER SALAD

This is a great winter salad when lettuce costs a fortune and still isn't very good. When I had it as part of a Middle Eastern mezze platter, the cauliflower was deep-fried, but I roast it instead and it is just as delicious.

Makes 6 servings

1 head cauliflower, trimmed
3 tbsp (45 mL) olive oil, divided
1 tsp (5 mL) chopped fresh thyme, or ¼ tsp (1 mL) dried
1 tsp (5 mL) salt, divided
1 tbsp (15 mL) white wine vinegar
1 tbsp (15 mL) lemon juice
½ tsp (2 mL) Dijon mustard
1 tsp (5 mL) honey
¼ cup (50 mL) chopped fresh chives

PER SERVING	
Calories	91
Protein	2 g
Fat	7 g
Saturates	1 g
Cholesterol	0 mg
Carbohydrate	6 g
Fibre	2 g
Sodium	415 mg
Potassium	184 mg
Excellent: Vitamin C; Folate	

1. Break cauliflower into florets (you should have about 6 cups/1.5 L).
2. In a large bowl, toss cauliflower with 1 tbsp (15 mL) oil, thyme and ½ tsp (2 mL) salt. Spread over a large baking sheet lined with parchment paper and bake in a preheated 400°F (200°C) oven for 25 to 30 minutes, or until lightly browned.
3. To prepare dressing, in a small bowl, whisk vinegar, lemon juice, mustard, honey, remaining ½ tsp (2 mL) salt and remaining 2 tbsp (25 mL) oil. Taste and adjust seasonings, adding more honey if necessary.
4. Toss cauliflower with dressing and sprinkle with chives. Serve at room temperature.

ROASTED CHERRY TOMATO SALAD

During most of the year the only good fresh tomatoes are cherry tomatoes, and they become sweet, crisp and incredibly tasty when roasted.

Spoon these tomatoes and their juices over greens, use as a sauce on pasta, risotto, pizza or polenta, or serve with grilled steak as a salsa.

Makes 6 servings

2 cups (500 mL) red cherry tomatoes
2 cups (500 mL) yellow or red cherry tomatoes
1 tbsp (15 mL) olive oil
1 tbsp (15 mL) balsamic vinegar
1 tbsp (15 mL) chopped fresh thyme, or ½ tsp (2 mL) dried
1 clove garlic, minced
½ tsp (2 mL) salt
¼ tsp (1 mL) pepper

1. In a large bowl, combine cherry tomatoes, oil, vinegar, thyme, garlic, salt and pepper. Spread on a baking sheet lined with parchment paper.
2. Roast in a preheated 400°F (200°C) oven for 10 to 12 minutes, or until tomatoes are just starting to burst. Taste and adjust seasonings if necessary.

Winter Caprese Salad

Break up ½ lb (250 g) bocconcini (fresh mozzarella) and combine with roasted cherry tomatoes. Drizzle with ⅓ cup (150 mL) balsamic dressing (page 141).

Makes 6 servings.

PER SERVING	
Calories	47
Protein	1 g
Fat	3 g
Saturates	trace
Cholesterol	0 mg
Carbohydrate	6 g
Fibre	1 g
Sodium	206 mg
Potassium	256 mg
Good: Vitamin C	

ASIAN COLESLAW WITH SWEET SUSHI GINGER

This coleslaw is great on top of a sandwich or burger. It is also a perfect dish to serve at a barbecue or with Asian-flavoured foods.

Makes 6 to 8 servings

8 cups (2 L) shredded Napa cabbage (about ½ cabbage)
4 carrots, coarsely shredded (about 2 cups/500 mL)
¼ cup (50 mL) sliced pickled ginger, slivered
4 green onions, thinly sliced
¼ cup (50 mL) chopped fresh cilantro
2 clove garlic, minced
¼ cup (50 mL) seasoned rice vinegar
2 tbsp (25 mL) soy sauce
1 tbsp (15 mL) honey
1 tsp (5 mL) dark sesame oil

1. In a large bowl, combine cabbage, carrots, pickled ginger, green onions and cilantro.
2. In a small bowl, whisk garlic, vinegar, soy sauce, honey and sesame oil.
3. Toss cabbage with dressing.

PER SERVING	
Calories	77
Protein	2 g
Fat	1 g
Saturates	0 g
Cholesterol	0 mg
Carbohydrate	15 g
Fibre	3 g
Sodium	625 mg
Potassium	172 mg
Excellent: Vitamin A; Vitamin C	

GRILLED TOMATO SALAD

This salad is spectacular when tomatoes are in season. It is worth using a good-quality balsamic vinegar, as you will require less oil. Instead of barbecuing, you could grill the tomatoes and onions in a grill pan or under the broiler.

Use leftovers as a pasta sauce, sandwich filling or bruschetta topping, or as a sauce on grilled foods. You could even puree the salad, add stock and turn it into a soup.

Makes 8 servings

6 large tomatoes (about 3 lb/1.5 kg), seeded and cut in
     1-inch (2.5 cm) slices
2 large onions, cut in ½-inch (1 cm) slices
2 tbsp (25 mL) olive oil, divided
1 cup (250 mL) fresh basil leaves, torn in pieces
¼ cup (50 mL) balsamic vinegar
1 clove garlic, minced
Salt and pepper to taste

1. Brush tomatoes and onions with a little olive oil. Grill tomatoes briefly on each side just until warm with grill marks. Grill onions until tender and browned. (They will take longer than tomatoes.)
2. Combine whole or cut-up tomatoes and onions in a bowl. Add basil.
3. In a small bowl, combine vinegar, garlic and remaining oil. Taste and add salt and pepper if necessary.
4. Combine tomatoes with dressing. Taste and adjust seasonings if necessary.

PER SERVING	
Calories	86
Protein	2 g
Fat	4 g
Saturates	1 g
Cholesterol	0 mg
Carbohydrate	13 g
Fibre	3 g
Sodium	15 mg
Potassium	424 mg
Good: Vitamin A; Vitamin C	

GRILLED VEGETABLE SALAD WITH GRILLED LEMON VINAIGRETTE

We first learned the trick of grilling lemons from Toronto chef Mark McEwan when he taught at my school. Grilling takes the sting out of the lemon juice. For a great potato salad, toss the dressing with potatoes, dill, green onions and mint.

Makes 8 servings

Grilled Lemon Vinaigrette

1 lemon
1 clove garlic, minced
1 tsp (5 mL) salt
1/4 cup (50 mL) olive oil
1 tsp (5 mL) chopped fresh thyme, or 1/4 tsp (1 mL) dried

Grilled Vegetables

1 bulb fennel, trimmed and cut in wedges
2 zucchini, sliced lengthwise
1/2 lb (250 g) asparagus, trimmed
2 portobello mushrooms, stems removed and gills scraped away
2 tbsp (25 mL) olive oil, optional
1/2 tsp (2 mL) salt
1 sweet red pepper
2 tbsp (25 mL) shredded fresh basil

PER SERVING	
Calories	92
Protein	2 g
Fat	7 g
Saturates	1 g
Cholesterol	0 mg
Carbohydrate	7 g
Fibre	3 g
Sodium	457 mg
Potassium	368 mg
Excellent: Vitamin C	
Good: Folate	

1. To prepare vinaigrette, cut lemon in half and place cut side down on a hot barbecue. Grill for about 5 minutes, or until well browned. Cool.
2. Squeeze lemon juice into a bowl. You should have about 1/4 cup (50 mL) juice. Whisk in garlic and salt. Whisk in oil and thyme. Taste and adjust seasonings, adding more oil if necessary.
3. To prepare vegetables, brush fennel, zucchini, asparagus and mushrooms with oil. Sprinkle with salt. Grill vegetables for a few minutes per side until just marked and slightly cooked. Slice mushrooms and arrange vegetables in a serving dish.
4. Meanwhile, grill pepper, turning often, until blackened. Cool and remove skin. Halve, seed and slice. Arrange over vegetables.
5. Pour dressing over salad and sprinkle with basil.

RAITA WITH TOMATOES AND CUCUMBER

Raitas are East Indian yogurt salads. They are usually served with East Indian meals to cool spicy tastes, but also make a refreshing addition to a picnic or barbecue. Traditionally the cucumber is peeled and seeded, but this is not absolutely necessary.

If you use yogurt cheese, you can make this salad a few hours ahead of time (if you use regular yogurt, combine the ingredients just before serving, as the salad may get watery if made too far in advance).

Makes 8 servings

1 English cucumber, peeled, seeded and grated
      (about 2 cups/500 mL)
1/2 tsp (2 mL) salt
1 cup (250 mL) yogurt cheese (page 391) or
      thick unflavoured low-fat yogurt
1 green onion, chopped
1/2 tsp (2 mL) ground cumin
Pinch cayenne
1 large tomato, seeded and diced (about 1 1/2 cups/375 mL)
2 tbsp (25 mL) chopped fresh cilantro
2 tbsp (25 mL) chopped fresh mint

1. In a colander or strainer, combine cucumber and salt. Allow to drain for 20 minutes. Rinse cucumber well. Wrap in a tea towel and squeeze out excess liquid.

2. In a large bowl, stir yogurt cheese until smooth. Stir in green onion, cumin and cayenne. Add cucumber, tomato, cilantro and mint and combine. Taste and adjust seasonings if necessary.

PER SERVING	
Calories	41
Protein	4 g
Fat	1 g
Saturates	1 g
Cholesterol	3 mg
Carbohydrate	5 g
Fibre	1 g
Sodium	173 mg
Potassium	208 mg
Good: Vitamin B12	

ROASTED VEGETABLE PASTA SALAD

This is an all-time favourite. Serve it warm or at room temperature.
Use a vegetable peeler to peel the peppers (page 146).

Makes 6 to 8 servings

8 plum tomatoes (about 2 lb/1 kg), quartered
2 sweet red peppers, preferably peeled and seeded, cut in chunks
2 sweet yellow peppers, preferably peeled and seeded, cut in chunks
4 Asian eggplants (about 1 lb/500 g), cut in 1-inch (2.5 cm) chunks
1 bulb fennel, trimmed and cut in wedges
1 large onion, peeled and cut in wedges
1 tbsp (15 mL) olive oil
1 tbsp (15 mL) chopped fresh rosemary, or 1/2 tsp (2 mL) dried
1 tbsp (15 mL) chopped fresh thyme, or 1/2 tsp (2 mL) dried
1/2 tsp (2 mL) salt
1/4 tsp (1 mL) pepper
2 heads garlic
1 lb (500 g) whole wheat or regular penne
2 tbsp (25 mL) chopped fresh mint

Balsamic Basil Dressing
3 tbsp (45 mL) balsamic vinegar
2 tbsp (25 mL) olive oil
1/2 tsp (2 mL) salt
1/4 tsp (1 mL) pepper
1/4 cup (50 mL) shredded fresh basil or chopped parsley

PER SERVING	
Calories	431
Protein	15 g
Fat	9 g
Saturates	1 g
Cholesterol	0 mg
Carbohydrate	82 g
Fibre	13 g
Sodium	423 mg
Potassium	983 mg

Excellent: Vitamin A;
Thiamine; Niacin;
Vitamin B6; Vitamin C;
Folate; Iron

1. Arrange tomatoes, cut side up, with peppers, eggplants, fennel and onion in a single layer on parchment-lined baking sheets. Sprinkle with oil, rosemary, thyme, salt and pepper.
2. Cut top quarter off heads of garlic. Wrap garlic heads in foil. Roast garlic and vegetables in a preheated 400°F (200°C) oven for 45 minutes, or until vegetables are tender and brown and garlic is soft.
3. Meanwhile, cook pasta in a large pot of boiling water just until tender. Drain well.
4. In a large bowl, combine vegetables, pasta and mint. Squeeze garlic out of cloves, add to vegetables and toss.
5. In a small bowl, combine vinegar, oil, salt and pepper. Stir in shredded basil. Toss vegetables and pasta with dressing. Taste and adjust seasonings if necessary.

GRILLED CORN SALAD

This recipe is a real winner. It is also the reason I now seldom cook for more than thirty people at a time. I once decided to make this salad for a wedding party of seventy-five people because I got a great price on a huge bag of corn. Just as I began grilling, it started to rain. It took my husband, Ray, and me ages to shuck and cook all the corn, and we were soaked by the end.

It's a good thing we loved the friends we were cooking for—and that they loved the salad!

Makes 6 to 8 servings

8 ears corn, husked
1 red onion, peeled and cut in $1/2$-inch (1 cm) slices
2 sweet red peppers
$1/2$ cup (125 mL) chopped fresh cilantro or parsley
$1/4$ cup (50 mL) chopped fresh chives or green onions
$1/3$ cup (75 mL) rice vinegar or cider vinegar
1 tbsp (15 mL) orange juice concentrate
1 clove garlic, minced
$1 1/2$ tsp (7 mL) chipotle puree (page 183)
1 tsp (5 mL) salt
$1/2$ tsp (2 mL) pepper
2 tbsp (25 mL) olive oil

1. Place corn, onion slices and peppers directly on grill and cook on all sides for about 5 minutes, or until corn is dotted with brown, onion slices are browned and peppers are blackened on all sides.
2. Break corn cobs in half and stand cut ends on a cutting board. Cut off kernels from top to bottom. Dice onion. Peel, seed and dice peppers.
3. In a large bowl, combine corn, onion, peppers, cilantro and chives.
4. In a small bowl, combine vinegar, orange juice concentrate, garlic, chipotle, salt and pepper. Whisk in oil.
5. Toss vegetables with dressing. Taste and adjust seasonings if necessary.

PER SERVING	
Calories	258
Protein	7 g
Fat	7 g
Saturates	1 g
Cholesterol	0 mg
Carbohydrate	51 g
Fibre	8 g
Sodium	413 mg
Potassium	598 mg

Excellent: Vitamin C; Thiamine; Folate
Good: Vitamin A; Niacin; Vitamin B6

CAESAR SALAD WITH CREAMY ROASTED GARLIC DRESSING

This Caesar dressing gets its richness from roasted garlic instead of from raw eggs, making it lower in fat but creamy and luscious. For a classic Caesar, add a few anchovies. You can also add grilled chicken or shrimp. The dressing is great served as a dip or used as a spread in sandwiches or quesadillas.

Makes 8 servings

1 head garlic
1 tsp (5 mL) Dijon mustard
1 tsp (5 mL) Worcestershire sauce
2 tbsp (25 mL) sherry vinegar
1 tbsp (15 mL) lemon juice
1/2 tsp (2 mL) salt
1/4 cup (50 mL) olive oil
1 tbsp (15 mL) grated Parmesan cheese
3 thick slices crusty whole wheat or white bread, cut in 1-inch
     (2.5 cm) cubes (about 2 cups/500 mL)
1 large head Romaine lettuce, cut or broken in 1-inch (2.5 cm)
     pieces (about 10 cups/2.5 L)
2 tomatoes, cut in wedges

1. To prepare dressing, cut top quarter off garlic, wrap garlic in foil and roast in a preheated 400°F (200°C) oven for 40 to 45 minutes, or until garlic is very tender. Squeeze garlic into a food processor or mash with a whisk.

2. Blend in mustard, Worcestershire, vinegar, lemon juice, salt, oil and cheese. Thin dressing with water if it is too thick. Taste and adjust seasonings if necessary.

3. To prepare croutons, spread bread cubes on a baking sheet. Bake in a preheated 375°F (190°C) oven for 10 to 12 minutes, or until crunchy. Stir once or twice during baking time.

4. Just before serving, toss lettuce with dressing and top with croutons. Garnish with tomatoes.

PER TBSP (15 mL) OF DRESSING

Calories	116
Protein	3 g
Fat	8 g
Saturates	1 g
Cholesterol	1 mg
Carbohydrate	10 g
Fibre	3 g
Sodium	250 mg
Potassium	324 mg

Excellent: Folate
Good: Vitamin A; Thiamine; Vitamin C

CARROT SALAD WITH MOROCCAN DRESSING

In Morocco this is usually served as a starter with other salads, but I often serve it as a side dish. It is so flavourful that it tastes great with any plain roast or grilled entree.

Makes 6 to 8 servings

2 lb (1 kg) carrots, cut on diagonal in 1/2-inch (1 cm) slices
1/3 cup (75 mL) orange juice
2 tbsp (25 mL) lemon juice
1 tbsp (15 mL) honey
1 tsp (5 mL) dark sesame oil
1 tsp (5 mL) paprika
1 tsp (5 mL) ground cumin
Pinch ground cinnamon
2 tbsp (25 mL) chopped fresh mint or parsley
2 tbsp (25 mL) chopped fresh cilantro or parsley
1 tsp (5 mL) sesame seeds, toasted (page 384)
Salt and pepper to taste

PER SERVING	
Calories	87
Protein	2 g
Fat	1 g
Saturates	trace
Cholesterol	o mg
Carbohydrate	18 g
Fibre	4 g
Sodium	85 mg
Potassium	337 mg
Excellent: vitamin A	
Good: vitamin B6	

1. Bring a large saucepan of water to a boil. Add carrots and cook for about 4 minutes. Drain, rinse with cold water and pat dry.
2. In a large bowl, combine orange juice, lemon juice, honey, sesame oil, paprika, cumin and cinnamon. Add carrots and toss. Sprinkle with mint, cilantro and sesame seeds. Season with salt and pepper.

ASIAN CHOPPED SALAD

Chopped salads are wonderful because every bite is full of different tastes and textures. In this recipe, the tofu is incognito, so for those who think they don't like tofu, this is a perfect introduction (you could also use grilled chicken, shrimp or steak). If you do not have or like all the salad ingredients, just use more of some or introduce new ones (e.g., grilled or roasted tomatoes and/or fennel would be great additions).

If you don't want to barbecue, just roast the vegetables and tofu on a baking sheet at 400°F (200°C) for 30 to 40 minutes, or until browned. Serve leftovers in pita bread or use in wraps or salad rolls (page 70).

Makes 8 to 10 servings

1 lb (500 g) extra-firm tofu
3 tbsp (45 mL) teriyaki sauce (page 290)
1 red onion, peeled and cut in 1/2-inch (1 cm) slices
2 zucchini, cut lengthwise in 1/2-inch (1 cm) slices
1 lb (500 g) asparagus, trimmed
2 Asian eggplants, cut lengthwise in 1/2-inch (1 cm) slices
2 ears corn, husked
2 tbsp (25 mL) olive oil, optional
2 sweet red peppers, halved and seeded
4 cups (1 L) chopped Romaine lettuce
1/2 cup (125 mL) chopped fresh herbs
     (e.g., parsley, cilantro, basil, mint or chives)

Orange Sesame Dressing

1 clove garlic, minced
3 tbsp (45 mL) orange juice
3 tbsp (45 mL) balsamic vinegar
1 tbsp (15 mL) soy sauce
1 tbsp (15 mL) honey
1 tbsp (15 mL) dark sesame oil
1/2 tsp (2 mL) hot Asian chili paste

PER SERVING

Calories	251
Protein	12 g
Fat	7 g
Saturates	1 g
Cholesterol	0 mg
Carbohydrate	41 g
Fibre	8 g
Sodium	439 mg
Potassium	895 mg

Excellent: Vitamin A;
Vitamin C; Thiamine;
Folacin
Good: Riboflavin;
Niacin; Vitamin B6;
Iron; Zinc

1. Cut tofu into slices about 1 inch (2.5 cm) thick. Place in a shallow dish and pour teriyaki sauce over top. Allow to marinate for at least 30 minutes.

2. Brush onion, zucchini, asparagus, eggplants and corn with oil. Grill vegetables on both sides until browned. Grill peppers, skin side down, until blackened. Pat tofu dry and brush or spray with oil. Grill for a few minutes per side until browned.

3. Cut onion, zucchini, asparagus and eggplants into 1/2-inch (1 cm) cubes and transfer to a large bowl. Cut corn off cobs (page 92). Peel peppers and dice. Dice tofu. Add corn, diced peppers and tofu to other vegetables. Reserve lettuce and herbs.

4. To prepare dressing, in a small bowl, whisk together garlic, orange juice, vinegar, soy sauce, honey, sesame oil and chili paste.

5. Combine tofu and vegetables with dressing. Just before serving, add lettuce and herbs. Taste and adjust seasonings if necessary.

GRILLED CHICKEN SALAD WITH PEANUT SAUCE

This salad is very easy to make. Instead of grilling the chicken you can use sliced leftover chicken or smoked chicken (use 3 to 4 cups/750 mL to 1 L). The servings look very generous because of all the lettuce, but don't worry—you'll get through it!

This salad can be served fresh and crisp, but it is also great when it gets a bit soggy. If you don't have corn tortillas, use about 1 cup (250 mL) broken commercial baked corn chips.

Makes 6 to 8 servings

Chicken

1 tbsp (15 mL) honey-style mustard
1 tsp (5 mL) dark sesame oil
1 clove garlic, minced
1 1/2 lb (750 g) boneless, skinless chicken breasts

Lime Honey Dressing

1/4 cup (50 mL) lime juice
2 tbsp (25 mL) honey
2 tbsp (25 mL) olive oil
2 tsp (10 mL) honey-style mustard
1 small clove garlic, minced
1/2 tsp (2 mL) pepper
Salt to taste

Peanut Sauce

2 tbsp (25 mL) peanut butter
2 tbsp (25 mL) honey
2 tbsp (25 mL) soy sauce
2 tbsp (25 mL) hot water

Salad

1 large head Romaine lettuce, shredded
1 head radicchio or 1/2 small red cabbage, shredded
2 carrots, grated
1 sweet red pepper, preferably roasted (page 146), seeded, peeled and cut in thin strips
4 corn tortillas
1 bunch fresh cilantro or parsley, chopped

PER SERVING	
Calories	328
Protein	31 g
Fat	11 g
Saturates	2 g
Cholesterol	70 mg
Carbohydrate	29 g
Fibre	4 g
Sodium	411 mg
Potassium	865 mg

Excellent: Vitamin A; Vitamin C; Niacin; Vitamin B6; Folate
Good: Thiamine; Riboflavin; Iron; Vitamin E

1. To prepare chicken, combine mustard, sesame oil and garlic. Rub into chicken. Grill chicken for 5 to 7 minutes per side, or until just cooked through. Cool and slice very thinly on diagonal.

2. To prepare dressing, in a small bowl, blend together lime juice, honey, olive oil, mustard, garlic, pepper and salt.

3. To prepare peanut sauce, in a small bowl, blend together peanut butter, honey, soy sauce and hot water.

4. In a large bowl, toss together lettuce, radicchio, carrots and red pepper.

5. Meanwhile, cut tortillas into thin strips (scissors work well) and spread on a baking sheet in a single layer. Bake in a preheated 400°F (200°C) oven for about 8 minutes, or until crisp.

6. Add tortilla strips, chicken and cilantro to salad. Toss with dressing. Drizzle peanut sauce over all.

FAUX PEANUT SAUCE

This is great for people who are allergic to peanuts, and it can be used any time a peanut sauce is called for. It does contain tahina, but you can omit it if you are also allergic to sesame seeds.

Puree 1/2 cup (125 mL) cooked chickpeas, 2 tbsp (25 mL) honey, 2 tbsp (25 mL) water, 2 tbsp (25 mL) soy sauce, 2 tbsp (25 mL) rice wine, 1 tbsp (15 mL) tahina and a dash of hot pepper sauce.

Makes about 3/4 cup (175 mL).

WHEAT BERRY AND FETA SALAD WITH DILL

We started out making this salad with farro, an ancient grain, but it was hard to find, so we now usually use wheat berries. Cook more than you need and freeze leftovers for future use. (If you can find farro, cook it as you would wheat berries.) You can also make this with brown rice or orzo (Italian pasta in the shape of rice).

As a side salad this will serve six to eight people, but it also makes a light lunch for four. It is very refreshing and clean tasting.

Makes 6 servings

1 cup (250 mL) wheat berries or farro
1/2 cup (125 mL) crumbled feta cheese
2 tbsp (25 mL) pine nuts, toasted (page 219)
3 tbsp (45 mL) black olives, pitted and halved

Lemon Dill Dressing

2 tbsp (25 mL) lemon juice
1 clove garlic, minced
1/2 tsp (2 mL) salt
1/4 tsp (1 mL) pepper
2 tbsp (25 mL) olive oil
1/4 cup (50 mL) chopped fresh dill
3 green onions, green part only, thinly sliced
2 tbsp (25 mL) chopped fresh parsley

1. Rinse wheat berries. In a large saucepan, cover wheat berries with 4 qt (4 L) cold water. Bring to a boil and cook for 1 to 1 1/2 hours, or until tender. Rinse with cold water and drain well. You should have about 2 1/2 cups (625 mL).
2. In a large bowl, combine wheat berries, feta, pine nuts and olives.
3. To prepare dressing, combine lemon juice, garlic, salt, pepper and oil. Stir in dill, green onions and parsley.
4. Combine wheat berries gently with dressing. Taste and adjust seasonings if necessary.

PER SERVING	
Calories	176
Protein	6 g
Fat	9 g
Saturates	3 g
Cholesterol	12 mg
Carbohydrate	20 g
Fibre	3 g
Sodium	376 mg
Potassium	121 mg

WHEAT BERRY AND GRILLED CORN SALAD

This is a perfect potluck dish, because wherever you take it, people always ask for the recipe. It has a wonderful flavour and is very healthful. Serve it as a vegetarian main course or as a side salad.

If you don't have wheat berries, use rice. If you don't have time to grill the corn, use frozen corn. Whatever you do, just make this salad—it's so good!

Makes 8 to 10 servings

2 cups (500 mL) wheat berries
4 ears corn, husked
2 sweet red peppers
1 lb (500 g) asparagus or green beans, trimmed
¹/₂ cup (125 mL) rice vinegar
2 tbsp (25 mL) orange juice concentrate
1 tbsp (15 mL) chipotle puree (page 183) or
        finely chopped jalapeño, optional
2 cloves garlic, minced
1 tsp (5 mL) salt
¹/₂ tsp (2 mL) pepper
3 tbsp (45 mL) olive oil
¹/₂ cup (125 mL) chopped fresh cilantro or shredded basil
¹/₄ cup (50 mL) chopped fresh chives

PER SERVING

Calories	277
Protein	8 g
Fat	7 g
Saturates	1 g
Cholesterol	0 mg
Carbohydrate	53 g
Fibre	9 g
Sodium	304 mg
Potassium	473 mg

Excellent: Vitamin C; Thiamine; Folacin
Good: Vitamin A; Niacin; Vitamin B6; Iron; Zinc

1. Rinse wheat berries. In a large saucepan, cover wheat berries with 4 qt (4 L) cold water. Bring to a boil and simmer gently for 1 to 1¹/₂ hours, or until tender. Rinse with cold water, drain well and transfer to a large bowl.

2. Meanwhile, grill corn on all sides for about 5 minutes, or until lightly browned. Cool. Cut corn in half, place cut side on a cutting board and cut kernels off cobs from top to bottom. Add corn to wheat berries.

3. Grill peppers on all sides until blackened. Cool. Peel, seed and dice and add to wheat berries and corn.

4. Grill asparagus until barely cooked. Dice. Add to wheat berries.

5. In a small bowl, combine vinegar, orange juice concentrate, chipotle, garlic, salt and pepper. Whisk in oil.

6. Toss wheat berries with dressing. Add cilantro and chives. Taste and adjust seasonings if necessary.

TABBOULEH SALAD WITH FRESH HERBS

This tabbouleh, made with lots of parsley, is similar to the traditional Middle Eastern version. If you can't find fresh mint, simply omit it; do not substitute dried.

This salad can also be made with couscous, rice or quinoa (page 349). Serve it as part of an appetizer mezze with your favourite hummos, carrot salad (page 122), cauliflower salad (page 113) and grilled pita. It also makes a great side dish.

Makes 6 to 8 servings

3/4 cup (175 mL) bulgur
3/4 cup (175 mL) boiling water
2 tomatoes, seeded and diced
1 small English cucumber, diced
3 green onions, chopped
4 cups (1 L) chopped fresh parsley
1/2 cup (125 mL) chopped fresh mint
1 clove garlic, minced
1/3 cup (75 mL) lemon juice
2 tbsp (25 mL) olive oil
1/2 tsp (2 mL) salt
1/2 tsp (2 mL) pepper

PER SERVING	
Calories	135
Protein	4 g
Fat	5 g
Saturates	1 g
Cholesterol	0 mg
Carbohydrate	21 g
Fibre	6 g
Sodium	220 mg
Potassium	462 mg
Excellent: Vitamin A; Vitamin C; Folate; Iron	

1. Place bulgur in an 8-inch (2 L) square baking dish. Cover with boiling water. Cover dish tightly with foil and let sit for 30 minutes. Fluff.

2. In a large bowl, combine bulgur, tomatoes, cucumber, green onions, parsley and mint.

3. To prepare dressing, in a small bowl, whisk together garlic, lemon juice, oil, salt and pepper. Toss with salad. Taste and adjust seasonings if necessary.

BLACK BEAN, CORN AND RICE SALAD

Each bite of this beautiful salad contains a burst of herbal flavours and a wonderful blend of textures. If you can't find fresh cilantro, basil or mint, just use more parsley and green onions. You can also use 2 cups (500 mL) canned beans instead of the dried beans.

Makes 8 servings

1 cup (250 mL) dried black beans
1 cup (250 mL) long-grain brown or white rice, preferably basmati
2 cups (500 mL) corn kernels
2 sweet red peppers, roasted (page 146), peeled, seeded and diced
1 jalapeño, seeded and diced
1 bunch arugula or watercress, trimmed and chopped
1/3 cup (75 mL) chopped fresh cilantro or parsley
1/3 cup (75 mL) shredded fresh basil
2 tbsp (25 mL) chopped fresh mint
2 tbsp (25 mL) chopped fresh chives or green onions
3 tbsp (45 mL) red wine vinegar
1/2 tsp (2 mL) pepper
1 clove garlic, minced
3 tbsp (45 mL) olive oil
Salt to taste

PER SERVING	
Calories	266
Protein	10 g
Fat	6 g
Saturates	1 g
Cholesterol	0 mg
Carbohydrate	45 g
Fibre	6 g
Sodium	10 mg
Potassium	485 mg

Excellent: Vitamin C; Folate
Good: Vitamin A; Thiamine; Vitamin B6

1. Soak beans in cold water for a few hours at room temperature or overnight in refrigerator. Rinse and drain well.
2. In a large saucepan, cover beans generously with water. Bring to a boil, reduce heat and cook gently for 1 to 1 1/2 hours, or until tender. Rinse and drain well. Transfer to a large bowl.
3. Meanwhile, wash rice well. Bring a large saucepan of water to a boil. Add rice and cook for 30 to 40 minutes, or until just tender (white rice should take about 15 to 20 minutes to cook). Drain well. Combine with beans.
4. Add corn, red peppers, jalapeño, arugula, cilantro, basil, mint and chives.
5. In a small bowl, whisk together vinegar, pepper and garlic. Whisk in oil. Taste and adjust seasonings, adding salt if necessary.
6. Toss salad with dressing.

CHOPPED GRILLED CHICKEN SALAD

You can use 1 lb (500 g) shrimp or 3/4 lb (375 g) steak instead of the chicken in this salad. You can also roast the chicken and vegetables instead of barbecuing them.

For an alternative dressing, use Sesame Ginger Dressing (page 145).

Makes 6 to 8 servings

1 tbsp (15 mL) Dijon mustard
1 tbsp (15 mL) soy sauce
1/4 tsp (1 mL) pepper
1 lb (500 g) boneless, skinless chicken breasts
2 sweet yellow peppers
2 sweet red peppers
1 lb (500 g) Asian eggplants, cut in 1/4-inch (5 mm) slices
2 small zucchini, halved lengthwise
1 large red onion, peeled and cut in 1/2-inch (1 cm) slices
2 ears corn, husked
1/2 lb (250 g) asparagus, trimmed
2 tomatoes, seeded and chopped
1/4 cup (50 mL) chopped black olives
1/4 cup (50 mL) shredded fresh basil or chopped parsley
1/4 cup (50 mL) chopped fresh chives or green onions

Dressing

3 tbsp (45 mL) red wine vinegar
3 tbsp (45 mL) balsamic vinegar
1 clove garlic, minced
1/2 tsp (2 mL) pepper
3 tbsp (45 mL) olive oil
Salt to taste
6 cups (1.5 L) chopped mixed salad greens (arugula, radicchio, red
    oak leaf, frisee, etc.)

1. In a shallow dish, combine mustard, soy sauce and pepper. Coat chicken with mixture and marinate overnight in refrigerator.
2. Grill peppers on all sides until blackened. Cool, peel, seed and cut into 1/2-inch (1 cm) pieces.
3. Grill chicken for 5 to 7 minutes per side, or until cooked through. Cut into 1/2-inch (1 cm) pieces.
4. Grill eggplants, zucchini, onion, corn and asparagus until just cooked. Cut eggplants, zucchini, onion and asparagus into

PER SERVING	
Calories	295
Protein	23 g
Fat	10 g
Saturates	1 g
Cholesterol	47 mg
Carbohydrate	34 g
Fibre	8 g
Sodium	232 mg
Potassium	1099 mg

Excellent: **Vitamin A; Vitamin C; Thiamine; Niacin; Vitamin B6; Folate**
Good: **Riboflavin; Iron**

¹/₂-inch (1 cm) pieces. Cut corn kernels from cob (page 92).

5. In a large bowl, combine chicken, grilled vegetables, tomatoes, olives, basil and chives.

6. In a small bowl, whisk together vinegars, garlic and pepper. Whisk in oil. Taste and adjust seasonings, adding salt if necessary.

7. Toss chicken and vegetables with dressing. Just before serving, add salad greens and toss again.

SUSHI SALAD

This homestyle version of sushi (called chirashi sushi) is full of delectable textures and tastes. There is absolutely no fat in the dressing, and the recipe can be varied in many ways. Add leftover chicken or shrimp, corn, zucchini, green beans, green onions, etc.

Makes 6 to 8 servings

1 ¹/₂ cups (375 mL) short-grain Japanese rice
1 ³/₄ cups (425 mL) cold water
¹/₄ lb (125 g) snow peas, trimmed
¹/₄ cup (50 mL) rice vinegar
2 large sheets toasted nori (about 8 x 7 inches/20 x 18 cm),
    broken up
2 tbsp (25 mL) chopped pickled ginger
1 carrot, grated
¹/₂ cup (125 mL) cooked peas
2 tbsp (25 mL) sesame seeds, toasted (page 384)
2 tbsp (25 mL) chopped fresh dill
2 tbsp (25 mL) chopped fresh chives or green onions
2 tbsp (25 mL) chopped fresh cilantro or parsley

PER SERVING	
Calories	226
Protein	6 g
Fat	2 g
Saturates	trace
Cholesterol	0 mg
Carbohydrate	46 g
Fibre	2 g
Sodium	20 mg
Potassium	189 mg
Excellent: Vitamin A	

1. Rinse rice until water runs clear. Place rice in a medium saucepan and add cold water. Cover. Bring to a boil and boil for 1 minute. Reduce heat to low and cook for 10 minutes. Remove saucepan from heat and let rest for 15 minutes. Do not remove lid at any time during cooking.

2. Meanwhile, blanch snow peas by immersing them in boiling water for 30 seconds. Drain and rinse with cold water. Slice peas on diagonal.

3. Transfer rice to a large bowl. Toss rice gently while fanning it, to prevent it from being too sticky. As you are fanning, gradually add vinegar, tossing gently, until all vinegar has been absorbed.

4. Add snow peas, nori, ginger, carrot, peas, sesame seeds, dill, chives and cilantro. Toss and serve at room temperature.

SPAGHETTI SALAD WITH TUNA

You can buy roasted peppers in jars to make this delicious salad even easier. If you cannot find fresh basil, just use more parsley or green onions. If you want to prepare this recipe ahead of time, refrigerate it and bring to room temperature before serving.

Makes 6 servings

3/4 lb (375 g) whole wheat or regular spaghetti
2 cloves garlic, minced
1/4 tsp (1 mL) hot red pepper flakes, optional
2 tbsp (25 mL) olive oil
1/2 tsp (2 mL) pepper
Salt to taste
2 tomatoes, seeded and diced
2 sweet red or yellow peppers, preferably roasted (page 146),
    peeled, seeded and diced
2 7-oz (198 mL) cans white tuna (water-packed),
    drained and flaked
2 tbsp (25 mL) chopped black olives
1/4 cup (50 mL) chopped fresh parsley
1/4 cup (50 mL) shredded fresh basil
2 green onions, chopped

1. Cook spaghetti in a large pot of boiling water until just tender.
2. Meanwhile, in a large bowl, combine garlic, hot pepper flakes, oil, pepper and salt. Stir in tomatoes, peppers, tuna and olives. Add parsley, basil and green onions.
3. Drain spaghetti well and toss with sauce. Taste and adjust seasonings if necessary. Serve warm or at room temperature.

PER SERVING	
Calories	331
Protein	23 g
Fat	7 g
Saturates	1 g
Cholesterol	22 mg
Carbohydrate	47 g
Fibre	6 g
Sodium	237 mg
Potassium	398 mg

Excellent: Niacin; Vitamin B12; Vitamin C
Good: Vitamin A; Vitamin B6; Folate; Iron

SPAGHETTI SALAD WITH ROASTED GARLIC AND TOMATO SALSA

This is a wonderful salad that can be served warm or at room temperature. If you make it ahead and refrigerate it, be sure to bring it to room temperature before serving. When tomatoes are not in season (most of the time), I use plum tomatoes or cherry tomatoes, as they seem to be decent all year. Instead of roasted garlic you can use two minced cloves fresh garlic.

Makes 6 to 8 servings

2 heads roasted garlic (page 67)
3 tbsp (45 mL) olive oil
3 tbsp (45 mL) balsamic vinegar
1/2 tsp (2 mL) salt
1/4 tsp (1 mL) pepper
1/4 tsp (1 mL) hot red pepper flakes, optional
1 lb (500 g) ripe plum tomatoes (4 to 6), halved, seeded and diced,
       or 2 cups (500 mL) cherry tomatoes, quartered
1/2 cup (125 mL) shredded fresh basil or chopped parsley
1/4 cup (50 mL) chopped fresh parsley
2 tbsp (25 mL) chopped fresh chives or green onions
3/4 lb (375 g) whole wheat or regular spaghetti

PER SERVING	
Calories	294
Protein	10 g
Fat	8 g
Saturates	1 g
Cholesterol	0 mg
Carbohydrate	50 g
Fibre	6 g
Sodium	211 mg
Potassium	322 mg

Good: Thiamine; Niacin; Vitamin B6; Vitamin C; Iron

1. In a large bowl, squeeze roasted garlic into oil and mash with a whisk until almost pureed. Add vinegar, salt, pepper and hot pepper flakes.
2. Add tomatoes, basil, parsley and chives. Combine well. Let salsa marinate while preparing pasta.
3. Cook pasta in a large pot of boiling water just until tender. Drain well. Combine with salsa and toss well. Taste and adjust seasonings if necessary.

THAI CHICKEN AND NOODLE SALAD

I make this salad with rice noodles or spaghettini. If you can't find all the fresh herbs, just use more parsley and green onions.

Makes 8 to 10 servings

1 lb (500 g) boneless, skinless chicken breasts
3 tbsp (45 mL) hoisin sauce
1 tbsp (15 mL) lime juice
1 tsp (5 mL) pepper
³/₄ lb (375 g) rice vermicelli or spaghettini
¹/₄ cup (50 mL) vegetable oil
6 cloves garlic, finely chopped
1 English cucumber
¹/₂ cup (125 mL) chopped fresh cilantro or parsley
¹/₂ cup (125 mL) chopped fresh mint
¹/₂ cup (125 mL) shredded fresh basil
6 green onions, chopped
1 sweet red pepper, preferably roasted (page 146), peeled, seeded and diced
Lettuce leaves, to serve

Thai Dressing

¹/₄ cup (50 mL) lemon juice
¹/₄ cup (50 mL) lime juice
¹/₄ cup (50 mL) water
2 tbsp (25 mL) Thai fish sauce or soy sauce
2 tbsp (25 mL) granulated sugar
¹/₄ tsp (1 mL) hot red pepper flakes
Salt to taste

1. Combine chicken, hoisin sauce, lime juice and pepper. Refrigerate for 6 hours or overnight.
2. Grill chicken for 5 to 7 minutes per side, or until just cooked through. Cool and slice thinly on diagonal.
3. If you are using rice noodles, soak in warm water for 15 minutes. Drain well (they do not need further cooking). If you are using spaghettini, cook noodles in a large pot of boiling water until tender but firm. Drain and cool under cold running water.
4. Meanwhile, heat oil in a small skillet over low heat. Add garlic and

THAI FISH SAUCE

Thai fish sauce is the Thai and Vietnamese equivalent of soy sauce, in that it is used in almost everything. It is made by layering fish (usually anchovies, but sometimes crab or shrimp) and salt. The Thai version is called nam pla and the Vietnamese nuoc nam. The sauce is inexpensive and keeps for a long time but, like soy sauce, it is high in sodium, so should be used sparingly (if you smell it, you'll understand why it is never used on its own).

PER SERVING	
Calories	348
Protein	22 g
Fat	9 g
Saturates	1 g
Cholesterol	48 mg
Carbohydrate	45 g
Fibre	2 g
Sodium	345 mg
Potassium	382 mg
Excellent: Vitamin C; Niacin; Vitamin B6	

cook gently for a few minutes until tender and fragrant, but not brown. Toss garlic/oil mixture with noodles.

5. Cut cucumber lengthwise into four pieces and slice thinly.

6. Combine chicken, cucumber, cilantro, mint, basil, green onions, red pepper and noodles and toss well.

7. To prepare dressing, whisk together lemon juice, lime juice, water, fish sauce, sugar and hot pepper flakes. Taste and adjust seasonings, adding salt if necessary.

8. Toss salad with dressing. Serve on a bed of lettuce leaves.

SPAGHETTINI WITH SALAD GREENS

This refreshing salad-style pasta dish can be served warm or at room temperature. I like to use organic baby arugula in this, but if you can't find it, use watercress or other greens. You'll need about 4 cups (1 L) chopped greens in total.

Makes 8 servings

1 lb (500 g) whole wheat or regular spaghettini
5 tomatoes, seeded and diced
1 bunch arugula or watercress, coarsely chopped
1 head radicchio or leaf lettuce, coarsely chopped
2 cloves garlic, minced
1/4 tsp (1 mL) hot red pepper flakes
1/2 tsp (2 mL) pepper
2 tbsp (25 mL) balsamic vinegar
2 tbsp (25 mL) olive oil
1/4 cup (50 mL) chopped black olives
Salt to taste

1. Cook spaghettini in a large pot of boiling water until tender but firm.

2. Meanwhile, in a large bowl, combine tomatoes, arugula and radicchio.

3. Whisk together garlic, hot pepper flakes, pepper, vinegar and oil.

4. Drain pasta well and combine immediately with tomatoes, dressing and olives. Taste and adjust seasonings, adding salt if necessary.

PER SERVING	
Calories	249
Protein	11 g
Fat	5 g
Saturates	1 g
Cholesterol	0 mg
Carbohydrate	46 g
Fibre	6 g
Sodium	53 mg
Potassium	387 mg

ROASTED SALMON SALAD NIÇOISE

This salad really looks like spring. Instead of salmon you could use halibut (cook like the salmon), fresh tuna (cook rare and slice thinly) or the traditional canned tuna. Roasted broccoli, green beans or sweet red or yellow peppers could be used instead of or in addition to the asparagus.

Makes 8 servings

4 tbsp (60 mL) olive oil, divided
1 tbsp (15 mL) chopped fresh rosemary, or 1/2 tsp (2 mL) dried
1/2 tsp (2 mL) salt
1/2 tsp (2 mL) pepper
2 lb (1 kg) baby potatoes, cleaned and halved
6 plum tomatoes, cut in wedges, or 2 cups (500 mL) cherry tomatoes
2 heads garlic
1 lb (500 g) asparagus, trimmed
2 lb (1 kg) salmon fillet in one piece, skin removed
1/3 cup (75 mL) balsamic vinegar
8 cups (2 L) mixed organic greens
2 tbsp (25 mL) chopped fresh tarragon or shredded basil, or
        1/2 tsp (2 mL) dried
4 hard-cooked egg whites, coarsely chopped
1 small bunch chives

1. Combine 2 tbsp (25 mL) oil, rosemary, salt and pepper. Toss potatoes with half this mixture.
2. Arrange tomato wedges, skin side down, and potatoes in a single layer on a parchment-lined baking sheet. Cut top quarter off heads of garlic and wrap in foil. Roast potatoes, tomatoes and garlic in a preheated 400°F (200°C) oven for 40 minutes. Remove baking sheet from oven and scatter asparagus over potatoes and tomatoes. Roast for 10 to 15 minutes longer, or until potatoes and garlic are tender and asparagus is bright green. Tomatoes should be browned on bottom.
3. Meanwhile, coat salmon with remaining oil/rosemary marinade. Place salmon on another baking sheet lined with parchment. About 20 minutes before vegetables are ready, place salmon in oven and roast for 15 to 18 minutes, or until just cooked through.
4. To prepare dressing, squeeze roasted garlic into vinegar and whisk until pureed. Whisk in remaining 2 tbsp (25 mL) oil. (You can also

PER SERVING	
Calories	407
Protein	29 g
Fat	20 g
Saturates	4 g
Cholesterol	64 mg
Carbohydrate	29 g
Fibre	4 g
Sodium	423 mg
Potassium	1173 mg

Excellent: Thiamine; Niacin; Vitamin B6; Vitamin B12; Vitamin C; Folate
Good: Vitamin A; Riboflavin; Iron

puree dressing in a food processor.)

5. Arrange greens over bottom of a large platter. Arrange potatoes down centre and tomatoes and asparagus along sides. With a large spatula, place salmon on top of potatoes. Drizzle dressing over salad. Sprinkle with tarragon and egg whites. Cut chives into 2-inch (5 cm) lengths and sprinkle over top.

ARUGULA SALAD WITH GRILLED SHRIMP, ASPARAGUS AND FENNEL

This delicious spring salad is great as an appetizer, light lunch or dinner. The dressing can be used on rice, pasta or potato salads or as a sauce for lamb or chicken.

Makes 6 servings

2 cloves garlic
1 bunch fresh basil, trimmed
2 tsp (10 mL) salt, divided
¼ cup (50 mL) olive oil
1 lb (500 g) extra-large shrimp, cleaned and butterflied
1 large bulb fennel (about 1 lb/500 g), trimmed and cut in wedges
1 lb (500 g) asparagus, trimmed
2 tbsp (25 mL) balsamic vinegar
1 tbsp (15 mL) lemon juice
¼ tsp (1 mL) pepper
4 cups (1 L) arugula, trimmed

PER SERVING	
Calories	181
Protein	15 g
Fat	10 g
Saturates	1 g
Cholesterol	112 mg
Carbohydrate	9 g
Fibre	4 g
Sodium	468 mg
Potassium	604 mg
Excellent: Vitamin B12; Folate	
Good: Niacin; Iron	

1. In a food processor, combine garlic, basil and 1 tsp (5 mL) salt and puree. Add oil and puree again. Combine 2 tbsp (25 mL) basil oil with shrimp, reserving remaining for dressing.

2. Grill shrimp, fennel and asparagus until browned and just cooked through, about 4 minutes in total. (This may have to be done in batches.)

3. To prepare dressing, whisk together vinegar, lemon juice, reserved basil oil, remaining 1 tsp (15 mL) salt and pepper.

4. Toss shrimp, fennel and asparagus with dressing. Taste and adjust seasonings if necessary. Serve salad on a bed of arugula.

ASIAN GRILLED STEAK SALAD

This is a stunning and delicious main course salad, which could also be made with shrimp or boneless, skinless chicken breasts. The dressing contains no fat at all and makes a wonderful dipping sauce for shrimp, salad rolls and satays.

Makes 6 servings

1/2 bunch fresh cilantro, including roots, stems and leaves
2 cloves garlic, chopped
1 tbsp (15 mL) chopped fresh ginger root
2 tbsp (25 mL) hoisin sauce
2 tbsp (25 mL) soy sauce
2 tbsp (25 mL) lemon juice
1 tsp (5 mL) hot Asian chili paste
1 lb (500 g) flank steak

Citrus Dipping Sauce

1/3 cup (75 mL) granulated sugar
1/3 cup (75 mL) water
2 tbsp (25 mL) rice vinegar or cider vinegar
2 tbsp (25 mL) orange juice
1 tbsp (15 mL) lemon juice
1 tbsp (15 mL) soy sauce
1 clove garlic, minced
1/2 tsp (2 mL) hot Asian chili paste
1 small carrot, grated or chopped (about 1/3 cup/75 mL)

Salad

10 cups (2.5 L) mixed salad greens
1 large English cucumber, thinly sliced
1/2 cup (125 mL) coarsely chopped fresh cilantro or parsley
1/4 cup (50 mL) chopped fresh mint
1/4 cup (50 mL) chopped fresh chives or green onions

1. To prepare marinade, in a food processor, puree cilantro, chopped garlic, ginger, hoisin sauce, soy sauce, lemon juice and hot chili paste.
2. Coat steak with marinade and marinate for 1 hour at room temperature, or overnight in refrigerator.
3. Grill steak for 4 to 5 minutes per side, or until medium-rare. Cool for at least 10 minutes. Slice thinly on diagonal.

CUCUMBERS

I prefer to use English cucumbers as they are not waxed, and I can use the skins if I wish. They also have fewer seeds than regular cucumbers.

If you are adding cucumbers to a salad dressing or dip like tzatziki (page 47), it is a good idea to salt them first so they will not ooze too much liquid and the dressing will not be too watery. Slice the cucumber and place in a colander or sieve. Toss with salt and let drain for about 30 minutes. Rinse and dry before using.

PER SERVING

Calories	210
Protein	20 g
Fat	6 g
Saturates	2 g
Cholesterol	29 mg
Carbohydrate	20 g
Fibre	2 g
Sodium	404 mg
Potassium	734 mg

Excellent: Vitamin A; Niacin; Folate; Vitamin B12
Good: Vitamin C; Riboflavin; Iron; Vitamin B6

4. Meanwhile, to prepare sauce, combine sugar and water in a small saucepan on high heat. Cook for a few minutes until sugar dissolves. Add vinegar, orange juice, lemon juice, soy sauce, minced garlic, chili paste and carrot. Taste and adjust seasonings if necessary. Cool.

5. Arrange salad greens on a flat dish. Arrange cucumber on top and sprinkle with chopped cilantro, mint and chives. Place steak slices on top and drizzle with sauce.

CHOPPED TUNA SALAD

Everyone seems to love tuna salad. (Many children don't even realize it's fish!) This version has lots of vegetables and looks beautiful.

Makes 4 to 6 servings

1 lb (500 g) asparagus, trimmed, cooked and diced
1 1/2 lb (750 g) potatoes, peeled, cooked and diced
1 1/2 cups (375 mL) corn kernels
2 7-oz (198 g) cans white tuna (water-packed), drained and flaked
4 cups (1 L) coarsely chopped ruby-tipped lettuce or Boston lettuce
1/3 cup (75 mL) shredded fresh basil or chopped parsley
4 green onions, chopped

Dressing

3 tbsp (45 mL) balsamic vinegar
1 clove garlic, minced
1/2 tsp (2 mL) salt
1/2 tsp (2 mL) pepper
2 tbsp (25 mL) olive oil

1. In a large bowl, combine asparagus, potatoes, corn, tuna, lettuce, basil and green onions.

2. To prepare dressing, in a small bowl, combine vinegar, garlic, salt and pepper. Whisk in oil.

3. Toss salad with dressing. Taste and adjust seasonings if necessary.

PER SERVING

Calories	391
Protein	29 g
Fat	10 g
Saturates	2 g
Cholesterol	33 mg
Carbohydrate	51 g
Fibre	7 g
Sodium	628 mg
Potassium	1259 mg

Excellent: Vitamin C; Thiamine; Niacin; Iron; Vitamin B6; Folate; Vitamin B12
Good: Vitamin A; Riboflavin

GREEK SALAD WITH GRILLED CHICKEN

Za'atar refers both to a Middle Eastern herb and a Middle Eastern herb mixture that includes thyme, oregano, salt and sesame seeds. If you don't have it, use dried oregano or thyme.

Makes 8 servings

4 boneless, skinless single chicken breasts
2 7-inch (18 cm) whole wheat or regular pita breads
2 tbsp (25 mL) olive oil
1 tbsp (15 mL) za'atar
2 large ripe tomatoes, seeded and cut in chunks
1 small English cucumber, peeled and cut in chunks
2 tbsp (25 mL) black olives, pitted and halved
2 oz (60 g) feta cheese, broken in small chunks
2 tbsp (25 mL) coarsely chopped fresh parsley
2 tbsp (25 mL) coarsely chopped green onions
2 tbsp (25 mL) coarsely chopped fresh cilantro
2 tbsp (25 mL) coarsely chopped fresh mint
1 small head Romaine lettuce, cut in chunks

Dressing

3 tbsp (45 mL) lemon juice
1 clove garlic, minced
1 tsp (5 mL) salt
1/4 tsp (1 mL) pepper
3 tbsp (45 mL) olive oil

1. Brush chicken and pita breads with oil and sprinkle with za'atar. Grill chicken for 5 to 7 minutes per side, or until just cooked through. Cut into chunks. Grill pita breads for 1 to 2 minutes per side, or until lightly browned. Cut into wedges.

2. In a large bowl, combine chicken, tomatoes, cucumber, olives, feta and herbs. Reserve lettuce and pita.

3. To prepare dressing, whisk together lemon juice, garlic, salt, pepper and oil. Gently combine chicken and vegetables with dressing.

4. About 30 minutes before serving, add pita. Just before serving add lettuce and toss. Taste and adjust seasonings if necessary.

PER SERVING	
Calories	241
Protein	20 g
Fat	12 g
Saturates	3 g
Cholesterol	48 mg
Carbohydrate	14 g
Fibre	3 g
Sodium	520 mg
Potassium	534 mg

Excellent: Niacin; Vitamin B6; Folate
Good: Vitamin A; Thiamine; Vitamin B12; Vitamin C

BALSAMIC SPA DRESSING

This dressing can also be made with other mild vinegars such as raspberry, sherry, Champagne or a good red wine vinegar.

Makes about 1³/4 cups (425 mL)

½ cup (125 mL) balsamic vinegar
2 tbsp (25 mL) lemon juice
2 tbsp (25 mL) olive oil
1 tbsp (15 mL) Dijon mustard
2 tsp (10 mL) Worcestershire sauce
1 clove garlic, minced
¼ tsp (1 mL) pepper
1 cup (250 mL) water
1 tsp (5 mL) honey, optional
¼ tsp (1 mL) salt, optional

PER TBSP (15 ML)	
Calories	10
Protein	trace
Fat	1 g
Saturates	trace
Cholesterol	0 mg
Carbohydrate	trace
Fibre	0 g
Sodium	12 mg
Potassium	8 mg

1. Whisk together vinegar, lemon juice, oil, mustard, Worcestershire, garlic and pepper. Whisk in water.
2. Taste and add honey and/or salt only if necessary.

BALSAMIC VINEGAR

Balsamic vinegar is traditionally made from the must of Trebbiano grapes. The vinegar is aged in different kinds of woods, and the woods (and how long and in which order the vinegar is kept in them) are the reason each balsamic tastes different.

There are basically three different types of balsamic. True balsamic vinegar has been aged for a long time and can cost more than $250 a bottle. Usually, the older the vinegar, the less acidic it is. The best balsamic is rarely used in salad dressings but is drizzled sparingly over Parmesan or grilled meat or fish.

Artisan balsamic vinegars have been made in the style of authentic balsamic but are not aged as long. They can be used in salad dressings and marinades and the good ones can be used straight on a salad without any oil. The harsh-tasting bottom-end balsamics (jokingly called overnight balsamics) are not balsamics at all but inexpensive vinegar with colour and flavouring added.

MUSTARD PEPPER DRESSING

This is a terrific all-purpose creamy dressing for green salads, roasted meats or potato salad (page 143).

Makes about 3/4 cup (175 mL)

2 tbsp (25 mL) red wine vinegar
1 tbsp (15 mL) Dijon mustard
1 clove garlic, minced
1 tsp (5 mL) pepper
Salt to taste
2 tsp (10 mL) honey
1/2 cup (125 mL) yogurt cheese (page 391), thick unflavoured
    low-fat yogurt, chicken stock or tomato juice
2 tbsp (25 mL) olive oil

1. Whisk together vinegar, mustard, garlic, pepper and salt.
2. Stir in honey, yogurt cheese and oil. Taste and adjust seasonings if necessary.

PER TBSP (15 ML)	
Calories	36
Protein	1 g
Fat	3 g
Saturates	1 g
Cholesterol	1 mg
Carbohydrate	2 g
Fibre	0 g
Sodium	26 mg
Potassium	39 mg

CREAMY GARLIC DRESSING

This unusual dressing is sweet and delicious, although most people would be shocked to know how much garlic is in it. Use it as a dressing on green salads or potato salads, as a topping for baked potatoes, as a dip for vegetables or as a sauce with roast meats, poultry or fish. You can also use the garlic puree (with or without the yogurt cheese) on bruschetta or pita with a little salsa on top.

Makes about ¹/₂ cup (125 mL)

1 head garlic (about 12 cloves), peeled
1 cup (250 mL) homemade chicken stock (page 109) or water
1 tsp (5 mL) honey
Pinch chopped fresh or dried rosemary
Pinch chopped fresh or dried thyme
2 tbsp (25 mL) balsamic vinegar
1 tbsp (15 mL) olive oil
¹/₄ tsp (1 mL) pepper
¹/₄ cup (50 mL) yogurt cheese (page 391), thick unflavoured low-fat
    yogurt, chicken stock or tomato juice
Salt to taste

1. In a small saucepan, combine garlic, stock, honey, rosemary and thyme. Bring to a boil. Reduce heat and cook gently for about 30 minutes, or until garlic is very tender and liquid has almost disappeared.
2. In a food processor, puree garlic with any juices. Blend in vinegar, oil, pepper and yogurt cheese. Taste and adjust seasonings, adding salt if necessary.

Potato Salad

Cook 2 lb (1 kg) potatoes and cut into cubes. Combine with ¹/₂ cup (125 mL) Creamy Garlic Dressing, Creamy Salsa (page 44), Mustard Pepper Dressing (page 142) or Goat Cheese Dip (page 48).
    Makes 4 to 6 servings.

Pasta with Creamy Garlic Dressing

Toss dressing with 3 oz (90 g) crumbled goat cheese, about 4 cups (1 L) cooked pasta and ¹/₄ cup (50 mL) shredded fresh basil or chopped parsley. Season with salt and pepper to taste.
    Makes 4 servings.

PER TBSP (15 ML)	
Calories	37
Protein	2 g
Fat	2 g
Saturates	trace
Cholesterol	1 mg
Carbohydrate	3 g
Fibre	trace
Sodium	11 mg
Potassium	71 mg

CITRUS VINAIGRETTE

Not only is this good on salad greens, it also adds glamour to poached or baked salmon or chicken.

Makes about 1 cup (250 mL)
1 small clove garlic, minced
1 tsp (5 mL) minced fresh ginger root
1 tbsp (15 mL) honey
2 tbsp (25 mL) rice vinegar
2 tbsp (25 mL) lemon juice
2 tbsp (25 mL) grapefruit juice
¼ cup (50 mL) orange juice
2 tbsp (25 mL) olive oil
1 tsp (5 mL) dark sesame oil
Dash hot red pepper sauce
2 tbsp (25 mL) chopped fresh cilantro or parsley
2 tbsp (25 mL) shredded fresh basil or chopped parsley
2 tbsp (25 mL) chopped fresh chives or green onions
Salt to taste

1. Whisk together garlic, ginger, honey, vinegar, lemon juice, grape-fruit juice and orange juice.
2. Whisk in olive oil, sesame oil and hot pepper sauce. Stir in cilantro, basil and chives. Taste and adjust seasonings, adding salt if necessary.

PER TBSP (15 ML)	
Calories	25
Protein	trace
Fat	2 g
Saturates	trace
Cholesterol	0 mg
Carbohydrate	2 g
Fibre	trace
Sodium	1 mg
Potassium	21 mg

SESAME GINGER DRESSING

This dressing explodes with the taste of fresh herbs. The small amount of sesame oil adds an exotic, mysterious flavour but only a minimal amount of fat. Buy it at Asian markets and keep it refrigerated after opening.

This dressing is good on mixed lettuces, grains and chicken or salmon salads. Or try it with the Chopped Grilled Chicken Salad (page 130).

Makes about $^2/_3$ cup (150 mL)

2 cloves garlic, minced
1 tbsp (15 mL) minced fresh ginger root
2 tsp (10 mL) honey-style mustard
2 tsp (10 mL) honey
1 tbsp (15 mL) soy sauce
2 tbsp (25 mL) lemon juice
2 tbsp (25 mL) balsamic vinegar
$^1/_4$ cup (50 mL) orange juice
1 tbsp (15 mL) olive oil
1 tsp (5 mL) dark sesame oil
$^1/_4$ tsp (1 mL) hot red pepper sauce, optional
$^1/_4$ cup (50 mL) chopped fresh cilantro or parsley
$^1/_4$ cup (50 mL) chopped fresh chives or green onions

1. Whisk together garlic, ginger, mustard, honey, soy sauce, lemon juice, vinegar, orange juice, olive oil, sesame oil and hot pepper sauce.
2. Stir in cilantro and chives. Taste and adjust seasonings if necessary.

PER TBSP (15 ML)	
Calories	29
Protein	trace
Fat	2 g
Saturates	trace
Cholesterol	0 mg
Carbohydrate	3 g
Fibre	trace
Sodium	79 mg
Potassium	37 mg

ROASTED RED PEPPER DRESSING

The pureed red pepper gives this dressing a thick texture, roasting the pepper adds a slightly earthy flavour, and the balsamic vinegar adds a tart sweetness. This dressing is particularly good on pasta salads, grain salads and chunky vegetable salads. You can also serve it as a sauce on plain grilled fish, chicken, lamb or steak.

When the dressing is refrigerated it gels slightly; add a little water before serving, if necessary.

Makes about 3/4 cup (175 mL)

1 sweet red pepper
1 clove garlic, chopped
1/4 cup (50 mL) balsamic vinegar
1/2 tsp (2 mL) pepper
2 tbsp (25 mL) chopped fresh basil or parsley
1 tbsp (15 mL) olive oil
2 tbsp (25 mL) water
Salt to taste

1. Cut red pepper in half and remove core and seeds. Arrange halves on a baking sheet, cut sides down. Broil until blackened and blistered. Cool and peel.
2. In a food processor, puree red pepper and garlic. Blend in vinegar, pepper, basil and oil. Whisk in water. Taste and adjust seasonings, adding salt if necessary.

PER TBSP (15 mL)	
Calories	14
Protein	trace
Fat	1 g
Saturates	trace
Cholesterol	0 mg
Carbohydrate	1 g
Fibre	trace
Sodium	0 mg
Potassium	25 mg

ROASTING AND PEELING PEPPERS

Roasting and peeling peppers, while not essential, gives them an earthy, smoky taste. It also makes them much sweeter and easier to digest. You can roast the peppers whole by placing them on a barbecue (grill a bunch at one time) and turning them every few minutes until all sides are blackened. Let the blackened peppers cool and then peel off the skins and remove the stems, ribs and seeds.

You can also cut the peppers in half, remove the ribs and seeds and place the peppers cut side down on a baking sheet. Place them under the broiler until they blacken, then cool and remove the charred skins. Or you can roast one pepper at a time over a gas element.

Roast peppers when they are in season and then freeze them for future use. Cut the peeled peppers into strips or chunks and place on a parchment- or waxed paper–lined baking sheet in a single layer. When the peppers are frozen, pack them into freezer bags or containers. The pieces will stay separate, allowing you to defrost a small amount at a time.

You can also peel raw peppers to make them sweeter and milder. Simply use a vegetable peeler (you will quickly learn to buy square-shaped peppers with smooth sides!).

REDUCING OIL IN SALAD DRESSINGS

In traditional salad dressings, the proportion of oil to vinegar is extremely high. But if you have a good-quality, sweet-tasting vinegar, you will need much less oil. Use mild vinegars such as vincotto (vinegar made from the cooked must of two varieties of dried grapes), balsamic, raspberry, rice and sherry vinegar. Use olive oil (other salad oils are unflavoured, but a small amount of flavourful olive oil goes a long way). You can also replace some of the oil with a puree of vegetables, orange juice, buttermilk, yogurt or soft yogurt cheese (page 391).

HONEY LIME VINAIGRETTE

My good friend Lynn Saunders loves this dressing and says she got it from me—I must give out more recipes than I can remember! She puts it on seafood salads and organic greens.

I always use freshly squeezed lemon and lime juice, but fresh lime juice makes an especially big difference in this dressing.

Makes about $^{1}/_{2}$ cup (125 mL)

$^{1}/_{4}$ cup (50 mL) lime juice
1 clove garlic, minced
$^{1}/_{2}$ tsp (2 mL) salt
Pinch pepper
1 tbsp (15 mL) honey
$^{1}/_{4}$ cup (50 mL) olive oil
3 tbsp (45 mL) chopped fresh cilantro

1. Whisk together lime juice, garlic, salt and pepper. Whisk in honey and olive oil. Stir in cilantro.

PER TBSP (15 ML)	
Calories	70
Protein	0 g
Fat	7 g
Saturates	1 g
Cholesterol	0 mg
Carbohydrate	3 g
Fibre	0 g
Sodium	147 mg
Potassium	17 mg

HEART SMART

PASTAS

PENNE WITH ROASTED CHERRY TOMATOES AND BOCCONCINI

Use a combination of red and yellow cherry tomatoes if you can find them. Serve this dish hot or at room temperature.

Makes 6 to 8 servings.

4 cups (1 L) cherry tomatoes
2 tbsp (25 mL) olive oil
2 cloves garlic, minced
1 tsp (5 mL) salt
1/4 tsp (1 mL) pepper
3/4 lb (375 g) whole wheat or regular penne
1/2 lb (250 g) bocconcini (fresh mozzarella), torn in chunks
2 tbsp (25 mL) pitted black olives
1/3 cup (75 mL) packed basil leaves, torn

1. Combine tomatoes with oil, garlic, salt and pepper. Spread in a shallow baking dish and roast in a preheated 400°F (200°C) oven for 10 minutes, or until tomatoes are starting to burst.

2. Meanwhile, cook pasta in a large pot of boiling water until tender but firm.

3. Drain pasta well and combine with hot cherry tomatoes and their juices, cheese, olives and basil. Taste and adjust seasonings if necessary.

SHREDDING BASIL

Fresh basil becomes bruised and turns black when it is chopped so, especially if I am using it as a garnish, I like to shred it. Stack the leaves or roll them, then slice, using a sharp knife.

PER SERVING

Calories	367
Protein	16 g
Fat	13 g
Saturates	5 g
Cholesterol	24 mg
Carbohydrate	51 g
Fibre	6 g
Sodium	363 mg
Potassium	327 mg

Good: Thiamine; Niacin; Vitamin C; Calcium; Iron

OLIVE OIL

I like to use olive oil. It is a monounsaturated fat (page 14) and it adds the delicious taste of olives to a dish. Extra-virgin olive oil has less acidity than regular olive oil; it is made with ripe olives without the use of heat or chemicals.

Buy olive oil in small quantities and, once it has been opened, use it within a few months. Otherwise, keep it in the refrigerator (the oil may firm up and become cloudy, but it will be fine when it returns to room temperature).

If I don't want the taste of olives in a dish, I usually use sunflower oil.

HOT PASTA

To serve piping-hot pasta, cook the sauce in a large deep skillet or saucepan. When the pasta is ready, add it to the skillet and toss with the sauce over low heat for a few minutes before serving.

If you are transferring the pasta to a serving bowl, the bowl should be hot (place it over the boiling pasta to heat), or serve the pasta directly into warmed individual bowls or plates. Rush the pasta to the table and tell guests to start eating right away!

MARK'S SPAGHETTI WITH TOMATO SAUCE

When my son, Mark, was growing up, he loved pasta, but only if it was served with an absolutely plain tomato sauce like this one. Over the years many people have told me their kids love it, too.

When I serve this I let everyone add their own grated cheese, chopped parsley and a pinch of hot pepper flakes if they wish. The sauce can be made ahead and reheated. It can also be frozen. I used to freeze it in ice-cube trays (two cubes make a perfect child-sized portion), but now I find it easier to freeze it flat in a zipper-style freezer bag and then just break off what I need.

You can also add leftover cooked chicken or vegetables to the sauce.

Makes 6 servings

1 28-oz (796 mL) can plum tomatoes, with juices, pureed
1 small onion, peeled and halved
2 cloves garlic, peeled but left whole
1 tbsp (15 mL) olive oil
Salt and pepper to taste
1 lb (500 g) whole wheat or regular spaghetti
¼ cup (50 mL) grated Parmesan cheese
2 tbsp (25 mL) shredded fresh basil or chopped parsley
Pinch hot red pepper flakes, optional

PER SERVING	
Calories	324
Protein	14 g
Fat	5 g
Saturates	1 g
Cholesterol	7 mg
Carbohydrate	62 g
Fibre	8 g
Sodium	298 mg
Potassium	416 mg
Good: Thiamine; Niacin	

1. In a saucepan, combine tomatoes, onion halves, garlic cloves and oil. Bring to a boil, reduce heat and simmer gently for 10 to 20 minutes, or until sauce cooks down and thickens slightly.
2. Remove and discard onion and garlic. Add salt and pepper.
3. Meanwhile, cook spaghetti in a large pot of boiling water until tender but firm. Drain well and toss with sauce. Taste and adjust seasonings if necessary. Serve and allow everyone to top pasta with cheese, basil and hot pepper flakes.

Spaghetti with Tomato Sauce and Arugula

Add a few handfuls of baby arugula or spinach to sauce a few minutes before end of cooking time. Cook just until wilted.

Makes 6 servings.

CRAZY LASAGNA

This is much easier than a traditional lasagna, and it is very versatile. You can omit the eggplant and double the zucchini and mushrooms, you can use cremini mushrooms instead of portobellos, or substitute almost any vegetables that you have in the refrigerator. If I use portobello mushrooms, I usually scrape out the gills for a cleaner look and taste.

This can be made a couple of days ahead and refrigerated, or it can be made a few weeks ahead and frozen. It is also wonderful served at room temperature.

Makes 8 to 10 servings

2 lb (1 kg) plum tomatoes, seeded and quartered (about 8)
1 lb (500 g) Asian eggplants (about 4), cut in ½-inch (1 cm) slices
1 lb (500 g) zucchini (about 2), cut in rounds
½ lb (250 g) portobello or cremini mushrooms,
      trimmed and cut in chunks
2 sweet red peppers, seeded and cut in chunks
1 large onion, peeled and cut in chunks
2 tbsp (25 mL) olive oil
1 tsp (5 mL) salt
¼ tsp (1 mL) pepper
2 heads garlic
¾ lb (375 g) whole wheat or regular lasagne noodles, broken up
2 cups (500 mL) pureed canned tomatoes
      (drained) or tomato sauce
1 lb (500 g) light ricotta cheese (about 2 cups/500 mL)
½ lb (250 g) bocconcini (fresh mozzarella), grated
      (about 2 cups/500 mL)
¼ cup (50 mL) chopped fresh basil or parsley
1 tbsp (15 mL) chopped fresh oregano, or ½ tsp (2 mL) dried
2 tbsp (25 mL) grated Parmesan cheese

PER SERVING	
Calories	438
Protein	22 g
Fat	15 g
Saturates	7 g
Cholesterol	37 mg
Carbohydrate	60 g
Fibre	10 g
Sodium	365 mg
Potassium	645 mg

Excellent: Vitamin A; Thiamine; Riboflavin; Niacin; Vitamin B6; Vitamin C; Folate; Calcium; Iron
Good: Vitamin B12

1. Arrange plum tomatoes, eggplants, zucchini, mushrooms, peppers and onion on two baking sheets lined with parchment paper. Drizzle with oil and sprinkle with salt and pepper. Cut top quarter off garlic heads and wrap heads in foil. Roast vegetables and garlic in a preheated 400°F (200°C) oven for 45 minutes, or until vegetables are browned.
2. Meanwhile, cook noodles in a large pot of boiling water until tender but firm. Drain and rinse with cold water.

3. In a large bowl, combine noodles with roasted vegetables. Squeeze in garlic. Add canned tomatoes, ricotta (leave it in blobs), bocconcini, basil and oregano. Taste and adjust seasonings if necessary.

4. Transfer mixture to a lightly oiled 13- x 9-inch (3.5 L) baking dish and sprinkle with Parmesan. Cover and bake at 350°F (180°C) for 30 minutes. Uncover and cook for 20 to 30 minutes longer, or until lightly browned. Allow to rest for 10 minutes before serving.

SPAGHETTI PUTTANESCA

This dish is so quick to make that one of the rumours of its origins is that the ladies of the night in Rome could whip it up for dinner between clients. Omit the anchovies if you are cooking this for vegetarians.

Makes 6 to 8 servings

1 tbsp (15 mL) olive oil
4 cloves garlic, finely chopped
1/4 tsp (1 mL) hot red pepper flakes
2 anchovies, minced, optional
1 28-oz (796 mL) can plum tomatoes, drained and chopped
1/4 cup (50 mL) black olives, halved
2 tbsp (25 mL) capers
1 lb (500 g) whole wheat or regular spaghetti
1/4 cup (50 mL) grated Parmesan cheese, optional
2 tbsp (25 mL) chopped fresh parsley

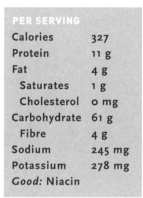

PER SERVING	
Calories	327
Protein	11 g
Fat	4 g
Saturates	1 g
Cholesterol	0 mg
Carbohydrate	61 g
Fibre	4 g
Sodium	245 mg
Potassium	278 mg
Good: Niacin	

1. Heat oil in large, deep non-stick skillet on medium heat. Add garlic and hot pepper flakes and cook gently for a few minutes until fragrant, but do not brown.

2. Stir in anchovies and tomatoes. Bring to a boil and cook for 5 minutes. Add olives and capers. Cook for 3 minutes longer.

3. Meanwhile, cook spaghetti in a large pot of boiling water until tender but firm. Drain well and toss with sauce, cheese and parsley. Taste and adjust seasonings if necessary.

PASTA WITH TOMATO SAUCE AND RICOTTA

The tomato sauce can be made ahead of time, but cook the pasta and toss with the sauce and ricotta just before serving. Although bacon and pancetta (unsmoked Italian bacon that can be found at Italian grocery stores) are both high in fat, a small amount adds a unique flavour. But you can omit it if you are making this for vegetarians.

Makes 6 servings

1 tbsp (15 mL) olive oil
1 oz (30 g) pancetta or bacon, diced, optional
1 onion, chopped
2 cloves garlic, finely chopped
1/4 tsp (1 mL) hot red pepper flakes
1 28-oz (796 mL) can plum tomatoes, with juices, pureed
1/2 tsp (2 mL) pepper
Salt to taste
1 lb (500 g) whole wheat or regular pasta spirals or penne
1/2 lb (250 g) light ricotta or pressed cottage cheese
      (about 1 cup/250 mL)
1/4 cup (50 mL) grated Parmesan cheese
1/4 cup (50 mL) shredded fresh basil or chopped parsley

1. Heat oil in a large, deep non-stick skillet on medium heat. Add pancetta and cook for about 5 minutes, or until crisp.
2. Add onion, garlic and hot pepper flakes to skillet. Cook gently for about 5 minutes.
3. Add tomatoes and cook for 15 minutes, or until sauce is reduced and thickens slightly. Add pepper and salt.
4. Meanwhile, cook pasta in a large pot of boiling water until tender but firm. Drain well and toss with sauce. Top with ricotta, Parmesan and basil. Taste and adjust seasonings if necessary. Toss well before serving.

PER SERVING	
Calories	370
Protein	18 g
Fat	7 g
Saturates	3 g
Cholesterol	7 mg
Carbohydrate	64 g
Fibre	8 g
Sodium	346 mg
Potassium	479 mg
Excellent: Iron	
Good: Thiamine; Niacin; Calcium	

PASTA WITH ROASTED CAULIFLOWER

When vegetables are roasted, their flavour intensifies and their sugars caramelize into a sweet, brown essence. This dish makes a great vegetarian main course or salad, and the roasted cauliflower can be served on its own as a side dish. You can also add four fresh plum tomatoes; cut them into quarters and roast them with the cauliflower.

Makes 4 to 6 servings

1 large head cauliflower (about 2 lb/1 kg)
2 tbsp (25 mL) olive oil, divided
1/2 tsp (2 mL) salt
1/2 lb (250 g) whole wheat penne or other medium pasta
2 tbsp (25 mL) red wine vinegar or balsamic vinegar
1 clove garlic, minced
Salt and pepper to taste
2 sweet red peppers, roasted (page 146), peeled, seeded and diced
2 tbsp (25 mL) chopped black olives
1/4 cup (50 mL) shredded fresh basil or chopped parsley

PER SERVING	
Calories	313
Protein	12 g
Fat	9 g
Saturates	1 g
Cholesterol	0 mg
Carbohydrate	53 g
Fibre	10 g
Sodium	336 mg
Potassium	727 mg
Excellent: Vitamin B6; Vitamin C; Folate	

1. Trim cauliflower and break into florets. In a large bowl, toss cauliflower with 1 tbsp (15 mL) oil and salt. Spread in a single layer on a parchment-lined baking sheet and roast in a preheated 400°F (200°C) oven for 25 to 30 minutes, or until cooked through and lightly browned. Stir occasionally.

2. Meanwhile, cook pasta in a large pot of boiling water until tender but firm. Drain well.

3. Whisk together vinegar, garlic and remaining 1 tbsp (15 mL) oil. Whisk in salt and pepper.

4. Toss pasta with cauliflower, peppers, olives, dressing and basil. Taste and adjust seasonings if necessary. Serve hot or at room temperature.

SPAGHETTI WITH ROASTED TOMATO SAUCE

You could have pasta with a different tomato sauce every night of the week. This one is very easy and has lots of flavour. It is also a good source of fibre and contains practically no fat! If you don't like things too spicy, omit the jalapeño.

Makes 6 servings

2 lb (1 kg) ripe plum tomatoes, quartered
1 onion, peeled and quartered
1 jalapeño, halved and seeded
1 head garlic
1 lb (500 g) whole wheat or regular spaghetti
1/2 cup (125 mL) shredded fresh basil or chopped cilantro
Salt and pepper to taste

1. Line a baking sheet with parchment paper or foil. Arrange tomatoes, onion and jalapeño on baking sheet. Cut top quarter off garlic head, wrap garlic in foil and place on baking sheet. Roast vegetables in a preheated 400°F (200°C) oven for 45 to 50 minutes, or until lightly browned.
2. Squeeze garlic out of skins into a food processor. Add tomatoes, onion and jalapeño and puree. Reheat sauce if necessary.
3. Meanwhile, cook spaghetti in a large pot of boiling water until tender but firm. Drain well and toss with vegetable puree and basil. Taste and season with salt and pepper.

PER SERVING	
Calories	278
Protein	14 g
Fat	2 g
Saturates	trace
Cholesterol	0 mg
Carbohydrate	64 g
Fibre	14 g
Sodium	20 mg
Potassium	493 mg

Excellent: Thiamine; Iron
Good: Vitamin A; Niacin; Vitamin B6; Vitamin C

COOKING PASTA

Use a large pot and lots of water so the noodles won't stick to the pot or to each other. Do not add oil to the cooking water. It adds unnecessary fat as well as preventing the pasta from absorbing the sauce properly.

Unless specified in the recipe (e.g., when you are cooking lasagna or cannelloni noodles ahead of time, to stop the pieces from sticking), do not rinse pasta after cooking; rinsing removes the outside starch that helps the sauce cling to the noodles.

Fresh homemade pasta takes only about 1 minute to cook. So-called "fresh" storebought pasta (that is often sold shrink-wrapped) usually takes about 6 minutes to cook. Dried commercial pasta takes 8 to 12 minutes.

No matter what kind of pasta you are cooking, never rely only on a timer to determine whether it is ready. Always taste it. If the pasta does not have an uncooked centre core, it is ready. Some people say you can tell whether pasta is cooked by throwing it against a wall, but this is not a good idea. The pasta will stick both before and after it is ready, and if you don't get it off the wall quickly, it will dry and the paint will come off with it. Finally, if your children see you do this, your kitchen will never be the same again!

PASTA WITH TOMATO AND RED PEPPER SAUCE

Adding a sweet vegetable like red pepper gives a wonderful flavour and great texture to tomato sauce.

You can add 1 cup (250 mL) cooked or smoked chicken or turkey to the sauce. Or, for a "creamy" version add 1 cup (250 mL) ricotta cheese at the end. Instead of using fresh basil, try topping each serving with 1 tbsp (15 mL) pesto (page 166).

Makes 6 to 8 servings

1 tbsp (15 mL) olive oil
1 onion, chopped
2 cloves garlic, finely chopped
Pinch hot red pepper flakes
1 1/2 lb (750 g) tomatoes, peeled, seeded and chopped
        (6 to 8 plum tomatoes), or 1 28-oz (796 mL) can
        plum tomatoes with juices, chopped
4 sweet red peppers, roasted (page 146),
        peeled, seeded and chopped
Salt and pepper to taste
1 lb (500 g) whole wheat or regular penne
1/4 cup (50 mL) grated Parmesan cheese, optional
1/4 cup (50 mL) shredded fresh basil or chopped parsley

1. Heat oil in a large, deep non-stick skillet on medium heat. Add onion, garlic and hot pepper flakes. Cook gently for 5 to 8 minutes, or until tender and fragrant.
2. Add tomatoes and peppers. Cook for 5 to 10 minutes, or until tomatoes cook down and become juicy. Add salt and pepper.
3. Meanwhile, cook pasta in a large pot of boiling water until tender but firm. Drain well and add to skillet with sauce. Toss well with Parmesan and basil. Taste and adjust seasonings if necessary.

PER SERVING	
Calories	320
Protein	12 g
Fat	4 g
Saturates	1 g
Cholesterol	0 mg
Carbohydrate	65 g
Fibre	9 g
Sodium	12 mg
Potassium	445 mg

Excellent: Vitamin A; Vitamin C
Good: Niacin; Vitamin B6; Folate

PASTA WITH RED PEPPERS AND EGGPLANT

Eggplant has a very "meaty" texture when it is used in this dish, and it gives the sauce body. The sauce can be made ahead and reheated, but cook the pasta just before serving.

Makes 6 servings

1 tbsp (15 mL) olive oil
1 red onion, chopped
3 cloves garlic, finely chopped
1/4 tsp (1 mL) hot red pepper flakes
1 lb (500 g) Asian eggplants (3 or 4), trimmed and diced
3 sweet red peppers, cut in 1 1/2-inch (4 cm) chunks
1 28-oz (796 mL) can plum tomatoes, with juices
Salt to taste
1 lb (500 g) whole wheat rigatoni or other tube pasta
1/2 cup (125 mL) grated Parmesan cheese
1/4 cup (50 mL) shredded fresh basil or chopped parsley

1. Heat oil in a large, deep non-stick skillet on medium heat. Add onion, garlic and hot pepper flakes and cook gently for 5 to 8 minutes, or until very tender and fragrant but not brown.
2. Add eggplants and sweet peppers and cook for 5 to 10 minutes, or until wilted slightly.
3. Add tomatoes and break up with a spoon. Cook for 10 to 15 minutes, or until sauce reduces and thickens slightly. Add salt.
4. Meanwhile, cook pasta in a large pot of boiling water until tender but firm. Drain well and toss with sauce. Taste and adjust seasonings if necessary. Sprinkle with cheese and basil. Toss well and serve immediately.

PER SERVING	
Calories	401
Protein	17 g
Fat	7 g
Saturates	2 g
Cholesterol	7 mg
Carbohydrate	75 g
Fibre	12 g
Sodium	381 mg
Potassium	778 mg
Excellent: Vitamin A; Thiamine; Niacin; Vitamin B6; Vitamin C; Iron	
Good: Folate; Calcium	

PASTA SHAPES

Although there are no hard and fast rules about which pasta to serve with which sauce, there is a reason for choosing one shape over another in a particular recipe. For example, tube pasta is good for catching all the little bits found in a sauce full of chopped ingredients. Pastas like rigatoni are traditionally used with chunky vegetable, seafood or chicken sauces so you can stab a piece of pasta and a chunk of something else at the same time. Long, thin pasta is used for smooth sauces or sauces with tiny pieces in them (big chunks would fall off when you twirl the strands). Tiny pasta is used in soups, so it can be spooned up easily.

If you want to use a few different pasta shapes in the same dish (kids especially love this), choose shapes that will take the same amount of time to cook, or add the shape that takes the longest to the pot first.

SPIRAL MACARONI WITH POTATOES AND RAPINI

Even if (like me) you do not like anchovies on their own, try them in this recipe. They add richness and body to the sauce without dominating the flavour. However, you can omit them for a vegetarian meal. (Any leftover anchovies can be frozen.)

This dish is traditionally made with ear-shaped pasta (orecchiette), but I like to use large macaroni or penne.

Makes 6 servings

1 baking potato, peeled and diced
3/4 lb (375 g) whole wheat spiral macaroni, penne or fusilli
1 large bunch rapini or broccoli (about 1 lb/500 g), cut in chunks
1/4 cup (50 mL) olive oil
3 anchovies, rinsed and minced
4 cloves garlic, finely chopped
1/4 tsp (1 mL) hot red pepper flakes
1/2 tsp (2 mL) pepper
1/2 cup (12 mL) hot pasta water

PER SERVING	
Calories	328
Protein	12 g
Fat	11 g
Saturates	2 g
Cholesterol	2 mg
Carbohydrate	50 g
Fibre	7 g
Sodium	125 mg
Potassium	466 mg

Excellent: Vitamin A; Niacin
Good: Thiamine; Vitamin B6; Vitamin C; Folate; Iron

1. Bring a large pot of water to a boil. Add potato and cook for 5 minutes. Add pasta and cook for 5 minutes longer.
2. Add rapini to pot with pasta and potatoes and continue to cook until pasta is tender. (It does not matter if potatoes fall apart; they will just become part of the sauce.) This will take another 7 to 10 minutes.
3. Meanwhile, heat oil in a large, deep non-stick skillet on medium heat. Add anchovies, garlic, hot pepper flakes and pepper and cook gently for a few minutes until fragrant, but do not brown garlic. Add 1/2 cup (125 mL) boiling water from pasta and cook for about 3 minutes.
4. When pasta and vegetables are ready, drain well. Add to garlic mixture and toss well. Taste and adjust seasonings if necessary.

MACARONI AND CHEESE WITH ROASTED BROCCOLI

For my lactose-intolerant family members, I make this using lactose-free milk and cheese. The casserole freezes well in individual servings (it's a great take-home treat for kids who live on their own).

Makes 8 to 10 servings

1 lb (500 g) broccoli, trimmed and cut in 1-inch (2.5 cm) pieces
1/2 lb (250 g) whole wheat macaroni (about 2 cups/500 mL)
3 tbsp (45 mL) vegetable oil
1/4 cup (50 mL) all-purpose flour
4 cups (1 L) milk, hot
1 tsp (5 mL) Worcestershire sauce
1/4 tsp (1 mL) hot red pepper sauce
2 tsp (10 mL) salt
1 tsp (5 mL) pepper
Pinch ground nutmeg
2 1/2 cups (625 mL) grated light Cheddar cheese, divided
1 cup (250 mL) fresh whole wheat or regular breadcrumbs

1. Spread broccoli on a large baking dish lined with parchment paper. Roast in a preheated 400°F (200°C) oven for 20 minutes, or until tender and slightly browned. Cool.

2. Meanwhile, cook macaroni in a large pot of boiling water until just tender (do not overcook). Drain well and rinse with cold water.

3. Heat oil in a large saucepan on medium heat. Add flour and cook for 3 minutes. Add hot milk and bring to a boil. Add Worcestershire, hot pepper sauce, salt, pepper and nutmeg. Reduce heat and cook gently for 5 minutes.

4. Add reserved macaroni, 2 cups (500 mL) cheese and roasted broccoli. Combine gently. Taste and adjust seasonings if necessary. Transfer macaroni mixture to a 13- x 9-inch (3.5 L) non-stick or lightly oiled baking dish.

5. Combine breadcrumbs with remaining 1/2 cup (125 mL) cheese and sprinkle on macaroni. Place on a baking sheet (to prevent spills) and bake in a preheated 350°F (180°C) oven for 30 minutes, or until hot and bubbling. Let sit for 5 to 10 minutes before serving.

PER SERVING	
Calories	344
Protein	19 g
Fat	15 g
Saturates	6 g
Cholesterol	30 mg
Carbohydrate	35 g
Fibre	4 g
Sodium	468 mg
Potassium	288 mg

Excellent: Calcium; Vitamin C; Riboflavin
Good: Vitamin A; Thiamine; Nicain; Folate

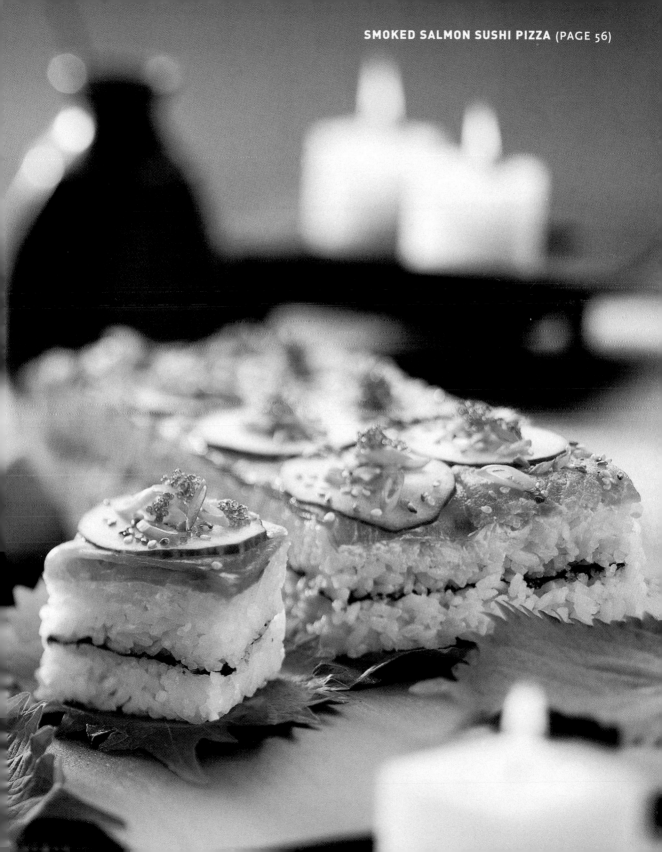

SMOKED SALMON SUSHI PIZZA (PAGE 56)

SMOKED TROUT SPREAD (PAGE 52)

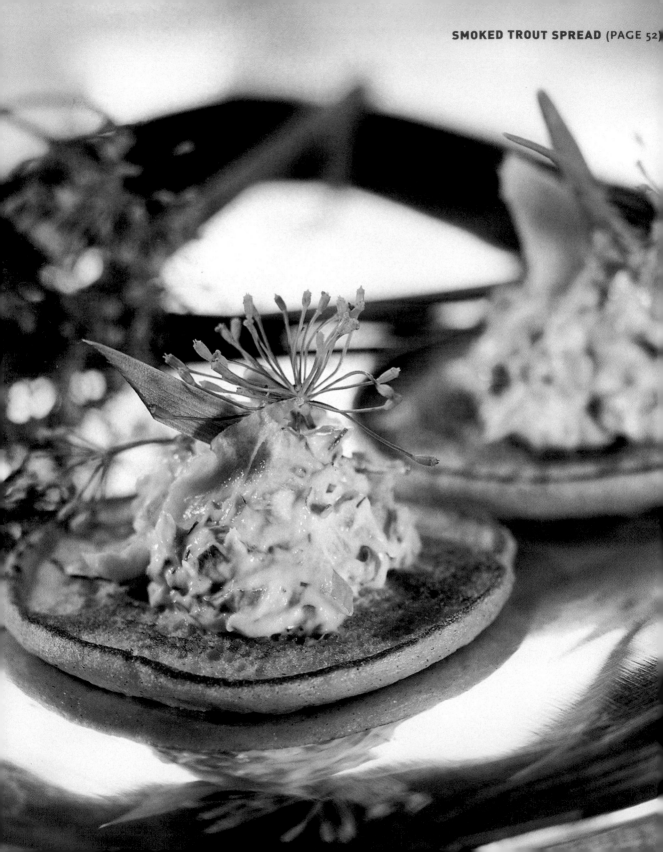

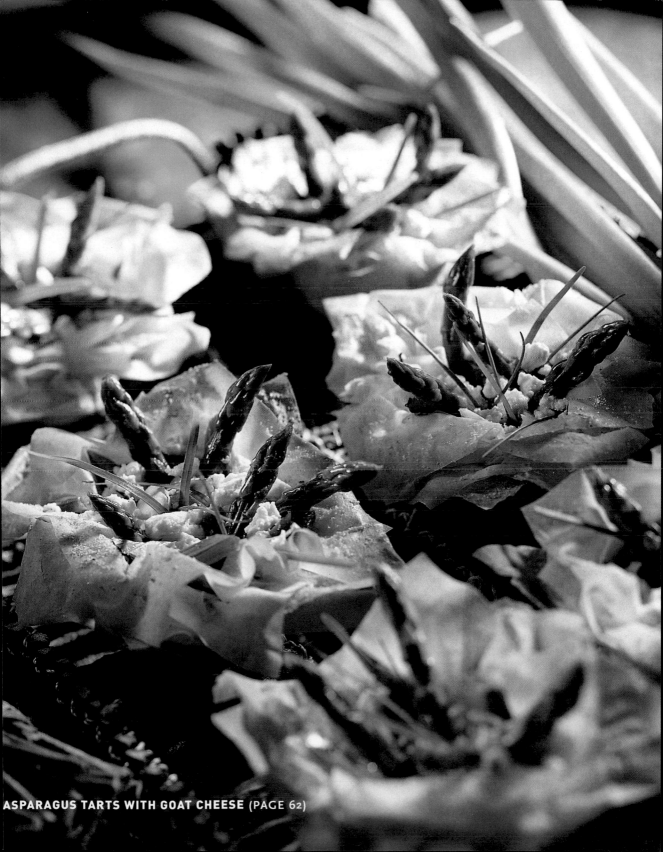

ASPARAGUS TARTS WITH GOAT CHEESE (PAGE 62)

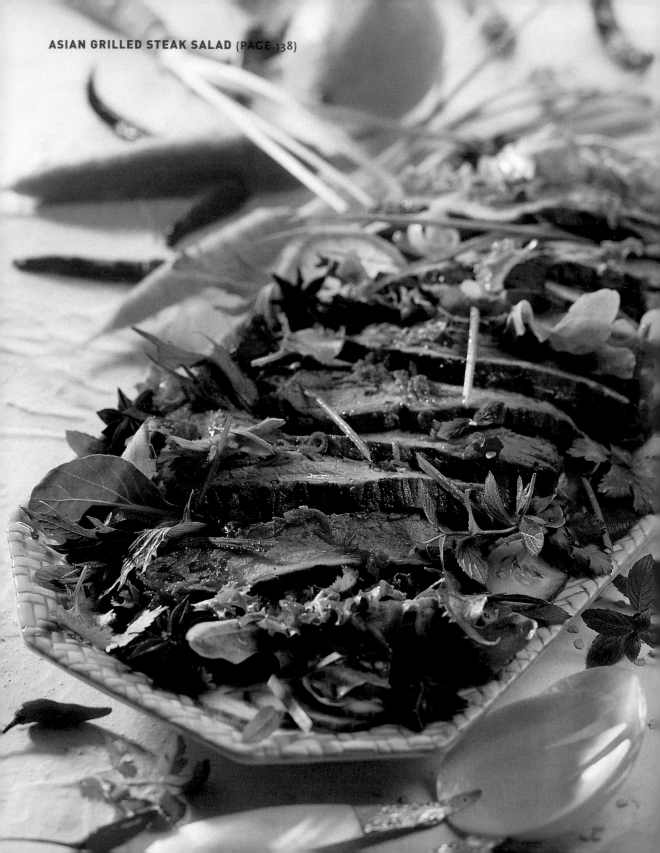

ASIAN GRILLED STEAK SALAD (PAGE 138)

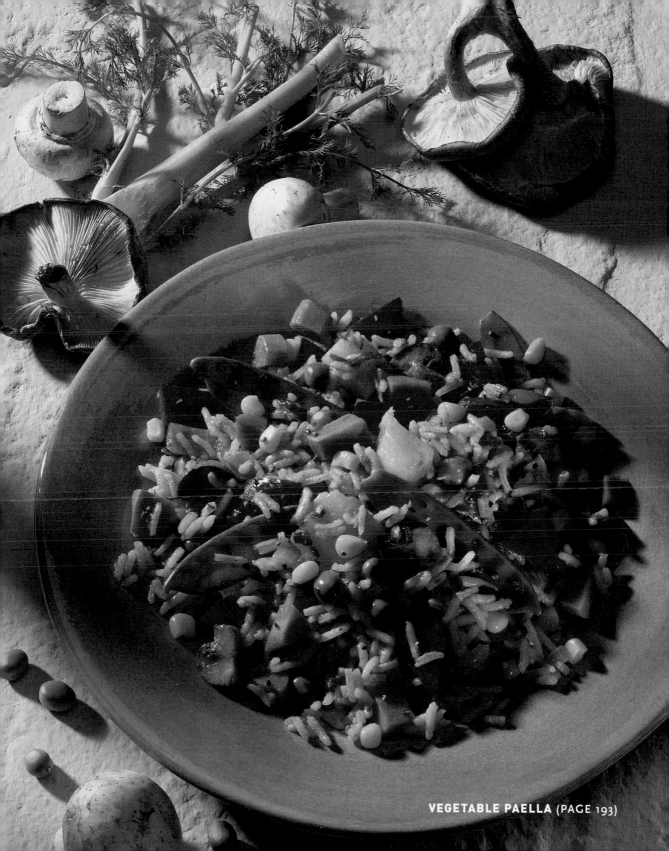

VEGETABLE PAELLA (PAGE 193)

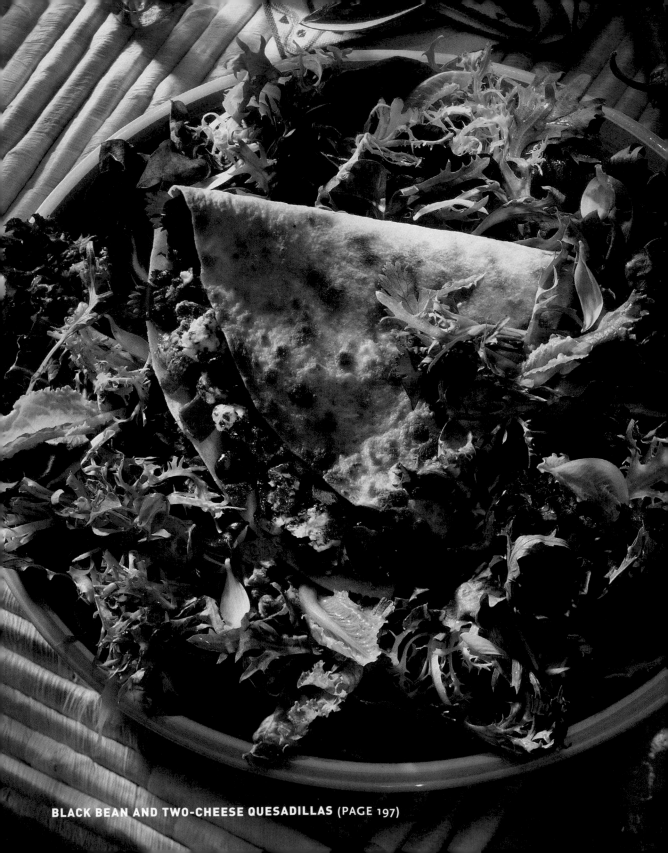

BLACK BEAN AND TWO-CHEESE QUESADILLAS (PAGE 197)

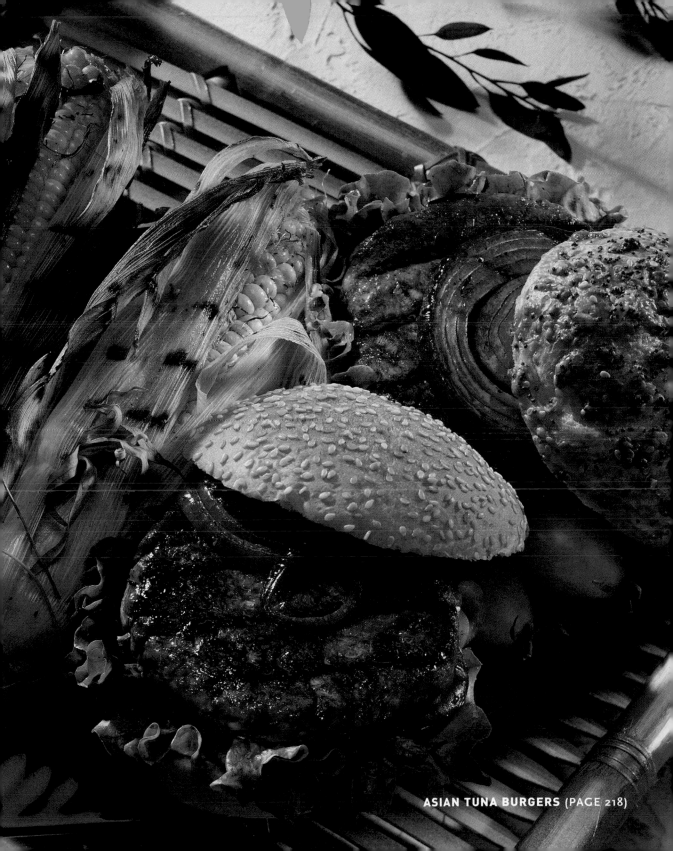

ASIAN TUNA BURGERS (PAGE 218)

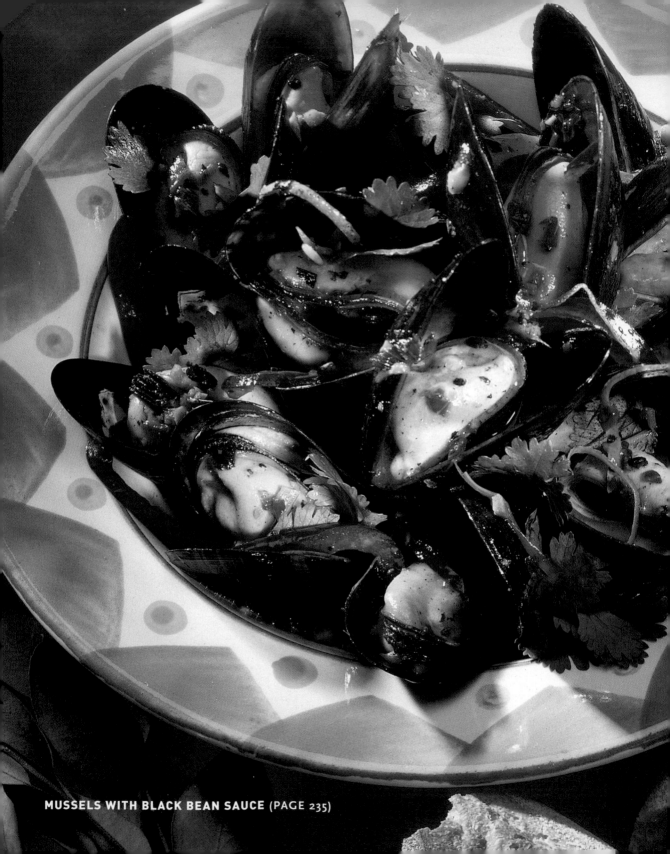

MUSSELS WITH BLACK BEAN SAUCE (PAGE 235)

SPAGHETTI RUSTICA

I adore the slightly bitter taste of rapini, a cross between broccoli and turnip greens. This is a great introduction to it, as rapini's unique flavour is mellowed a bit by the pasta.

If you cannot find wild mushrooms (page 289), just use regular brown (cremini) mushrooms.

Makes 6 to 8 servings

1 tbsp (15 mL) olive oil
4 cloves garlic, finely chopped
Pinch hot red pepper flakes
$1/4$ lb (125 g) fresh wild mushrooms, trimmed and sliced
      (about 1 $1/2$ cups/375 mL)
1 cup (250 mL) cooked red kidney beans
1 tsp (5 mL) salt
$1/4$ tsp (1 mL) pepper
1 lb (500 g) whole wheat or regular spaghetti
1 bunch rapini or broccoli, trimmed and chopped
      (about 1 lb/500 g)
$1/4$ cup (50 mL) pitted black olives, chopped
$1/4$ cup (50 mL) chopped fresh parsley

PER SERVING	
Calories	374
Protein	16 g
Fat	5 g
Saturates	1 g
Cholesterol	0 mg
Carbohydrate	67 g
Fibre	9 g
Sodium	480 mg
Potassium	539 mg

Excellent: Vitamin A; Thiamine; Riboflavin; Niacin; Folate; Iron
Good: Vitamin B6; Vitamin C

1. Heat oil in a large, deep non-stick skillet on medium heat. Add garlic and hot pepper flakes and cook gently for a few minutes until tender and fragrant but not brown.
2. Add mushrooms and cook for 5 to 10 minutes, or until softened. Add kidney beans, salt and pepper and cook for a few minutes longer.
3. Meanwhile, cook spaghetti in a large pot of boiling water for 5 minutes. Add rapini and cook for 5 minutes longer. Drain well, reserving $1/2$ cup (125 mL) pasta cooking water.
4. Add reserved water and olives to skillet. Heat thoroughly. Toss with drained pasta, rapini and parsley. Taste and adjust seasonings if necessary.

PASTA WITH GRILLED SALMON AND STIR-FRIED VEGETABLES

This makes an unusual and elegant Asian-flavoured main course. If you cannot grill the salmon, roast it (page 225) or cook it in a non-stick skillet.

Makes 6 servings

Salmon

1 tbsp (15 mL) honey
1 tsp (5 mL) dark sesame oil
1/2 tsp (2 mL) hot Asian chili paste
1 lb (500 g) salmon fillet, skin removed, cut in 6 pieces

Sauce

1 tbsp (15 mL) olive oil
2 tbsp (25 mL) finely chopped fresh ginger root
3 cloves garlic, finely chopped
1/4 tsp (1 mL) hot red pepper flakes
2 leeks or small onions, trimmed and cut in 1-inch (2.5 cm) pieces
1 carrot, thinly sliced on diagonal
1 sweet red pepper, seeded and cut in 1-inch (2.5 cm) pieces
1 bunch bok choy, spinach or Swiss chard, chopped
1/4 cup (50 mL) rice vinegar
1 tbsp (15 mL) dark sesame oil
1 tbsp (15 mL) honey
1/2 tsp (2 mL) pepper
Salt to taste
1 lb (500 g) whole wheat or regular penne or other tube pasta
6 green onions, cut in 1-inch (2.5 cm) pieces
1/4 cup (50 mL) chopped fresh cilantro or parsley

1. In a small bowl, combine honey, sesame oil and chili paste. Rub into salmon.

2. To prepare sauce, heat olive oil in a large, deep non-stick skillet or wok on medium heat. Add ginger, garlic and hot pepper flakes. Cook gently for a few minutes until fragrant, but do not brown.

3. Add leeks and carrot. Cook, stirring constantly, for 5 minutes. If mixture looks dry, add 1/4 cup (50 mL) water.

4. Add red pepper and bok choy. Cook for 5 minutes, or until just wilted. Add vinegar, sesame oil, honey, pepper and salt. Cook for another 5 minutes.

PER SERVING	
Calories	473
Protein	28 g
Fat	12 g
Saturates	2 g
Cholesterol	7 mg
Carbohydrate	72 g
Fibre	10 g
Sodium	104 mg
Potassium	1191 mg

Excellent: Thiamine; Riboflavin; Niacin; Vitamin B12; Vitamin C; Folate; Iron
Good: Calcium

PER SERVING

Calories	342
Protein	15 g
Fat	7 g
Saturates	2 g
Cholesterol	7 mg
Carbohydrate	61 g
Fibre	8 g
Sodium	575 mg
Potassium	419 mg

Good: Thiamine; Niacin; Calcium

5. Grill salmon for 3 to 5 minutes per side, or until just cooked through.

6. Meanwhile, cook pasta in a large pot of boiling water until tender but firm. Drain well.

7. Add green onions to sauce and reheat sauce if necessary. Toss drained pasta with sauce. Add cilantro. Taste and adjust seasonings if necessary. Top each serving of pasta with a piece of salmon.

PENNE ARRABIATA

This spicy pasta sauce (*arrabiata* means angry) is easy and very quick to make. Use more or less of the hot pepper flakes, depending on how feisty you and your guests like your food.

Makes 6 servings

1 tbsp (15 mL) olive oil
4 cloves garlic, finely chopped
1/2 tsp (2 mL) hot red pepper flakes
1 28-oz (796 mL) can plum tomatoes, with juices, pureed
1/2 tsp (2 mL) salt
1/2 tsp (2 mL) pepper
1/3 cup (75 mL) shredded fresh basil or chopped parsley, divided
1 lb (500 g) whole wheat or regular penne or other tube pasta
1/2 cup (125 mL) grated Parmesan cheese

1. Heat oil in a large, deep non-stick skillet on medium heat. Add garlic and hot pepper flakes. Cook gently for a few minutes until fragrant, but do not brown.

2. Add tomatoes, salt and pepper and cook for 10 to 15 minutes, or until sauce thickens slightly. Add half the basil.

3. Meanwhile, cook pasta in a large pot of boiling water until tender but firm. Drain well. Pour sauce over top and sprinkle with remaining basil and cheese. Toss well. Taste and adjust seasonings if necessary. Serve immediately.

SPAGHETTI AND SEAFOOD CASSEROLE

This is a great one-dish meal. You can vary the pasta, fish or herbs depending on your taste and what you have on hand.

Makes 8 servings

1 tbsp (15 mL) olive oil
1 onion, finely chopped
4 cloves garlic, finely chopped
1/4 tsp (1 mL) hot red pepper flakes
1 28-oz (796 mL) can plum tomatoes, with juices, pureed
1 lb (500 g) whole wheat or regular spaghetti or linguine, broken in
       2-inch (5 cm) pieces
4 cups (1 L) homemade fish stock (page 109), vegetable stock
       or water
3/4 lb (375 g) halibut or other thick white-fleshed fish fillets, skin
       removed, cut in 2-inch (5 cm) cubes
3/4 lb (375 g) salmon fillets, skin removed, cut in 2-inch (5 cm)
       cubes
1/2 lb (250 g) cleaned shrimp
1/2 lb (250 g) mussels in shells, cleaned
Salt and pepper to taste
2 tbsp (25 mL) chopped fresh parsley

1. Heat oil in a large saucepan or Dutch oven on medium heat. Add onion, garlic and hot pepper flakes and cook gently for 5 to 8 minutes, or until tender.

2. Add tomatoes and bring to a boil. Cook for 10 to 15 minutes, or until sauce has thickened and reduced slightly.

3. Add pasta and stir well. Add stock and bring to a boil. Cook for 10 minutes, stirring often.

4. Bury halibut and salmon in pasta, cover and cook for 3 minutes. Add shrimp and mussels, cover and cook for 5 to 10 minutes longer, or until fish is cooked, shrimp are pink and curled and mussels have opened. Season with salt and pepper and sprinkle with parsley.

PER SERVING	
Calories	406
Protein	35 g
Fat	10 g
Saturates	2 g
Cholesterol	82 mg
Carbohydrate	47 g
Fibre	5 g
Sodium	294 mg
Potassium	879 mg

Excellent: Thiamine; Niacin; Vitamin B6; Vitamin B12; Folate; Iron
Good: Riboflavin

PASTA WITH SWORDFISH AND OLIVES

This swordfish dish (page 217), a lower-fat adaptation of a delicious Giuliano Bugialli recipe, is easy and flavourful. It could also be made with fresh tuna, halibut, cod or any thick, meaty-textured fish. You could also grill the swordfish separately, cut it into cubes and add it to the sauce at the end for a smoky, grilled taste.

Makes 6 to 8 servings

1 tbsp (15 mL) olive oil
1 onion, finely chopped
4 cloves garlic, finely chopped
1/4 tsp (1 mL) hot red pepper flakes
1 carrot, diced
1 stalk celery, diced
1 28-oz (796 mL) can plum tomatoes, with juices,
    pureed or broken up
3 tbsp (45 mL) green or black olives, pitted and coarsely chopped
2 tbsp (25 mL) capers
1 1/2 lb (750 g) swordfish, cut in 1 1/2-inch (4 cm) chunks
1 lb (500 g) whole wheat or regular penne
1/4 cup (50 mL) chopped fresh parsley
1/4 cup (50 mL) shredded fresh basil or chopped parsley
Salt and pepper to taste

1. Heat oil in a large, deep non-stick skillet on medium heat. Add onion, garlic and hot pepper flakes and cook gently for a few minutes.
2. Add carrot and celery and cook for 5 minutes longer. If vegetables begin to stick or burn, add a little water.
3. Add tomatoes and bring to a boil. Reduce heat and simmer for 10 minutes, until reduced and slightly thickened. Add olives, capers and swordfish and cook for 5 to 7 minutes, or until fish is just cooked through.
4. Meanwhile, cook pasta in a large pot of boiling water until tender but firm. Drain well and toss with sauce, parsley and basil. Taste and season with salt and pepper if necessary.

PER SERVING	
Calories	459
Protein	35 g
Fat	9 g
Saturates	2 g
Cholesterol	44 mg
Carbohydrate	64 g
Fibre	9 g
Sodium	476 mg
Potassium	822 mg

Excellent: Vitamin A; Niacin; Vitamin B6; Vitamin B12; Iron
Good: Vitamin C; Folate

LINGUINE WITH GRILLED SEAFOOD AND PESTO TOMATO SAUCE

This dish is so delicious that every bite explodes with flavour. My fashionable cousin Barbara, who eats out all over the world, came in when we were testing this recipe and said she had to have the recipe to make for friends. She called the day after the dinner to say it had been a huge success. "I felt just like you," she said, which is funny, because I always want to feel just like her!

If you do not want to use shellfish, use fresh halibut, salmon, monkfish or tuna. The tomato sauce and pesto can be made ahead, but cook the pasta and seafood at the last minute. The linguine with just the tomato and pesto is perfect for vegetarians.

Makes 6 to 8 servings

1/2 lb (250 g) cleaned large shrimp, butterflied and cut in half
1/2 lb (250 g) scallops, trimmed and cut in two rounds
2 tbsp (25 mL) olive oil, divided
1/3 cup (75 mL) tomato pesto or regular pesto, divided
1 onion, chopped
3 cloves garlic, finely chopped
Pinch hot red pepper flakes
1 28-oz (796 mL) can plum tomatoes, with juices
3/4 lb (375 g) whole wheat or regular linguine or spaghetti
Salt and pepper to taste

1. In a large bowl, combine shrimp and scallops with 1 tbsp (15 mL) oil and 1 tbsp (15 mL) pesto.
2. Heat remaining 1 tbsp (15 mL) oil in a large, deep non-stick skillet on medium heat. Add onion, garlic and hot pepper flakes and cook gently for a few minutes without browning.
3. Add tomatoes and bring to a boil. Cook gently for 10 to 15 minutes, or until thickened, breaking up tomatoes as you stir. (Puree sauce at this point if desired.)
4. Grill seafood just until almost cooked. Add seafood to tomato sauce and combine gently. Do not overcook. (Seafood can also be cooked directly in sauce without grilling.)
5. Meanwhile, cook pasta in a large pot of boiling water until tender but firm. Drain well.
6. Toss pasta with sauce. Add salt and pepper. Top each serving with about 1 tsp (5 mL) pesto, or to taste.

TOMATO PESTO

In a food processor, chop 2 peeled cloves garlic. Add 2 cups (500 mL) packed fresh basil leaves and 1 tbsp (15 mL) toasted pine nuts (page 219). Chop. Add 1/4 cup (50 mL) V-8 or tomato juice and 1/2 tsp (2 mL) pepper and puree.

Makes about 1/2 cup (125 mL).

PER SERVING

Calories	353
Protein	23 g
Fat	7 g
Saturates	1 g
Cholesterol	66 mg
Carbohydrate	54 g
Fibre	6 g
Sodium	363 mg
Potassium	627 mg

Good: Thiamine; Niacin; Vitamin B6; Vitamin B12; Iron

PESTO

This is a great all-purpose pesto. Use it on pizzas, in sandwiches and salad dressings, or combine it with goat cheese for a great spread.

In a food processor, chop 2 peeled cloves garlic and 2 tbsp (25 mL) toasted pine nuts. Add 1¹/₂ cups (375 mL) packed fresh basil leaves, ¹/₂ tsp (2 mL) salt and ¹/₄ tsp (1 mL) pepper and chop finely. Blend in ¹/₄ cup (50 mL) olive oil and puree.

Makes about ¹/₂ cup (125 mL).

SHANGHAI NOODLES WITH PORK TENDERLOIN

You can use boned and skinned chicken or turkey breasts or diced extra-firm tofu in this instead of pork tenderloin.

Makes 6 servings

4 cups (1 L) cooked whole wheat spaghetti or
    round Chinese wheat noodles (no eggs)
1 tbsp (15 mL) dark sesame oil
2 tbsp (25 mL) vegetable oil, divided
³/₄ lb (375 g) pork tenderloin,
    cut in slices ¹/₄ inch (5 mm) thick and then cut in half
3 cloves garlic, finely chopped
¹/₂ tsp (2 mL) hot Asian chili paste
¹/₄ lb (125 g) fresh shiitake mushrooms, trimmed and thinly sliced
    (about 1 ¹/₂ cups/375 mL)
2 carrots, thinly sliced on diagonal
³/₄ lb (375 g) bok choy or broccoli, trimmed and coarsely chopped
1 ¹/₂ cups (375 mL) homemade chicken stock (page 109), or water
¹/₄ cup (50 mL) hoisin sauce or oyster sauce
1 tbsp (15 mL) soy sauce
1 tbsp (15 mL) water
3 green onions, sliced on diagonal

1. Toss cooked noodles with sesame oil.
2. Heat 1 tbsp (15 mL) vegetable oil in a large non-stick skillet or wok on medium-high heat. Add pork slices and cook for 1 to 2 minutes, or until browned. Remove from pan.
3. Heat remaining 1 tbsp (15 mL) vegetable oil in skillet. Add garlic and chili paste and cook for 15 seconds, or until fragrant but not brown.
4. Add mushrooms and carrots to skillet and cook for 2 minutes. Add bok choy and cook for a few minutes longer, just until greens start to wilt. Add stock, hoisin, soy sauce and water. Bring to a boil.
5. Add cooked noodles and pork. Reduce heat to low and cook for about 3 minutes, tossing gently until noodles have absorbed liquid and everything is very hot. If sauce is not thick enough, combine 1 tbsp (15 mL) cornstarch with 2 tbsp (25 mL) cold water and add to skillet. Cook for 1 to 2 minutes, or until liquid thickens just enough to coat noodles. Stir in green onions.

PER SERVING

Calories	407
Protein	25 g
Fat	11 g
Saturates	2 g
Cholesterol	32 mg
Carbohydrate	56 g
Fibre	7 g
Sodium	418 mg
Potassium	628 mg

Excellent: Vitamin A; Thiamine; Niacin; Vitamin B6; Iron
Good: Riboflavin; Vitamin C; Folate

SWEET AND SPICY CHICKEN LO MEIN

This is a favourite one-dish dinner. It can be prepared with turkey breast, flank steak, lamb or pork strips. You can also make a vegetarian version by using strips of extra-firm tofu instead of the meat, and water instead of chicken stock.

According to Jenny Cheng Burke, a great cook who works with me at the cooking school, *lo mein* means mixing noodles—any kind of noodle that is cooked and mixed into a dish.

If you are using up leftover cooked meat, add it at the end with the noodles just to reheat.

Makes 6 servings

3/4 lb (375 g) whole wheat or regular linguine or Chinese noodles
1 lb (500 g) boneless, skinless chicken breasts, thinly sliced
1/4 cup (50 mL) soy sauce, divided
2 tbsp (25 mL) cornstarch, divided
1 cup (250 mL) homemade chicken stock (page 109) or water
1/3 cup (75 mL) rice vinegar
2 tbsp (25 mL) rice wine
3 tbsp (45 mL) brown sugar
2 tbsp (25 mL) molasses
1 tbsp (15 mL) dark sesame oil
1 tbsp (15 mL) vegetable oil
1 tbsp (15 mL) chopped fresh ginger root
5 green onions, chopped
3 cloves garlic, finely chopped
1 tsp (5 mL) hot Asian chili paste
1 leek or small onion, trimmed and thinly sliced
1 carrot, grated
1 sweet red pepper, seeded and thinly sliced
1/4 lb (125 g) snow peas, sliced
1/4 cup (50 mL) chopped fresh cilantro or parsley

1. Cook linguine in a large pot of boiling water until tender but firm. (If you are using Chinese noodles, cook in boiling water for about 2 minutes.) Rinse noodles with cold water and drain well.
2. Meanwhile, combine chicken with 1 tbsp (15 mL) soy sauce and 1 tbsp (15 mL) cornstarch.
3. Combine stock, vinegar, rice wine, brown sugar, molasses, sesame

PER SERVING	
Calories	428
Protein	30 g
Fat	7 g
Saturates	1 g
Cholesterol	47 mg
Carbohydrate	64 g
Fibre	7 g
Sodium	767 mg
Potassium	681 mg

Excellent: Vitamin A; Thiamine; Niacin; Vitamin B6; Vitamin C; Iron
Good: Riboflavin; Folate

oil, remaining 3 tbsp (45 mL) soy sauce and remaining 1 tbsp (15 mL) cornstarch.

4. Just before serving, heat vegetable oil in a large, deep non-stick skillet or wok on medium-high heat. Add chicken and stir-fry for a few minutes, or just until it loses its raw appearance.

5. Add ginger, green onions, garlic and chili paste. Stir-fry for 1 minute. Add leek, carrot and red pepper. Cook for 3 to 4 minutes, or just until vegetables wilt.

6. Stir up sauce and add to skillet. Bring to a boil and cook for 1 minute. Add snow peas and cooked noodles and heat thoroughly. Add cilantro. Taste and adjust seasonings if necessary.

SPAGHETTI WITH SHRIMP AND CHERRY TOMATOES

It is amazing that something this delicious could be so quick and easy.

Makes 4 to 6 servings

3 tbsp (45 mL) olive oil
3 cloves garlic, finely chopped
Pinch hot red pepper flakes
2 cups (500 mL) cherry tomatoes
3/4 lb (375 g) cleaned shrimp, diced
1 tsp (5 mL) salt
3/4 lb (375 g) whole wheat or regular spaghetti
2 tbsp (25 mL) shredded fresh basil

1. Heat oil in a large, deep non-stick skillet on medium heat. Add garlic and hot pepper flakes and cook for a few minutes, but do not brown.

2. Add tomatoes and cook, stirring often, for 5 to 8 minutes, or until tomatoes just begin to split their skins and give off some juices.

3. Add shrimp and cook for 3 to 5 minutes, or until shrimp are cooked through and tomatoes are quite juicy. Add salt.

4. Meanwhile, cook spaghetti in a large pot of boiling water until tender but still firm. Drain well and add to sauce. Cook for 1 to 2 minutes on low heat, tossing well, until pasta has absorbed juices. Add basil. Taste and adjust seasonings if necessary.

PER SERVING	
Calories	484
Protein	27 g
Fat	12 g
Saturates	2 g
Cholesterol	121 mg
Carbohydrate	71 g
Fibre	8 g
Sodium	738 mg
Potassium	402 mg

Excellent: Niacin; Vitamin B12; Iron
Good: Thiamine; Vitamin B6

SPICY SINGAPORE NOODLES

This is a spicy vegetarian dish containing tofu, but shrimp or strips of chicken can be used instead. If you do not like your food too spicy, omit the hot chili paste and use only half the curry powder.

Makes 4 to 6 servings

1/2 lb (250 g) thin rice vermicelli or angelhair or spaghettini pasta
1/3 cup (75 mL) homemade vegetable stock (page 109) or water
2 tbsp (25 mL) soy sauce
1 tbsp (15 mL) granulated sugar
1 tbsp (15 mL) dark sesame oil
1 tbsp (15 mL) rice wine
1 tbsp (15 mL) vegetable oil
1/4 lb (125 g) tofu, cut in sticks, patted dry
1 tbsp (15 mL) chopped fresh ginger root
3 green onions, finely chopped
2 cloves garlic, finely chopped
1 tbsp (15 mL) curry powder or paste
1/2 tsp (2 mL) hot Asian chili paste
2 leeks, trimmed and thinly sliced
1 carrot, grated
1 sweet red pepper, seeded and thinly sliced
1/4 lb (125 g) very fresh bean sprouts

1. Cover rice noodles with warm water and soak for 15 minutes. (If you are using regular pasta, cook in a large pot of boiling water until tender.) Drain noodles well.

2. In a small bowl, combine stock, soy sauce, sugar, sesame oil and rice wine.

3. Heat vegetable oil in a large, deep non-stick skillet or wok on medium-high heat. Add tofu and stir-fry for a few minutes until slightly browned. Remove from pan.

4. Add ginger, green onions and garlic to skillet. Cook for 30 seconds. Add curry powder and chili paste and cook for 10 to 20 seconds longer. Add leeks, carrot and red pepper. Cook for a few minutes, or until barely wilted.

5. Add bean sprouts and reserved sauce and bring to a boil. Add tofu and noodles and cook together until hot and well combined. Taste and adjust seasonings if necessary.

COOKING PASTA AHEAD

Although pasta tastes best when it is cooked at the last minute, you can cook it ahead the way many restaurants do. When the pasta is cooked, chill it in cold water, drain well and toss with 1 tbsp (15 mL) oil per pound (500 g) of pasta. Reheat the pasta in boiling water or directly in the sauce just before serving.

PER SERVING

Calories	364
Protein	9 g
Fat	9 g
Saturates	1 g
Cholesterol	0 mg
Carbohydrate	62 g
Fibre	4 g
Sodium	451 mg
Potassium	377 mg

Excellent: Vitamin A; Vitamin C; Vitamin B6; Iron
Good: Niacin; Folate

SPAGHETTI WITH CHICKEN MEATBALLS

Everybody loves this dish. You can add grilled or roasted vegetables and/or hot red pepper sauce. You can also use ground beef, turkey, pork, veal or a combination for the meatballs.

Serve this with a salad and you are set. Leftover meatballs make great sandwiches. Serve with the sauce and sliced pickled jalapeños.

Makes 6 servings

1 tbsp (15 mL) olive oil
1 onion, chopped
1 carrot, finely chopped
1 stalk celery, finely chopped
2 cloves garlic, finely chopped
Pinch hot red pepper flakes
1 28-oz (796 mL) can plum tomatoes, with juices, pureed
1 lb (500 g) lean ground chicken breast
1 egg, beaten
3/4 cup (175 mL) fresh whole wheat or regular breadcrumbs
1 tsp (5 mL) salt
1/4 tsp (1 mL) pepper
1 lb (500 g) whole wheat or regular spaghetti
3 tbsp (45 mL) chopped fresh parsley

PER SERVING

Calories	427
Protein	31 g
Fat	6 g
Saturates	1 g
Cholesterol	80 mg
Carbohydrate	66 g
Fibre	9 g
Sodium	699 mg
Potassium	705 mg

Excellent: Vitamin A; Vitamin B6
Good: Thiamine; Niacin; Vitamin B12; Folate

1. Heat oil in a large, deep non-stick skillet on medium-high heat. Add onion, carrot, celery, garlic and hot pepper flakes. Cook for about 5 minutes, or until tender.
2. Add tomatoes and bring to a boil. Reduce heat and cook gently, uncovered, for about 10 minutes.
3. Meanwhile, to prepare meatballs, in a large bowl, combine ground chicken, egg, breadcrumbs, salt and pepper. Shape into about 24 small meatballs.
4. Add meatballs to skillet and spoon some sauce over meatballs. Cook on low heat, covered, for about 20 minutes, and then uncovered for about 10 minutes. Taste and adjust seasonings if necessary.
5. Meanwhile, cook pasta in a large pot of boiling water until tender. Drain well.
6. Serve sauce over pasta and sprinkle with parsley.

Butternut Frittata
Roesti Potato Pizza
Grilled Vegetarian Pizza
Pizza Salad with Roasted Garlic Hummos
Polenta with Roasted Ratatouille
Baked Polenta Casserole
Polenta with Wild Mushrooms
Vegetarian Pad Thai Noodles
Nasi Goreng with Tofu
Fried Rice with Grilled Tofu
Stir-fried Tofu and Broccoli with Sweet and Sour Sauce
Risotto with Tomatoes and Beans
Mixed Bean Chili
Portobello Mushroom Burgers with Roasted Garlic
    Mayonnaise
Vegetable Paella
Baked Beans in Brewmaster's Barbecue Sauce
Tortilla Rolls with Hummos and Grilled Eggplant
Ribollita
Black Bean and Two-Cheese Quesadillas
Vegetarian Burgers with Tomato Salsa

HEART

SMART

MEATLESS MAIN COURSES

BUTTERNUT FRITTATA

I got the idea for a butternut frittata from a quiche I had at a stylish Cape Town cafe called Melissa's. A frittata is like a crustless quiche— much less rich but very delicious. You can serve it for brunch or lunch with a salad, or cut it into small squares and serve it as a hot or cold hors d'oeuvre.

Makes 8 servings

2 lb (1 kg) peeled butternut or buttercup squash
1 tbsp (15 mL) chopped fresh rosemary, or
　　　½ tsp (2 mL) dried, divided
1 tbsp (15 mL) chopped fresh thyme, or
　　　½ tsp (2 mL) dried, divided
1½ cups (375 mL) crumbled soft unripened goat cheese or
　　　grated light Cheddar cheese
6 eggs
¼ cup (50 mL) water
½ tsp (2 mL) salt
¼ tsp (1 mL) pepper
Pinch ground nutmeg

1. Cut squash into 1-inch (2.5 cm) chunks (you should have about 4 cups/1 L). Sprinkle with half the rosemary and thyme. Spread on a baking sheet lined with parchment paper and roast in a preheated 400°F (200°C) oven for about 30 minutes, or until lightly browned and tender. Cool.

2. Place squash in a lightly oiled 9-inch (2.5 L) square baking dish. Sprinkle cheese over top.

3. Beat eggs with water, salt, pepper, remaining rosemary and thyme and nutmeg. Pour over squash.

4. Place dish on a baking sheet and bake in a preheated 350°F (180°C) oven for 30 to 35 minutes, or until centre is just firm. Cool for 10 minutes before serving.

PER SERVING	
Calories	209
Protein	12 g
Fat	12 g
Saturates	7 g
Cholesterol	162 mg
Carbohydrate	15 g
Fibre	2 g
Sodium	342 mg
Potassium	462 mg

Excellent: Vitamin A; Riboflavin; Vitamin B12
Good: Niacin; Vitamin C; Folate

ROESTI POTATO PIZZA

When you are in the food business it is hard to turn your culinary imagination off, even when you are on holiday. Potato-crusted pizza was an idea I got from a restaurant called The Bistro that we visited when we took the kids snowboarding in Banff. Use the suggested toppings, or try roasted tomatoes with or without pesto, or roasted or grilled fennel, zucchini or eggplant. You can also add roasted garlic and/or roasted red peppers to the topping.

If you prefer a thicker crust, add an extra potato and cook a little longer. The crust can be baked a few hours ahead. Add the toppings and bake for the final 15 minutes just before serving.

Serve as an appetizer, light main course or brunch dish.

Makes 6 servings

3 large Yukon Gold or baking potatoes, peeled and grated (about
        4 cups/1 L)
1 tsp (5 mL) salt
2 tbsp (25 mL) olive oil
1/2 cup (125 mL) tomato sauce (page 151)
1/2 cup (125 mL) grated part-skim mozzarella or smoked
        mozzarella cheese
1/4 cup (50 mL) crumbled soft unripened goat cheese
1/2 cup (125 mL) shredded fresh basil, divided

PER SERVING	
Calories	172
Protein	6 g
Fat	8 g
Saturates	3 g
Cholesterol	9 mg
Carbohydrate	19 g
Fibre	2 g
Sodium	525 mg
Potassium	412 mg
Good: Vitamin B6	

1. Pat potatoes dry with a tea towel or paper towels. In a large bowl, toss potatoes with salt.

2. Brush a 12-inch (30 cm) metal pizza pan with a little of the oil. Press potatoes into pan and brush with remaining oil. Bake in a preheated 425°F (220°C) oven for 30 minutes, or until potatoes are cooked and crusty.

3. Spread tomato sauce over potatoes. Sprinkle with mozzarella, goat cheese and 1/4 cup (50 mL) basil.

4. Reduce heat to 375°F (190°C) and bake pizza for 15 minutes, or until cheese is bubbling. Sprinkle with remaining basil.

GRILLED VEGETARIAN PIZZA

It is hard to believe that pizza dough wouldn't fall through the grates when you grill it, but it doesn't. (You can also simply roll out the dough, place it on an oiled baking sheet, add toppings and bake in a 450°F/230°C oven for 15 to 20 minutes.)

If you don't want to make your own crust, buy uncooked dough at the supermarket. Add grilled onions, sliced tomatoes or other vegetables to the topping if you wish.

Makes 8 servings

Crust

1 cup (250 mL) warm water
1 tbsp (15 mL) granulated sugar
1 envelope dry yeast (1 tbsp/15 mL)
1 cup (250 mL) all-purpose flour
1 cup (250 mL) whole wheat flour
2 tbsp (25 mL) cornmeal
1 tsp (5 mL) salt
2 tbsp (25 mL) olive oil, divided

Topping

1 cup (250 mL) packed fresh basil leaves
3 tbsp (45 mL) olive oil
1/2 tsp (2 mL) salt
1/2 cup (125 mL) tomato sauce (page 151) or
     Cherry Tomato Sauce
4 oz (125 g) part-skim mozzarella or bocconcini cheese
     (fresh mozzarella), thinly sliced

1. To prepare crust, in a large bowl, combine warm water and sugar. Sprinkle with yeast and let stand for 10 minutes, or until yeast bubbles up.

2. Stir in all-purpose flour, whole wheat flour, cornmeal, salt and 1 tbsp (15 mL) oil. (This can be done by hand or in a food processor.) If necessary, add more all-purpose flour until dough is still very soft but does not stick to your fingers or counter.

3. Knead dough for 5 to 8 minutes, form into a ball and place in a large bowl with remaining 1 tbsp (15 mL) oil. Roll dough in oil. Cover and let rise for 1 to 1 1/2 hours, or until dough doubles in volume.

CHERRY TOMATO SAUCE

Use this sauce for pastas or omelettes.

Heat 1 tbsp (15 mL) olive oil in a large, deep non-stick skillet on medium heat. Add 4 chopped cloves garlic and a pinch hot red pepper flakes and cook gently for a few minutes until fragrant. Add 4 cups (1 L) whole cherry tomatoes, 1 tsp (5 mL) salt, 1/4 tsp (1 mL) pepper and 2 tbsp (25 mL) shredded fresh basil and cook for 5 to 10 minutes, or until tomatoes split and deflate and sauce becomes somewhat thick. If pan becomes dry, add 1/4 cup (50 mL) water.

Makes about 3 cups (750 mL).

PER INDIVIDUAL PIZZA	
Calories	226
Protein	8 g
Fat	9 g
Saturates	2 g
Cholesterol	8 mg
Carbohydrate	28 g
Fibre	3 g
Sodium	477 mg
Potassium	199 mg
Good: Niacin; Folate	

4. Meanwhile, to prepare topping, in a food processor, puree basil, oil and salt.

5. Punch dough down and cut into 8 pieces. Roll out or stretch each piece of dough until very thin (about 6 inches/15 cm in diameter). Do not worry if pieces are oddly shaped. Spray with non-stick cooking spray or brush with a little olive oil.

6. Place dough on a hot grill and grill for 1 to 2 minutes per side. Reduce heat to low.

7. Top pizzas with tomato sauce and mozzarella, close lid and cook for about 5 minutes, or until cheese bubbles and crust is crispy on bottom (check occasionally to make sure bottom is not browning too much). You can also transfer grilled dough to a baking sheet, add toppings and bake in a preheated 400°F/200°C oven for 10 minutes.

8. Drizzle each pizza with 1 tsp (5 mL) basil oil. (Freeze any remaining basil oil.)

MEATLESS MAIN COURSE SOUPS
- French Onion Soup (page 82)
- Hot and Sour Soup (page 93)
- Pasta e Fagioli (page 95)
- Mexican Green Lentil Soup (page 96)
- Israeli Red Lentil Soup (page 97)
- White Bean Soup with Salad Salsa (page 98)
- Mushroom, Bean and Barley Soup (page 99)
- Moroccan Mixed Bean Soup with Pasta (page 100)
- Black Bean Soup with Yogurt and Spicy Salsa (page 101)
- Split Pea Soup with Dill (page 102)
- Green Minestrone with Parmesan Cheese Crisps (page 103)
- Chickpea and Spinach Soup (page 104)
- Quick Miso Soup (page 107)

PIZZA SALAD WITH ROASTED GARLIC HUMMOS

This is fun to serve and delicious to eat. Serve it with a knife and fork, as the spinach salad tends to fall off.

The garlic hummos makes a wonderful spread on its own. The foccacia can also be topped with ratatouille (pages 180 and 330).

Makes 8 servings

1 10-inch (25 cm) whole wheat or regular foccacia
2 tbsp (25 mL) olive oil
1 clove garlic, minced
$\frac{1}{4}$ tsp (1 mL) salt
$\frac{1}{4}$ tsp (1 mL) pepper

Roasted Garlic Hummos

1 19-oz (540 mL) can chickpeas, rinsed and drained, or 2 cups
     (500 mL) cooked chickpeas
1 head roasted garlic (page 67), or 2 cloves minced raw garlic
3 tbsp (45 mL) lemon juice
1 tbsp (15 mL) dark sesame oil
$\frac{1}{2}$ tsp (2 mL) ground cumin
$\frac{1}{2}$ tsp (2 mL) hot red pepper sauce
Salt and pepper to taste

Salad

1 lb (500 g) fresh baby spinach
1 lb (500 g) tomatoes, seeded and diced, or 2 cups (500 mL)
     cherry tomatoes, halved
$\frac{1}{4}$ cup (50 mL) shredded fresh basil, optional
3 tbsp (45 mL) balsamic vinegar
1 clove garlic, minced
$\frac{1}{2}$ tsp (2 mL) salt
$\frac{1}{2}$ tsp (2 mL) pepper
2 tbsp (25 mL) olive oil

1. Slice foccacia in half horizontally. Place cut side up on a baking sheet.
2. In a small bowl, combine olive oil and minced garlic. Brush over cut surfaces of bread. Sprinkle with salt and pepper. Bake in a preheated 400°F (200°C) oven for 10 minutes, or until warm and crusty.
3. Meanwhile, to prepare hummos, place chickpeas in a food

MEATLESS MAIN COURSE SALADS
- Roasted Squash, Baby Spinach and Bocconcini Salad (page 112)
- Grilled Vegetable Salad with Grilled Lemon Vinaigrette (page 117)
- Roasted Vegetable Pasta Salad (page 119)
- Asian Chopped Salad (page 123)
- Wheat Berry and Feta Salad with Dill (page 126)
- Wheat Berry and Grilled Corn Salad (page 127)
- Tabbouleh Salad with Fresh Herbs (page 128)
- Black Bean, Corn and Rice Salad (page 129)
- Sushi Salad (page 131)
- Spaghetti Salad with Roasted Garlic and Tomato Salsa (page 133)
- Spaghettini with Salad Greens (page 135)

PER SERVING

Calories	297
Protein	10 g
Fat	12 g
Saturates	2 g
Cholesterol	0 mg
Carbohydrate	42 g
Fibre	8 g
Sodium	665 mg
Potassium	683 mg

Excellent: Vitamin A;
Vitamin C; Folate; Iron
Good: Thiamine;
Riboflavin; Niacin;
Vitamin B6

processor. Squeeze roasted garlic out of skins and blend with chick-peas. Add lemon juice, sesame oil, cumin and hot pepper sauce and blend in. Taste and season with salt and pepper if necessary.

4. In a large bowl, combine spinach, tomatoes and basil.

5. In a small bowl, combine vinegar, garlic, salt and pepper. Whisk in olive oil. Toss salad with dressing.

6. To assemble, spread hummos over toasted foccacia (add a little water if mixture is too thick to spread). Spoon salad over top of bread. Cut each foccacia half into quarters to serve.

DRIED BEANS

Beans are becoming more and more popular, partly for health reasons, but also because people are realizing how delicious they are. Beans are high in fibre, are a source of protein and contain little fat.

- Cannellini, white kidney and great northern beans are all similar and can be used interchangeably.
- Navy beans or pea beans are white, small and round. I like to use them in baked beans, bean soups and salads.
- Red kidney beans are often used in chili dishes and bean salads.
- Black turtle beans (page 197) are used in chili dishes, soups and salads.

To cook beans, cover with cold water and soak overnight in the refrigerator (I prefer not to use the quick-soak method, which can make the beans tough). Rinse and drain the soaked beans, then place in a large pot with lots of cold water. Bring to a boil, skim off any scum that rises to the surface, reduce the heat and simmer gently for 1 to 1½ hours, or until tender. Make a big batch and freeze them; 1 cup (250 mL) dried beans should make about 2 cups (500 mL) cooked.

To save time, you can substitute canned beans for dried beans. Recipes will take less preparation and cooking time, but the texture of the dish may suffer, and canned beans are higher in sodium. I always rinse canned beans to remove as much salt as possible.

Some people find beans hard to digest. Here are some tips:

- Soaking dried beans in cold water overnight in the refrigerator and discarding the soaking liquid before cooking seems to reduce the gas.
- Cook beans thoroughly; beans cooked *al dente* are harder to digest.
- If you are not used to eating beans, start with small amounts.
- Beano is available in many drugstores and supermarkets, in pills or drops; it is an enzyme that helps most people digest beans. Follow the package instructions; some need more than others.

POLENTA WITH ROASTED RATATOUILLE

Polenta is to Italians what oatmeal or Red River cereal is to Canadians and what grits are to the Southern states.

Polenta is quickly becoming more common in North America. It is simply cooked cornmeal, and it can be served with any number of sauces. Creamy-style polenta dishes are served in wide soup bowls with a topping immediately after cooking. Polenta can also be chilled, cut into squares and grilled or pan-fried before being served with the topping. The squares can even be served as a kind of hors d'oeuvre, topped with pesto or another spread.

Ratatouille is a savoury vegetable stew that is usually cooked on the stove, but when the vegetables are roasted, the flavours really intensify. I learned about roasting at high heat at my cottage, where the forty-year-old oven seemed to cook everything at about 650°F! But when roasted dishes turned out great, I began to crank up my oven at home, too (though not quite that high).

For a main course, serve this with salad and crusty bread. As a side dish, the ratatouille can be served on its own or topped with crumbled goat cheese.

Makes 6 servings
4 cups (1 L) water (use 6 cups/1.5 L for creamy polenta)
1 tsp (5 mL) salt
1/2 tsp (2 mL) pepper
1 cup (250 mL) cornmeal (regular or quick-cooking)
1/4 cup (50 mL) pesto (page 167), optional

Roasted Ratatouille
1 large onion, peeled and cut in 12 wedges
12 cloves garlic, peeled but left whole
3/4 lb (375 g) Asian eggplants (about 3), cut in chunks
1/2 lb (250 g) zucchini (about 2 medium),
          cut in 1/2-inch (1 cm) rounds
1 lb (500 g) plum tomatoes, cut in 4 wedges
1 bulb fennel (1 to 1 1/2 lb/500 to 750 g),
          trimmed and cut in 12 wedges
1/4 lb (125 g) shiitake mushrooms, stemmed, or
          portobello mushrooms, with stems, cut in quarters

PER SERVING	
Calories	189
Protein	5 g
Fat	3 g
Saturates	trace
Cholesterol	0 mg
Carbohydrate	38 g
Fibre	7 g
Sodium	619 mg
Potassium	818 mg
Excellent: Vitamin C	
Good: Vitamin A; Niacin; Vitamin B6; Folate	

1 sweet red pepper, seeded and cut in strips
1 sweet yellow pepper, seeded and cut in strips
1 tbsp (15 mL) chopped fresh rosemary, or 1/2 tsp (2 mL) dried
1 tbsp (15 mL) chopped fresh thyme, or 1/2 tsp (2 mL) dried
1/2 tsp (2 mL) salt
1/2 tsp (2 mL) pepper
1/4 cup (50 mL) shredded fresh basil or chopped fresh parsley
1 tbsp (15 mL) olive oil
1 tbsp (15 mL) balsamic vinegar

1. To prepare polenta, bring water to a boil in a large saucepan. Add salt and pepper. Very slowly whisk in cornmeal. If you are using regular cornmeal, cook, stirring often, on low heat for about 30 minutes. If you are using quick-cooking cornmeal, cook for about 5 minutes.

2. When polenta is ready, stir in pesto. Taste and adjust seasonings if necessary. Spread polenta in a non-stick or parchment paper-lined 13- x 9-inch (3.5 L) baking dish. Cool and refrigerate until ready to use.

3. Meanwhile, to prepare ratatouille, spread onion, garlic, eggplant, zucchini, tomatoes, fennel, mushrooms and sweet peppers in a single layer in a large lightly oiled roasting pan. Sprinkle with rosemary, thyme, salt and pepper.

4. Roast vegetables in a preheated 400°F (200°C) oven for 45 minutes, or until tender and browned. Stir occasionally. Toss with basil, oil and vinegar. Taste and adjust seasonings if necessary.

5. Cut polenta into 12 3-inch (7.5 cm) squares. Grill or pan-fry in a lightly oiled non-stick skillet until lightly browned. Serve topped with ratatouille.

BAKED POLENTA CASSEROLE

Prepare the polenta and tomato sauce in advance and assemble the casserole before serving.

When you are making polenta, it is a good idea to stir it with a long-handled wooden spoon, as it tends to spit at you from the pot. To protect yourself even further, wear an oven mitt on your stirring hand.

Makes 8 to 10 servings

Polenta

5 cups (1.25 L) water
1/2 tsp (2 mL) salt
1/4 tsp (1 mL) pepper
1 1/2 cups (375 mL) cornmeal (regular or quick-cooking)

Tomato Sauce

1 tbsp (15 mL) olive oil
1 onion, chopped
2 cloves garlic, finely chopped
Pinch hot red pepper flakes
2 28-oz (796 mL) cans plum tomatoes, with juices
1/2 tsp (2 mL) pepper
Salt to taste
2 tbsp (25 mL) chopped fresh parsley
1/2 lb (250 g) light ricotta cheese, broken up
1/4 cup (50 mL) tomato pesto (page 166)
3/4 cup (175 mL) grated part-skim mozzarella cheese
2 tbsp (25 mL) grated Parmesan cheese

1. In a large saucepan, bring water to a boil. Add salt and pepper. Very slowly add cornmeal to boiling water in a thin stream, whisking constantly. Reduce heat and cook on low heat for about 30 minutes for regular cornmeal and 5 minutes for quick-cooking, until thickened and tender. Stir occasionally. Taste and adjust seasonings if necessary.
2. Pour polenta into an 8- x 4-inch (1.5 L) loaf pan that has been lined with waxed paper. Chill for a few hours or overnight.
3. To prepare sauce, heat oil in a large, deep non-stick skillet on medium heat. Add onion, garlic and hot pepper flakes and cook gently for 5 to 8 minutes, or until mixture is very fragrant and tender.
4. Add tomatoes and cook for 20 to 30 minutes, or until thick. Puree sauce. Add pepper, salt and parsley. Taste and adjust seasonings if necessary.

PER SERVING	
Calories	231
Protein	11 g
Fat	7 g
Saturates	3 g
Cholesterol	16 mg
Carbohydrate	33 g
Fibre	4 g
Sodium	611 mg
Potassium	588 mg

Good: Vitamin A;
Vitamin C; Niacin;
Calcium; Vitamin B6

5. To assemble, unmould polenta and cut loaf into ½-inch (1 cm) slices. Cut each slice in half on diagonal. Spoon about 1 cup (250 mL) tomato sauce in bottom of a 13- x 9-inch (3.5 L) baking dish. Arrange overlapping slices of polenta on top of sauce. Dot with ricotta and pesto. Spoon remaining tomato sauce on top and sprinkle with mozzarella and Parmesan.

6. Bake in a preheated 375°F (190°C) oven for 30 to 35 minutes, or until top is slightly golden and casserole is bubbling. Allow to rest for 5 to 10 minutes before serving.

FRESH CHILES

Even though there are guidelines on how to tell the difference between a hot and mild chile (in general, the smaller and pointier the chile, the hotter it is), be careful. Where the chile is grown, how much water and sunlight the plant receives, and even where the individual chile is located on the plant can all make a difference, so never trust a chile!

Usually, however, poblanos are mild, jalapeños and banana peppers are medium hot, the small green serranos are slightly hotter, and Scotch bonnets (sometimes called habañeros or cascabels) are very, very hot (they are small and round and can be green, yellow or red). If you prefer a milder taste, remove the ribs and seeds, which are the hottest parts.

Jalapeños are thumb-shaped and dark green. Fresh, canned and pickled can be used interchangeably, although the flavours may be slightly different. Individual jalapeños vary greatly, so taste them before adding them to a dish.

Chipotles are jalapeños that have been dried and smoked. They have a sensational smoky taste but are very hot, so use them cautiously. If you can't find them, substitute a jalapeño or chipotle Tabasco. Dried chipotles need to be reconstituted in hot water. Canned chipotles, which come packed in hot adobo sauce, can be pureed and transferred to a jar after being opened, and refrigerated for up to a few months. They can also be frozen (page 300).

Be careful when you handle fresh chiles, as it is hard to tell exactly how hot they are before it is too late. If you have sensitive skin, wear plastic gloves (or just cover your hands with plastic bags), and never touch your eyes, mouth or nose during or after handling chiles. There are many cures for "chile fingers," such as washing your hands in salt or soaking them in milk, but time and lots of washing will also work in the end.

POLENTA WITH WILD MUSHROOMS

In this recipe the polenta is made ahead, cooled until firm and reheated, but the mushrooms can also be served on the creamy polenta as soon as it is cooked. Leftover polenta can be cut up and used as "croutons" in salads, or you can use it as a base for canapes or pizza toppings (serve it hot or cold). Use leftover mushrooms as a topping for pizza or bruschetta, or add them to a pasta sauce.

White truffle oil will add an intense flavour to this dish. (You can buy it in specialty stores.)

Makes 8 servings

10 cups (2.5 L) water or milk, or a combination
2 tsp (10 mL) salt
¹/₂ tsp (2 mL) pepper
2 cups (500 mL) cornmeal (regular or quick-cooking)
1 tbsp (15 mL) white truffle oil, optional
2 tbsp (25 mL) olive oil
1 onion, thinly sliced
3 cloves garlic, finely chopped
1 lb (500 g) portobello mushrooms, trimmed and sliced
Salt and pepper to taste
¹/₄ cup (50 mL) fresh parsley leaves

1. In a large, deep saucepan, bring water to a boil. Add salt and pepper. Slowly whisk in cornmeal. Reduce heat to low and cook, stirring, for about 30 minutes for regular cornmeal and 5 minutes for quick-cooking. Stir in truffle oil. Taste and adjust seasonings if necessary.
2. Pour polenta into two 8- or 9-inch (1.5 or 2 L) round baking dishes lined with parchment paper. Cool.
3. Before serving, brush polenta with a little of the olive oil and reheat in a preheated 400°F (200°C) oven for 20 to 30 minutes. Cut into wedges. (You could also remove polenta from pans, cut into wedges and barbecue or cook in a grill pan or non-stick skillet until browned and crisp.)
4. Meanwhile, heat remaining olive oil in a large, deep non-stick skillet on medium-high heat. Add onion and garlic and cook for a few minutes until wilted. Add mushrooms and cook for 10 to 15 minutes, or until any liquid evaporates. Season with salt and pepper.
5. Spoon mushrooms over polenta and garnish with parsley.

PER SERVING	
Calories	177
Protein	4 g
Fat	4 g
Saturates	1 g
Cholesterol	0 mg
Carbohydrate	31 g
Fibre	3 g
Sodium	597 mg
Potassium	259 mg
Excellent: Folate	
Good: Niacin	

VEGETARIAN PAD THAI NOODLES

Pad Thai is one of Thailand's most popular dishes. It is easy to prepare at home and everyone always loves it, even most kids. (Though my own daughter thinks it is best served perfectly plain. No egg, no peanuts, no bean sprouts—just noodles and sauce!) Serve it as a side dish or appetizer as part of an Asian meal.

You can add diced grilled tofu to this or, for a non-vegetarian version, grilled chicken or shrimp. Be sure to use really fresh bean sprouts.

Makes 6 servings

½ lb (250 g) rice noodles (about ¼ inch/5 mm wide)
⅓ cup (75 mL) ketchup or tomato sauce
3 tbsp (45 mL) soy sauce or Thai fish sauce
3 tbsp (45 mL) lime juice
3 tbsp (45 mL) rice vinegar
3 tbsp (45 mL) brown sugar
½ tsp (2 mL) hot Asian chili paste
1 tbsp (15 mL) vegetable oil
1 small onion, thinly sliced
3 cloves garlic, finely chopped
2 eggs, lightly beaten
1 cup (250 mL) very fresh bean sprouts
3 tbsp (45 mL) chopped peanuts
2 green onions, chopped
⅓ cup (75 mL) chopped fresh cilantro

PER SERVING	
Calories	270
Protein	8 g
Fat	7 g
Saturates	1 g
Cholesterol	72 mg
Carbohydrate	46 g
Fibre	2 g
Sodium	728 mg
Potassium	280 mg
Good: Vitamin B6	

1. In a large bowl, soak noodles in warm water for 15 minutes, or until softened but still firm. Drain well. If not using immediately, rinse with cold water and drain again.

2. Combine ketchup, soy sauce, lime juice, vinegar, brown sugar and chili paste.

3. Heat oil in a large, deep non-stick skillet or wok on medium-high heat. Add onion and garlic. Stir-fry for a few minutes, or until lightly browned and tender. Add ketchup mixture and bring to a boil. Add eggs. When they start to set, stir mixture together.

4. Add noodles and heat thoroughly. Add bean sprouts and cook for 1 minute. Sprinkle with peanuts, green onions and cilantro.

NASI GORENG WITH TOFU

Nasi goreng is Indonesian fried rice. It is traditionally served with fried egg, cucumber and prawn crackers.

Makes 4 to 6 servings
½ lb (250 g) extra-firm tofu
¼ cup (50 mL) soy sauce, divided
2 tbsp (25 mL) rice vinegar
1 tbsp (15 mL) brown sugar
1 egg
1 tbsp (15 mL) water
1 tbsp (15 mL) vegetable oil, divided
1 large onion or 4 shallots, chopped
3 cloves garlic, chopped
1 tbsp (15 mL) finely chopped fresh ginger root
1 tbsp (15 mL) curry powder or paste, or more to taste
5 cups (1.25 L) cooked rice
½ English cucumber, thinly sliced
¼ cup (50 mL) chopped fresh cilantro
4 green onions, chopped
1 cup (250 mL) yogurt cheese (page 391) or
       thick unflavoured low-fat yogurt

1. Cut tofu into 1-inch (2.5 cm) slices and pat dry.
2. In a small bowl, combine 2 tbsp (25 mL) soy sauce with vinegar and sugar. Pour over tofu and turn to coat. Marinate for 10 minutes or up to a few hours in refrigerator.
3. In a small bowl, beat egg with water.
4. Heat 1 tsp (5 mL) oil in a large, deep non-stick skillet on medium-high heat and add egg. Cook like a flat pancake, lifting edges so that uncooked egg can spread underneath and cook. Flip and cook second side. Remove from pan, roll up and slice into thin ribbons.
5. Heat 1 tsp (5 mL) oil in same skillet. Drain tofu, pat dry and cook for a few minutes per side, or until browned. Remove from pan and dice.
6. In a bowl or food processor, combine onion, garlic, ginger and curry powder.
7. Heat remaining 1 tsp (5 mL) oil in skillet. Add paste from food processor and cook until fragrant, about 2 to 3 minutes. Add rice and cook for about 5 minutes, or until hot. Add tofu and stir in remaining

PER SERVING
Calories   472
Protein   21 g
Fat   11 g
  Saturates   2 g
  Cholesterol 60 mg
Carbohydrate   74 g
  Fibre   3 g
Sodium   1118 mg
Potassium   615 mg
Excellent: Niacin; Folate; Vitamin B12; Calcium; Zinc
Good: Riboflavin; Iron

2 tbsp (25 mL) soy sauce. Taste and adjust seasonings if necessary.
8. Transfer rice to a serving bowl and garnish with egg strips, cucumber, cilantro and green onions. Serve yogurt cheese on the side for guests to stir in themselves.

FRIED RICE WITH GRILLED TOFU

Both the tofu and rice are delicious on their own, but together they make a perfect meatless main course.

Makes 4 to 6 servings
1/2 lb (250 g) extra-firm tofu
1 tbsp (15 mL) hoisin sauce
1 tsp (5 mL) dark sesame oil
1/4 tsp (1 mL) hot Asian chili paste
1 tbsp (15 mL) vegetable oil
1 onion, chopped
1 sweet red pepper, seeded and chopped
4 cups (1 L) cooked rice
3 tbsp (45 mL) rice vinegar or cider vinegar
2 tbsp (25 mL) orange juice concentrate
1 tbsp (15 mL) soy sauce
1/4 cup (50 mL) chopped fresh cilantro or parsley
4 green onions, chopped

1. Pat tofu dry. Cut into 3 or 4 slices about 1 inch (2.5 cm) thick.
2. In a small bowl, combine hoisin sauce, sesame oil and chili paste. Spread over tofu. Marinate for 10 to 60 minutes.
3. Cook tofu on a lightly oiled hot grill or skillet for a few minutes per side, or until brown. Dice.
4. Meanwhile, heat vegetable oil in large, deep non-stick skillet or wok on medium heat. Add onion and red pepper and cook gently for about 5 minutes, or until tender. Add rice and break up. Cook, stirring, for 5 minutes, or until hot. Stir in vinegar, orange juice concentrate and soy sauce.
5. Gently fold in tofu, cilantro and green onions.

PER SERVING

Calories	398
Protein	12 g
Fat	8 g
Saturates	1 g
Cholesterol	0 mg
Carbohydrate	70 g
Fibre	3 g
Sodium	306 mg
Potassium	350 mg

Excellent: Vitamin C; Iron
Good: Niacin; Vitamin B6; Folate

STIR-FRIED TOFU AND BROCCOLI WITH SWEET AND SOUR SAUCE

This recipe may sound too healthy to be delicious, but it has converted a lot of people to tofu. The tofu can be added uncooked at the end, but it does enhance the colour and texture to cook it separately. It could also be grilled in large pieces and then diced. If you are introducing people to tofu, try substituting chicken or shrimp for half the tofu.

Makes 4 to 6 servings.

2 tbsp (25 mL) hoisin sauce
2 tbsp (25 mL) rice wine
1 tsp (5 mL) hot Asian chili paste
³/₄ lb (375 g) extra-firm tofu, cut in 2-inch (5 cm) pieces and patted dry
1¹/₂ cups (375 mL) chopped or pureed canned or fresh tomatoes
¹/₄ cup (50 mL) ketchup or tomato sauce
2 tbsp (25 mL) rice vinegar or cider vinegar
2 tbsp (25 mL) honey
2 tbsp (25 mL) soy sauce
¹/₄ tsp (1 mL) five-spice powder, optional
2 tbsp (25 mL) cornstarch
2 tbsp (25 mL) cold water
1 tsp (5 mL) dark sesame oil
1 tbsp (15 mL) vegetable oil
3 green onions, chopped
1 tbsp (15 mL) finely chopped fresh ginger root
3 cloves garlic, finely chopped
¹/₂ lb (250 g) shiitake mushrooms, stemmed and sliced (about 3 cups/750 mL)
1 sweet red pepper, seeded and thinly sliced
1 bunch broccoli, trimmed and cut in 1-inch (2.5 cm) pieces
¹/₄ cup (50 mL) chopped fresh cilantro, basil or parsley

1. Combine hoisin sauce, rice wine and chili paste. Add tofu and turn to coat well. Marinate for up to 20 minutes.
2. In a large bowl, combine tomatoes, ketchup, vinegar, honey, soy sauce and five-spice powder.
3. In a small bowl, whisk together cornstarch, cold water and sesame oil until smooth.

FIVE-SPICE POWDER
Five-spice powder is a slightly anise- or licorice-flavoured aromatic spice mixture used in Asian cooking. In many recipes, curry powder can be used instead, although the taste will be quite different.

To make your own five-spice powder, grind together equal amounts of star anise, fennel seeds, cinnamon, cloves and Sichuan peppercorns.

PER SERVING

Calories	287
Protein	15 g
Fat	11 g
Saturates	1 g
Cholesterol	0 mg
Carbohydrate	38 g
Fibre	6 g
Sodium	905 mg
Potassium	917 mg

Excellent: Vitamin A; Vitamin C; Folate; Iron
Good: Thiamine; Riboflavin; Niacin; Vitamin B6; Calcium; Zinc

4. To cook, heat vegetable oil in a large, deep non-stick skillet or wok on medium-high heat. Add tofu and cook for a few minutes until lightly browned. Remove from pan and reserve. There should still be a teaspoon or two of oil in pan; add oil if necessary.

5. Add green onions, ginger and garlic to skillet. Stir-fry for 30 seconds. Add mushrooms and red pepper. Cook for 2 minutes.

6. Add broccoli, tofu and tomato mixture and bring to a boil. Cook for 3 minutes.

7. Stir up cornstarch mixture, add half to skillet and cook for 30 to 60 seconds, or until thickened. If sauce is not thick enough, add a bit more. Transfer to a platter and sprinkle with cilantro.

COOKING WITH TOFU

Tofu, or bean curd, is curded soybean milk that has been pressed into custard-like cakes. Look for whole pieces covered with water and check the expiry date before buying. I like to buy organic tofu if it's available.

Japanese silken tofu is often sold in tubs or Tetra Paks. It can be soft or firm but is more fragile than Chinese tofu. Extra-firm can be easily used in pureed dishes and salad dressings and must be handled gently. Pat it dry with paper towels but do not press it, as it breaks up easily.

Chinese tofu can also be purchased in different degrees of firmness. Extra-firm can be easily used in stir-fried and grilled dishes. If you don't have extra-firm tofu, you can press regular or firm tofu to make it less watery. Place the tofu on a plate lined with paper towels, cover with more towels and press down with a kitchen brick, frying pan or cans of tomatoes for about 30 minutes.

Keep tofu in the refrigerator, and change the water once a day. Drain well and pat dry before using.

RISOTTO WITH TOMATOES AND BEANS

Although many people say you have to use a lot of butter or oil to make a good risotto, I think the rice is so creamy anyway that in some cases you hardly miss the extra fat.

This is a very hearty risotto that makes an excellent meatless main course. Serve it with a salad. Since half my family is lactose-intolerant, I've become accustomed to adding the cheese at the table, but you can stir it in if you prefer.

Makes 6 to 8 servings

1 tbsp (15 mL) olive oil
1 onion, finely chopped
3 cloves garlic, finely chopped
1/2 tsp (2 mL) hot red pepper flakes
2 cups (500 mL) short-grain Italian rice
1 28-oz (796 mL) can plum tomatoes, with juices,
    pureed or broken up, hot
3 cups (750 mL) homemade vegetable stock (page 109) or
    water, hot
2 cups (500 mL) cooked navy beans or white kidney beans, or
    1 19-oz (540 mL) can beans, rinsed and drained
Salt and pepper to taste
1/4 cup (50 mL) chopped fresh parsley
1/2 cup (125 mL) grated Parmesan cheese

1. Heat oil in a large saucepan over medium heat. Add onion, garlic and hot pepper flakes. Cook gently for 5 to 8 minutes, or until very fragrant and tender.
2. Add rice to onion mixture and combine well. Cook for 1 minute.
3. Add 1/2 cup (125 mL) hot tomatoes and cook on medium to medium-high heat, stirring, until all liquid has been absorbed. Keep adding tomatoes about 1/2 cup (125 mL) at a time. Cook, stirring, until liquid is gone before adding more.
4. After all tomatoes have been added, start adding hot stock. After adding about 2 cups (500 mL) stock, stir in beans. Heat thoroughly. Continue adding stock until rice is tender but still slightly firm.
5. Stir in salt, pepper, parsley and cheese.

PER SERVING	
Calories	431
Protein	15 g
Fat	6 g
Saturates	2 g
Cholesterol	7 mg
Carbohydrate	79 g
Fibre	7 g
Sodium	401 mg
Potassium	657 mg

Excellent: Folate
Good: Thiamine;
Niacin; Vitamin B6;
Calcium; Iron

MIXED BEAN CHILI

This is delicious made with only one type of bean, but my favourite is a combination of black turtle beans, white navy beans, white kidney beans and/or black-eyed peas. You can also use 4 cups (1 L) cooked or canned beans instead of dried.

I usually serve this plain or with steamed brown or white rice and a salad. Provide bowls of yogurt, diced tomatoes, grated Cheddar or Monterey Jack cheese, chopped cilantro and diced jalapeño and let guests add their own garnishes. If you like your chili hot, add more chipotles.

Makes 8 to 10 servings

2 cups (500 mL) mixed dried beans
1 tbsp (15 mL) vegetable oil
2 onions, chopped
4 cloves garlic, finely chopped
3 tbsp (45 mL) chili powder
1 tsp (5 mL) ground cumin
1 tsp (5 mL) paprika
1 tsp (5 mL) dried oregano
1 28-oz (796 mL) can plum tomatoes, with juices, pureed
2 tbsp (25 mL) chipotle puree, or 2 jalapeños, seeded and diced
1/2 tsp (2 mL) pepper
Salt to taste
2 tbsp (25 mL) chopped fresh cilantro or parsley

PER SERVING	
Calories	215
Protein	12 g
Fat	3 g
Saturates	trace
Cholesterol	0 mg
Carbohydrate	38 g
Fibre	12 g
Sodium	198 mg
Potassium	797 mg

Excellent: Iron; Folate
Good: Vitamin A; Vitamin C; Thiamine; Niacin; Vitamin B6

1. Cover beans generously with cold water and soak overnight in refrigerator. Drain beans well and place in a large pot. Cover with water, bring to a boil, reduce heat and cook gently for 30 minutes.
2. Meanwhile, heat oil in a large heavy saucepan or Dutch oven on medium heat. Add onions and garlic and cook gently for 5 minutes, or until tender and fragrant.
3. Add chili powder, cumin, paprika and oregano. Cook, stirring, for about 30 seconds, or until well combined. Stir in tomatoes and chipotle. Cook for 10 minutes.
4. Rinse and drain beans well and add to sauce mixture. Add water if necessary so beans are covered by about 1 inch (2.5 cm) liquid. Cook, covered, for 1 to 2 hours, or until beans are tender and mixture is quite thick. (Uncover if necessary to reduce liquid.) Add pepper, salt and cilantro.

PORTOBELLO MUSHROOM BURGERS WITH ROASTED GARLIC MAYONNAISE

Even meat eaters love these, because portobello mushrooms have a wonderful meaty taste and texture. They even look like burgers!

Instead of the garlic mayonnaise, you could use any of the dips or spreads in the Appetizers chapter. Serve the burgers with roasted potatoes and coleslaw (page 268). You could also use tomato slices instead of the red peppers.

Makes 4 servings

2 tbsp (25 mL) lemon juice
1 tbsp (15 mL) olive oil
2 cloves garlic, minced
1 tbsp (15 mL) chopped fresh rosemary, or 1/2 tsp (2 mL) dried
1/2 tsp (2 mL) salt
1/2 tsp (2 mL) pepper
4 large (4-inch/10 cm) portobello mushrooms
1 large red onion, cut in 4 slices
2 sweet red peppers
4 kaiser rolls or hamburger buns, preferably whole wheat
12 leaves fresh basil or 4 lettuce leaves

Roasted Garlic Mayonnaise

1 head roasted garlic (page 67)
1/3 cup (75 mL) yogurt cheese (page 391)
2 tbsp (25 mL) light mayonnaise
1 tbsp (15 mL) lemon juice
1/4 tsp (1 mL) pepper
Salt to taste

1. To prepare mushrooms, in a large bowl, combine lemon juice, oil, minced garlic, rosemary, salt and pepper.

2. Cut stems off mushrooms and reserve for another use. Marinate mushroom caps and onion slices in oil mixture.

3. Grill peppers on all sides until blackened. Cool, peel, seed and cut into large pieces.

4. Grill mushrooms and onion until browned on both sides, about 5 to 8 minutes. Reserve mushrooms, onion slices and red peppers with buns and basil leaves.

5. To prepare mayonnaise, squeeze garlic out of skins into a food

PER SERVING	
Calories	372
Protein	13 g
Fat	10 g
Saturates	2 g
Cholesterol	6 mg
Carbohydrate	62 g
Fibre	7 g
Sodium	749 mg
Potassium	863 mg

Excellent: Riboflavin; Niacin; Vitamin B6; Vitamin C; Folate; Iron
Good: Vitamin A; Thiamine

processor (or squeeze into a bowl and mash with a fork). Blend in yogurt cheese, mayonnaise, lemon juice and pepper. Taste and season with salt if necessary.

6. Assemble sandwiches by placing mushrooms on bottom halves of buns. Top with grilled onion, pieces of pepper and basil leaves. Smear top of buns with garlic mayonnaise. Serve burgers hot or cold.

VEGETABLE PAELLA

Although traditionally paella contains morsels of chicken, sausage and/or seafood, this version is also delicious. Add 2 cups (500 mL) cooked chickpeas (one 19-oz/540 mL can) if you wish.

Makes 8 servings

1 tbsp (15 mL) olive oil
2 onions, diced
2 cloves garlic, finely chopped
1 tsp (5 mL) smoked paprika
2 carrots, diced
1 large bulb fennel or celery, trimmed and cut in chunks
1 sweet red pepper, seeded and cut in chunks
1/4 lb (125 g) mushrooms, trimmed and quartered
1 28-oz (796 mL) can plum tomatoes, drained and chopped
2 cups (500 mL) brown or white short-grain rice
1 tsp (5 mL) salt
1/4 tsp (1 mL) pepper
Pinch crushed saffron or turmeric
3 cups (750 mL) vegetable stock (page 109) or water, hot
1 cup (250 mL) corn kernels
1 cup (250 mL) peas

PER SERVING	
Calories	279
Protein	7 g
Fat	4 g
Saturates	1 g
Cholesterol	0 mg
Carbohydrate	56 g
Fibre	8 g
Sodium	474 mg
Potassium	665 mg

Excellent: Vitamin A; Vitamin B6; Vitamin C
Good: Thiamine; Niacin; Folate; Iron

1. Heat oil in a large ovenproof saucepan or Dutch oven on medium heat. Add onions, garlic and paprika and cook gently for 5 minutes.

2. Add carrots, fennel, red pepper and mushrooms. Cook for about 5 minutes. Add 1/4 cup (50 mL) water at any time if pot seems dry. Stir in tomatoes and rice. Cook for a few minutes.

3. Add salt, pepper and saffron to hot stock. Add stock to rice and bring to a boil. Cover and baked in a preheated 350°F (180°C) oven for 1 hour (if you are using white rice, bake for only 45 minutes).

4. Sprinkle top of rice with corn and peas. Cover and bake for 5 minutes longer. Toss gently. Taste and adjust seasonings if necessary.

BAKED BEANS IN BREWMASTER'S BARBECUE SAUCE

I used to think that if you cooked beans in barbecue sauce, the beans would absorb even more of the flavour. But in fact, beans take much longer to soften if they are cooked in a very acidic or sugary mixture, so cook them to a tender state before adding them to the sauce.

Makes 8 servings

2 cups (500 mL) dried navy beans

Barbecue Sauce

2 tsp (10 mL) vegetable oil

2 onions, diced

1 clove garlic, finely chopped

1 1/2 cups (375 mL) pureed plum tomatoes or tomato sauce

1 28-oz (796 mL) can plum tomatoes, with juices, broken up

1 12-oz (341 mL) bottle beer

1/3 cup (75 mL) molasses

1/4 cup (50 mL) red wine vinegar

2 tbsp (25 mL) maple syrup or brown sugar

1 tbsp (15 mL) chopped fresh sage, or 1/2 tsp (2 mL) dried

1 tbsp (15 mL) Dijon mustard

2 tsp (10 mL) chipotle puree (page 183), or 1 jalapeño, seeded and chopped

1/2 tsp (2 mL) salt

1/2 tsp (2 mL) pepper

1. Soak beans in plenty of cold water in refrigerator overnight. Drain well. Place beans in a large pot and cover with cold water. Bring to a boil, reduce heat and simmer gently, uncovered, for 1 to 1 1/2 hours, or until tender. Rinse and drain well.

2. Meanwhile, heat oil in a large, deep non-stick skillet on medium heat. Add onions and garlic. Cook gently for 5 to 8 minutes, or until tender and fragrant.

3. Add pureed tomatoes, canned tomatoes, beer, molasses, vinegar, maple syrup, sage, mustard, chipotle, salt and pepper. Bring to a boil, reduce heat and simmer for 5 minutes.

4. Stir in beans. Transfer mixture to a casserole dish. Cover and bake in a preheated 350°F (180°C) oven for 2 hours, stirring occasionally. Remove cover for last 20 minutes of cooking time. Allow to rest for 10 minutes before serving.

PER SERVING	
Calories	303
Protein	14 g
Fat	2 g
Saturates	trace
Cholesterol	0 mg
Carbohydrate	60 g
Fibre	12 g
Sodium	631 mg
Potassium	1083 mg

Excellent: Thiamine; Folate; Iron
Good: Niacin; Vitamin B6; Calcium

EGGPLANT

I usually prefer to use the thin, zucchini-shaped Asian or Japanese eggplants, as they do not need to be peeled or salted (some recipes call for eggplants to be sprinkled with salt to extract liquid and bitterness). If you can only find large eggplants, choose the longer, thinner ones, because they contain fewer seeds.

TORTILLA ROLLS WITH HUMMOS AND GRILLED EGGPLANT

This is a great idea for an appetizer, but these rolls can also be served whole as sandwiches. Instead of the hummos you can use white bean spread (page 50), or try fillings like caramelized onions (page 44) or sauteed wild mushrooms (page 60). The filling can be as simple or as complex as you wish. The hummos can also be served on its own as a dip.

Makes 32 pieces

1 lb (500 g) Asian eggplants or zucchini (about 4)
3 sweet red peppers
1 19-oz (540 mL) can chickpeas, rinsed and drained, or
    2 cups (500 mL) cooked chickpeas
3 tbsp (45 mL) lemon juice
1 tbsp (15 mL) dark sesame oil
2 cloves garlic, minced
1/2 tsp (2 mL) ground cumin
1/2 tsp (2 mL) hot red pepper sauce
3 tbsp (45 mL) unflavoured low-fat yogurt or
    yogurt cheese (page 391)
4 10-inch (25 cm) whole wheat or regular flour tortillas
1/2 cup (125 mL) shredded fresh basil or chopped parsley

1. Cut eggplants lengthwise into 1/4-inch (5 mm) slices. Grill until browned on both sides.
2. Grill peppers until blackened on all sides. Cool, peel, seed and cut peppers into strips.
3. To prepare hummos, in a food processor, combine chickpeas, lemon juice, sesame oil, garlic, cumin and hot pepper sauce. Add enough yogurt to make hummos spreadable. Taste and adjust seasonings if necessary.
4. Spread hummos over tortillas. Arrange strips of eggplant and peppers over two-thirds of each tortilla, leaving clear edge at top. Sprinkle eggplant and tortillas with basil. Roll up tortillas tightly. Wrap individually in plastic wrap and refrigerate.
5. Slice rolls on diagonal to serve (the cook gets to eat the ragged ends of the rolls!).

PER PIECE	
Calories	49
Protein	2 g
Fat	1 g
Saturates	0 g
Cholesterol	0 mg
Carbohydrate	8 g
Fibre	1 g
Sodium	45 mg
Potassium	88 mg
Good: **Vitamin C**	

RIBOLLITA

Ribollita, which is like a recooked minestrone, is a favourite dish in Tuscany, where it is made with leftover minestrone and the famous unsalted Tuscan bread. But many people like it better than the minestrone itself.

I usually make this like a casserole, a method I learned from my friend Luigi Berra.

Makes 8 to 10 servings

1 tbsp (15 mL) olive oil
1 onion, chopped
3 cloves garlic, finely chopped
Pinch hot red pepper flakes
1 carrot, diced
1 stalk celery, diced
1 zucchini, diced
3 cups (750 mL) chopped cabbage
4 cups (1 L) homemade vegetable stock (page 109) or water
2 28-oz (796 mL) cans plum tomatoes, with juices
1 19-oz (540 mL) can white kidney beans, rinsed and drained, or
        2 cups (500 mL) cooked beans
1 bunch Swiss chard or rapini, chopped
1 cup (250 mL) whole wheat or regular macaroni or soup pasta
1/2 tsp (2 mL) pepper
1/4 cup (50 mL) chopped fresh basil or parsley
Salt to taste
12 thick slices whole wheat or regular Italian bread
1/2 cup (125 mL) grated Parmesan cheese

1. Heat oil in a large Dutch oven on medium heat. Add onion, garlic and hot pepper flakes. Cook gently for 5 to 8 minutes, or until tender.
2. Add carrot, celery, zucchini and cabbage. Cook for about 5 minutes to wilt vegetables slightly.
3. Add stock and tomatoes and bring to a boil, breaking up tomatoes with a spoon. Cook for 30 minutes, or until vegetables are tender.
4. Add beans, Swiss chard and pasta and cook for 15 minutes longer. Stir in pepper and basil. Taste and add salt if necessary.
5. Line a 13- x 9-inch (3.5 L) baking dish with half the bread. Spoon soup over top and sprinkle with cheese. Repeat layers.
6. Bake in a preheated 350°F (180°C) oven for 20 to 25 minutes, or until golden brown and bubbling.

PER SERVING	
Calories	322
Protein	15 g
Fat	5 g
Saturates	2 g
Cholesterol	5 mg
Carbohydrate	57 g
Fibre	10 g
Sodium	757 mg
Potassium	1038 mg

Excellent: Vitamin A; Niacin; Vitamin C; Folate; Iron
Good: Thiamine; Riboflavin; Vitamin B6; Calcium

BLACK BEANS

Black turtle beans are often used in South-western and Mexican dishes, soups and salads. You can use canned beans or cook dry ones.

To cook, soak 1 lb (500 g) dried beans (about 2 cups/500 mL) in cold water overnight in the refrigerator. Rinse, drain and place in a large saucepan. Cover generously with cold water. Bring to a boil, skim off scum and cook gently, covered, for 1 to 1½ hours, or until tender. Rinse beans and drain well. You should have about 4 cups (1 L).

Do not confuse turtle beans with the fermented Asian black beans (page 73).

BLACK BEAN AND TWO-CHEESE QUESADILLAS

Cut these into wedges and serve them as appetizers, or place wedges on top of a lightly dressed green salad with your favourite tomato salsa and serve as a lunch or light supper.

These can be made ahead and reheated. (I like to barbecue them for extra flavour, or I make them in a panini maker or sandwich grill.) They can also be made open-faced and served like a pizza.

Makes 6 servings

1 cup (250 mL) cooked black beans
1 tomato, seeded and chopped
1 sweet red pepper, preferably roasted (page 146),
        peeled, seeded and chopped
1 tbsp (15 mL) chipotle puree (page 183), or
        1 jalapeño, seeded and chopped, optional
1 clove garlic, minced
½ cup (125 mL) chopped fresh cilantro or parsley
2 tbsp (25 mL) chopped fresh chives or green onions
2 tbsp (25 mL) shredded fresh basil
1½ cups (375 mL) grated light Monterey Jack or
        Cheddar cheese
½ cup (125 mL) crumbled soft unripened goat cheese or feta
6 10-inch (25 cm) whole wheat or regular flour tortillas or
        8-inch (20 cm) pita breads, split

1. Combine black beans, tomato, red pepper, chipotle, garlic, cilantro, chives, basil, Monterey Jack and goat cheese.
2. Place tortillas on counter in a single layer. Spread filling evenly over half of each tortilla.
3. Fold unfilled half of tortilla over filled side and press together.
4. Grill quesadillas for 2 to 3 minutes per side, or until lightly browned. You can also bake them in a single layer on a baking sheet in a preheated 400°F (200°C) oven for 7 to 10 minutes, or cook for a few minutes per side in a lightly oiled non-stick skillet or grill pan.

PER SERVING	
Calories	331
Protein	18 g
Fat	11 g
Saturates	6 g
Cholesterol	27 mg
Carbohydrate	38 g
Fibre	5 g
Sodium	467 mg
Potassium	342 mg
Excellent: Vitamin C; Calcium	
Good: Niacin	

VEGETARIAN BURGERS WITH TOMATO SALSA

Although there are many frozen vegetarian patties on the market, a good one is hard to find. These burgers take a while to prepare but they are easy, and you could make a double batch and freeze them so you have them on hand. Serve with any salsa or tomato sauce or garlic mayonnaise (page 192). Or just top with lettuce, tomato slices and/or avocado slices. Vegans should omit the egg. If you wish, you can coat the burgers in 1 ½ cups (375 mL) breadcrumbs after forming the patties and cook in a large non-stick skillet brushed with a little oil.

Makes 8 burgers

1 cup (250 mL) barley
1 tbsp (15 mL) olive oil
1 small onion, finely chopped
2 cloves garlic, finely chopped
1 small carrot, finely chopped
1 stalk celery, finely chopped
½ lb (250 g) mushrooms, trimmed and chopped
2 tbsp (25 mL) chopped fresh parsley
1 tsp (5 mL) chopped fresh rosemary, or pinch dried
1 tsp (5 mL) grated lemon peel
1 tsp (5 mL) salt
½ tsp (2 mL) pepper
Dash hot red pepper sauce
½ cup (125 mL) fresh whole wheat or regular breadcrumbs
1 egg, optional

Tomato Salsa

4 tomatoes, seeded and chopped
1 jalapeño, seeded and chopped
¼ cup (50 mL) chopped fresh cilantro
2 tbsp (25 mL) chopped fresh chives or green onions
1 clove garlic, minced

8 whole wheat or regular kaiser buns

1. Cook barley in a large pot of boiling water for 45 to 55 minutes, or until very tender. Drain well. Spread in a large bowl or shallow dish to cool. You should have about 4 cups (1 L).

PER SERVING	
Calories	201
Protein	6 g
Fat	4 g
Saturates	1 g
Cholesterol	0 mg
Carbohydrate	38 g
Fibre	4 g
Sodium	448 mg
Potassium	288 mg
Good: Vitamin A; Thiamine; Niacin; Folate; Iron	

2. Meanwhile, heat oil in a large, deep non-stick skillet on medium heat. Add onion and garlic and cook gently for 5 to 8 minutes, or until tender. Add carrot and celery and cook for a few minutes longer. Add mushrooms, increase heat and cook until any liquid evaporates. Add parsley, rosemary, lemon peel, salt, pepper and hot pepper sauce.

3. Combine vegetable mixture with barley. Taste and adjust seasonings if necessary. Stir in breadcrumbs and egg.

4. Transfer mixture to a food processor and process on/off until mixture holds together well but you can still see shape of barley (you may have to do this in batches).

5. Shape mixture into 8 patties. Refrigerate until ready to cook.

6. Meanwhile, to prepare salsa, combine tomatoes, jalapeño, cilantro, chives and garlic.

7. To cook burgers, spray patties on both sides with non-stick cooking spray or brush with olive oil. Place on a baking sheet lined with parchment paper and bake in a preheated 400°F (200°C) oven for 20 to 25 minutes, or until very hot and slightly crispy. Serve burgers in buns and top with salsa.

Arctic Char with Oatmeal Crust
Fish Steaks with Rosemary
Oven-baked Fish and Chips
Steamed Fish with Spinach and Black Bean Sauce
Halibut with Thai Red Curry Sauce
Cilantro-roasted Halibut
Oven-poached Halibut with Herb Vinaigrette
Grilled Halibut on Lemon Slices
Catfish with Capers and Lemon
Cod Baked in Tomato Sauce with Onions
Roasted Red Snapper with Hot Chiles
Cape Malay Pickled Fish and Onions
Gefilte Fish Loaf
Seared Tuna with Olive and Tomato Salsa
Grilled Tuna with Japanese Noodle Salad
Asian Tuna or Swordfish Burgers
Swordfish Sicilian
Cedar-planked Salmon
Sesame-crusted Salmon on Greens
Steamed Salmon with Korean Dressing
Hoisin-glazed Salmon
Tandoori Salmon
Roasted Salmon with Lentils

Halibut with Couscous Crust and Tomato Olive Vinaigrette
Roasted Halibut with Balsamic Vinegar
Chreime (Fish in Spicy Cherry Tomato Sauce)
Oven-steamed Seafood Dinner
Risotto with Seafood and Peppers
Warm Sea Scallops Wrapped in Prosciutto on Greens
Spicy Thai Shrimp
Grilled Butterflied Shrimp with Salsa Verde
Mussels Provençale
Mussels with Black Bean Sauce

HEART SMART

FISH AND SEAFOOD

ARCTIC CHAR WITH OATMEAL CRUST

This fish has a crunchy and delicious coating. Use salmon or salmon trout if you can't find Arctic char.

Makes 6 to 8 servings

2 lb (1 kg) Arctic char fillet, skin removed
1 tsp (5 mL) salt
$^1/_4$ tsp (1 mL) pepper
$^3/_4$ cup (175 mL) large-flake rolled oats
$^1/_4$ cup (50 mL) dry whole wheat or panko breadcrumbs (page 204)
2 tbsp (25 mL) chopped fresh parsley
2 tbsp (25 mL) olive oil
1 lemon, cut in wedges

1. Pat fish dry and season with salt and pepper. Place fish, fleshy side up, on a baking sheet lined with parchment paper.
2. In a small bowl, combine rolled oats, breadcrumbs, parsley and oil. Pat mixture gently on fish.
3. Bake in a preheated 425°F (220°C) oven for 12 to 14 minutes, depending on thickness of fish, until just cooked through. Serve with lemon.

PER SERVING	
Calories	262
Protein	32 g
Fat	10 g
Saturates	1 g
Cholesterol	0 mg
Carbohydrate	11 g
Fibre	1 g
Sodium	473 mg
Potassium	899 mg
Excellent: Thiamine; Riboflavin; Niacin	

FISH STEAKS WITH ROSEMARY

Many people like to cook fish fillets because they have no bones, but there's a lot to be said for fish steaks. Not only are they easier to turn; they are also more flavourful because they are cooked on the bone.

This simple recipe works with any fish that barbecues or broils well, such as halibut, salmon, tuna, red snapper, monkfish or swordfish. (If you are using tuna, cook it for half the time so it remains rare inside.) To jazz it up a little, serve with Spicy Corn Salsa.

PER SERVING

Calories	155
Protein	24 g
Fat	6 g
Saturates	1 g
Cholesterol	36 mg
Carbohydrate	trace
Fibre	0 g
Sodium	348 mg
Potassium	513 mg

Excellent: Niacin; Vitamin B12
Good: Vitamin B6

Makes 4 servings

4 fish steaks or fillets (about 6 oz/175 g each), 1 inch (2.5 cm) thick
1 tbsp (15 mL) olive oil
1 tbsp (15 mL) chopped fresh rosemary, or 1/2 tsp (2 mL) dried
1/2 tsp (2 mL) pepper
1/2 tsp (2 mL) salt

1. Pat fish dry. Brush fish with oil and sprinkle with rosemary and pepper. Marinate in refrigerator for up to 8 hours.
2. Just before cooking, sprinkle salt over both sides of fish. Grill fish for 4 to 5 minutes per side. (You can also cook fish in a hot non-stick skillet or grill pan brushed with olive oil.)

SPICY CORN SALSA

Use this as a dip, garnish for soups, topping for bruschetta or pizza, or as a sauce with plain grilled lamb, fish or chicken. If you don't want the sauce to be at all spicy, leave out the hot pepper; for a slightly milder sauce, remove the ribs and seeds. You can also add 1 cup (250 mL) cooked black turtle beans.

In a food processor, combine 2 cups (500 mL) corn kernels, 1 roasted, seeded and peeled sweet red pepper, 1 1/2 tsp (7 mL) minced chipotle or jalapeño and 1 minced clove garlic. Process on/off until mixture is slightly pasty and sticks together. Add 1 tbsp (15 mL) balsamic vinegar or rice vinegar, 1/4 cup (50 mL) chopped fresh cilantro or parsley, 2 tbsp (25 mL) chopped fresh chives or green onions and 1/4 tsp (1 mL) salt. Process just until mixed.

Makes about 2 cups (500 mL).

OVEN-BAKED FISH AND CHIPS

This dish is healthful and delicious, with a crisp breading and "light" French fries (you can use sweet potatoes, too). Use any white-fleshed fish fillets. Serve with coleslaw (page 268).

Makes 4 servings

1 1/2 lb (750 g) Yukon Gold or baking potatoes
3 tbsp (45 mL) olive oil, divided
1 tsp (5 mL) salt, divided
1/2 tsp (2 mL) pepper, divided
4 tsp (20 mL) chopped fresh thyme, or
      3/4 tsp (4 mL) dried, divided
1 1/2 lb (750 g) white-fleshed fish fillets, in 4 pieces, skin removed
1 cup (250 mL) dry whole wheat or panko breadcrumbs

1. Peel or scrub potatoes and cut into thick French-fry shapes. Pat dry and toss with 1 tbsp (15 mL) oil, 1/2 tsp (2 mL) salt, 1/4 tsp (1 mL) pepper and 1 tsp (5 mL) thyme. Arrange in a single layer on a baking sheet lined with parchment paper. Bake in a preheated 425°F (220°C) oven for 40 to 45 minutes, or until browned, crispy and tender.

2. Meanwhile, pat fish dry and arrange fleshy side up on a separate baking sheet lined with parchment paper.

3. In a small bowl, combine breadcrumbs with remaining 1 tbsp (15 mL) thyme, 1/2 tsp (2 mL) salt, 1/4 tsp (1 mL) pepper and 2 tbsp (25 mL) oil. Gently pat evenly onto top of fish.

4. When chips have been cooking for about 35 minutes, place fish in oven. Bake for 10 to 12 minutes, depending on thickness of fish, just until cooked.

PER SERVING	
Calories	419
Protein	27 g
Fat	8 g
Saturates	1 g
Cholesterol	49 mg
Carbohydrate	58 g
Fibre	4 g
Sodium	486 mg
Potassium	1089 mg

Excellent: Thiamine; Niacin; Vitamin B6; Vitamin B12
Good: Folate; Iron

BREADCRUMBS

If you have extra bread, make your own breadcrumb. For fresh bread-crumbs, chop the bread (with or without the crusts) in the food processor and freeze the crumbs. For dry breadcrumbs, spread the crumbs on a baking sheet and bake in a 250°F (120°C) oven for about an hour. Then process again if you want really fine crumbs.

If you do not have a food processor, freeze the chunk of bread and grate it.

Panko breadcrumbs are flakes made from bread with the crusts cut off; the flakes have been puffed under pressure to crisp them. Because they are extra dry and crisp, they make a wonderful coating for breaded foods. Look for them in Japanese and Asian markets and some super-markets.

STEAMED FISH WITH SPINACH AND BLACK BEAN SAUCE

This is quick, easy, low in fat and perfectly delicious. I like it best made with halibut or salmon, but any thick fish fillet will be good. Serve it with steamed rice and stir-fried vegetables.

To oven-steam, bake the fish, tightly covered, at 425°F (220°C) for 10 to 12 minutes, until just cooked through.

Makes 4 servings

1 lb (500 g) fresh baby spinach
4 halibut fillets (about 4 oz/125 g each), 1 inch (2.5 cm) thick,
    skin removed
2 tbsp (25 mL) black bean sauce
1 tbsp (15 mL) lemon juice
1 tbsp (15 mL) dark sesame oil
1 tbsp (15 mL) chopped fresh ginger root
½ tsp (2 mL) pepper
¼ cup (50 mL) water
2 green onions, chopped
2 tbsp (25 mL) chopped fresh cilantro or parsley

PER SERVING	
Calories	160
Protein	19 g
Fat	6 g
Saturates	1 g
Cholesterol	24 mg
Carbohydrate	9 g
Fibre	3 g
Sodium	237 mg
Potassium	923 mg

Excellent: Vitamin A; Niacin; Vitamin B6; Folate; Vitamin B12; Iron
Good: Riboflavin; Calcium

1. Press spinach into bottom of a 10-inch (25 cm) deep pie pan (spinach will wilt when cooked). Pat fish dry and place on spinach in a single layer.
2. In a small bowl, combine black bean sauce, lemon juice, sesame oil, ginger, pepper and water. Pour over fish.
3. Set up steaming unit by placing a small rack or crisscrossed pairs of chopsticks in bottom of a wok or large deep skillet. Fill with water up to bottom of rack and bring water to a boil. Set dish with fish on top. Cover wok tightly (use foil if wok does not have a lid).
4. Steam fish for 12 to 15 minutes, or until just cooked through. Transfer to a serving dish and sprinkle with green onions and cilantro.

HALIBUT WITH THAI RED CURRY SAUCE

This Thai-influenced dish has become a classic in many restaurants. The sauce can be made ahead. The fish can be roasted, grilled or sauteed, but cook it just before serving.

Makes 6 servings

Thai Red Curry Sauce

1 tbsp (15 mL) vegetable oil
1 tbsp (15 mL) chopped fresh ginger root
1 tbsp (15 mL) chopped fresh lemongrass
1/2 cup (125 mL) fresh basil leaves
1 tbsp (15 mL) Thai red curry paste
1/4 cup (50 mL) light coconut milk
1 cup (250 mL) tomato puree or sauce (not tomato paste)
1 tbsp (15 mL) sweet Thai chili sauce
1/4 cup (50 mL) fresh cilantro leaves
1 tbsp (15 mL) granulated sugar
1 tbsp (15 mL) lime juice

Fish

2 tbsp (25 mL) soy sauce
2 tbsp (25 mL) lime juice
1 tsp (5 mL) honey
1 tsp (5 mL) ground coriander
1 clove garlic, minced
1 tbsp (15 mL) chopped fresh cilantro
6 halibut fillets (about 6 oz/175 g each), 1 inch (2.5 cm) thick,
    skin removed

1. To prepare sauce, heat oil in a large saucepan on medium heat. Add ginger, lemongrass, basil and curry paste and cook, stirring, for a few minutes. Add coconut milk, tomato puree, sweet chili sauce and cilantro leaves. Bring almost to a boil, reduce heat and cook gently for 15 minutes.
2. Strain sauce. Return to saucepan and add sugar and lime juice.
3. Just before serving, prepare fish by combining soy sauce, lime juice, honey, coriander, garlic and chopped cilantro. Pat fish dry and rub marinade on fish.
4. Place fish on a baking sheet lined with parchment paper and roast in a preheated 425°F (220°C) oven for 10 to 15 minutes, or until just cooked through. To serve, drizzle sauce over fish.

COCONUT MILK

Often used in Asian cooking, coconut milk is high in fat, so only use a little, or buy light coconut milk (available at health food stores and specialty shops). Freeze any extra, as it is very perishable (freeze flat in a zipper-style plastic bag so you can snap off what you need.)

PER SERVING

Calories	269
Protein	37 g
Fat	8 g
Saturates	1 g
Cholesterol	54 mg
Carbohydrate	11 g
Fibre	2 g
Sodium	369 mg
Potassium	1094 mg

Excellent: Niacin; Vitamin B6; Vitamin B12
Good: Vitamin A; Iron

CILANTRO-ROASTED HALIBUT

I had a cooking show for a couple of years on WTN. The crew would eat everything after we had shot each segment, and while they tended to be a bit fussy when it came to fish, they all loved this.

This cilantro pesto works equally well on salmon, shrimp or black cod. Use the cilantro stems and roots as well as the leaves for a more intense flavour.

Makes 6 to 8 servings

1 clove garlic, chopped
1 1/2 cups (375 mL) fresh cilantro leaves, stems and roots
2 tbsp (25 mL) hoisin sauce
1 tbsp (15 mL) Thai fish sauce or soy sauce
1 tbsp (15 mL) lime juice or lemon juice
1 tbsp (15 mL) rice vinegar
1/2 tsp (2 mL) hot Asian chili paste
2 lb (1 kg) halibut, in one piece, about 2 inches (5 cm) thick,
    skin removed

Asian Sesame Salad

2 tbsp (25 mL) rice vinegar
1 tsp (5 mL) honey-style mustard
1/2 tsp (2 mL) hot Asian chili paste
1/2 tsp (2 mL) dark sesame oil
1 tbsp (15 mL) olive oil
8 cups (2 L) mixed salad greens

PER SERVING	
Calories	223
Protein	33 g
Fat	7 g
Saturates	1 g
Cholesterol	49 mg
Carbohydrate	6 g
Fibre	2 g
Sodium	453 mg
Potassium	1013 mg

Excellent: Vitamin A; Niacin; Vitamin B6; Vitamin B12; Folate *Good:* ; Thiamine; Riboflavin; Vitamin C

1. In a food processor, chop garlic and cilantro. Add hoisin sauce, fish sauce, lime juice, rice vinegar and chili paste. Process to form a paste.
2. Pat halibut dry, place in a shallow dish and smear with marinade, turning to coat well. Refrigerate for 30 minutes.
3. Place fish on a baking sheet lined with parchment paper. Roast in a preheated 425°F (220°C) oven for 25 to 35 minutes, or until cooked through.
4. Meanwhile, to prepare salad, combine vinegar, mustard, chili paste, sesame oil and olive oil.
5. Toss greens with dressing. Serve fish on a bed of greens.

OVEN-POACHED HALIBUT WITH HERB VINAIGRETTE

I once had a dish like this in a posh New York restaurant. I was with five friends and we all ordered different things so that we could sample as many dishes as possible. It was one of those "take a bite and pass it on" meals. A poached halibut with herb vinaigrette was the best item we tried that night, but I didn't get enough of it. So now I make it at home and eat a whole portion by myself.

This dish can be served warm or cold.

Makes 6 servings

Herb Vinaigrette

1/4 cup (50 mL) Champagne vinegar or sherry vinegar, or
     lemon juice
1/4 cup (50 mL) water
1/2 tsp (2 mL) granulated sugar
1/2 tsp (2 mL) dry mustard
1/2 tsp (2 mL) pepper
1 shallot, minced, optional
2 tbsp (25 mL) olive oil
1/4 tsp (1 mL) hot red pepper sauce
2 tbsp (25 mL) chopped fresh cilantro or parsley
2 tbsp (25 mL) chopped fresh chives or green onions
2 tbsp (25 mL) chopped fresh parsley
2 tbsp (25 mL) chopped fresh basil

Fish

6 halibut fillets (about 4 oz/125 g each), skin removed
1 tbsp (15 mL) lemon juice
1/4 tsp (1 mL) pepper
4 large carrots, grated
1 bunch watercress, optional

1. To prepare vinaigrette, whisk together vinegar, water, sugar, mustard, pepper and shallot. Whisk in oil, hot pepper sauce, cilantro, chives, parsley and basil.

2. Pat halibut dry and sprinkle with lemon juice and pepper. Marinate for about 10 minutes.

PER SERVING	
Calories	181
Protein	24 g
Fat	6 g
Saturates	1 g
Cholesterol	36 mg
Carbohydrate	6 g
Fibre	1 g
Sodium	96 mg
Potassium	649 mg

Excellent: Vitamin A; Niacin; Vitamin B6; Vitamin B12

3. Line a baking dish with parchment paper. Spread carrots over paper. Arrange fish on top. Cover with a second piece of parchment.

4. Bake fish in a preheated 400°F (200°C) oven for 8 to 10 minutes, or until fish just begins to flake when separated with a knife.

5. Remove fish from oven and place carefully on a serving platter. Scatter with carrots. Pour vinaigrette over top. Arrange watercress around edge of platter.

GRILLED HALIBUT ON LEMON SLICES

Halibut has a sweet, mild flavour that makes it very popular. Try to use fresh halibut rather than frozen for the silkiest texture, and do not overcook it as it dries out easily.

I learned about this technique for cooking fish on lemon slices from our popular guest teacher Hugh Carpenter, who wrote a fantastic book called *Fast Fish*. The lemon prevents the fish from sticking and infuses it with a delicious flavour.

Makes 4 servings

4 halibut fillets (about 6 oz/175 g each), 1 inch (2.5 cm) thick, skin removed
1 tbsp (15 mL) olive oil
1/2 tsp (2 mL) salt
1/4 tsp (1 mL) pepper
2 tbsp (25 mL) chopped fresh thyme, or 1 tsp (5 mL) dried
2 lemons, cut in 1/4-inch (5 mm) slices

1. Pat halibut dry and place in a shallow baking dish. In a small bowl, combine oil, salt, pepper and thyme. Rub mixture into fish. Marinate in refrigerator until ready to cook.

2. Arrange lemon slices on grill in a square or strip with slices touching each other. Arrange fish on lemon slices. Close barbecue and grill on medium-high heat for 12 to 15 minutes, or until fish is just cooked through. Do not turn fish. If you are doing this in an open grill pan, or if your barbecue does not have a cover, invert a metal baking pan over fish to create a makeshift cover.

3. Lift fish off lemon slices. Squeeze lemon over fish before serving.

PER SERVING	
Calories	217
Protein	36 g
Fat	7 g
Saturates	1 g
Cholesterol	54 mg
Carbohydrate	0 g
Fibre	0 g
Sodium	384 mg
Potassium	774 mg

Excellent: Niacin; Vitamin B6; Vitamin B12

CATFISH WITH CAPERS AND LEMON

Catfish is the number one farmed fish in North America. It is quickly becoming more popular as the industry takes care to make sure the product is consistent and well regulated.

You can also use tilapia or any thin white-fleshed fish in this recipe. Garnish with lemon wedges and sprigs of parsley.

Makes 4 servings

1 lb (500 g) catfish fillets, about ½ inch (1 cm) thick,
    skin removed
½ tsp (2 mL) salt
¼ tsp (1 mL) pepper
½ cup (125 mL) all-purpose flour
1 tbsp (15 mL) olive oil
½ cup (125 mL) dry white wine, fish stock or
    chicken stock (page 00)
2 tbsp (25 mL) lemon juice
2 tbsp (25 mL) homemade fish stock (page 109),
    chicken stock or water
2 tbsp (25 mL) capers
2 tbsp (25 mL) chopped fresh parsley

1. Pat fish dry. Season with salt and pepper. Dip lightly into flour just before cooking.

2. Heat oil in a large non-stick skillet on medium-high heat. Cook catfish for 3 to 4 minutes per side, depending on thickness, until browned and cooked through.

3. Remove fish from skillet and place on a serving platter. Wipe out pan and return to heat. Add wine and cook down to a few tablespoons. Add lemon juice, stock, capers and parsley. Pour sauce over fish.

CAPERS

Capers are the buds of the caper plant, which grows in the Mediterranean, usually near water. For some reason, many people think capers are "fishy," perhaps because they are often served with fish. They have a piquant flavour that cuts the richness of things like smoked salmon. They can be bought packed in either vinegar or salt, and should be rinsed well before using.

PER SERVING	
Calories	263
Protein	19 g
Fat	11 g
Saturates	2 g
Cholesterol	60 mg
Carbohydrate	10 g
Fibre	1 g
Sodium	500 mg
Potassium	362 mg

Excellent: Thiamine; Niacin; Vitamin B12

COD BAKED IN TOMATO SAUCE WITH ONIONS

This is a wonderfully easy and quick way to prepare fish, but if you prefer to assemble the dish ahead, you can bake it in a casserole. Pour the cooked tomato sauce over the fish and bake at 400°F (200°C) for 15 to 20 minutes, or until the fish is cooked through.

Use any thick white-fleshed fillet in this recipe.

Makes 6 servings

1 tbsp (15 mL) olive oil
2 onions, sliced
4 cloves garlic, finely chopped
Pinch hot red pepper flakes
1 28-oz (796 mL) can plum tomatoes, with juices, or
        4 cups (1 L) cherry tomatoes
1 tbsp (15 mL) chopped fresh thyme, or 1/2 tsp (2 mL) dried
2 tbsp (25 mL) pitted black olives, optional
Salt and pepper to taste
6 pieces cod (about 4 oz/125 g each), 1 inch (2.5 cm) thick,
        skin removed
1/4 cup (50 mL) chopped fresh parsley

PER SERVING	
Calories	152
Protein	21 g
Fat	3 g
Saturates	1 g
Cholesterol	46 mg
Carbohydrate	10 g
Fibre	2 g
Sodium	285 mg
Potassium	572 mg

Excellent: Niacin; Vitamin B12
Good: Vitamin C; Vitamin B6

1. Heat oil in a large, deep non-stick skillet on medium heat. Add onions, garlic and hot pepper flakes. Cook gently for a few minutes, until onions wilt.

2. Add tomatoes and thyme. Break tomatoes up with a spoon. Bring to a boil and cook, stirring often, until thick, about 5 to 7 minutes. Stir in olives, salt and pepper.

3. Pat cod dry and add to skillet, spooning sauce over top. Cover and cook for 5 to 8 minutes, depending on thickness, until fish is just cooked through. Sprinkle with parsley before serving.

ROASTED RED SNAPPER WITH HOT CHILES

So many restaurants are serving whole grilled fish that more people are comfortable cooking a whole fish at home. If my baking pan is large enough to accommodate the whole fish, I leave the head and tail on, because the fish looks much more important that way!

You can prepare this ahead of time and bake it just before serving, or bake it ahead and serve it cold or at room temperature.

Makes 4 to 6 servings

1 4-lb (2 kg) red snapper, cleaned
2 tbsp (25 mL) chopped fresh ginger root
2 cloves garlic, chopped
1 tbsp (15 mL) hot Asian chili paste
1 tsp (5 mL) dark sesame oil
1/4 cup (50 mL) chopped fresh cilantro or parsley
3 green onions, chopped
1/2 tsp (2 mL) salt
1 tbsp (15 mL) olive oil
1 lemon, sliced, optional
Sprigs fresh cilantro or parsley, optional

1. If fish is too large for baking dish, cut off head and tail. Pat fish dry inside and out. Cut 4 diagonal slits in each side of fish.
2. In a food processor, blend together ginger, garlic and chili paste. Add sesame oil, cilantro, green onions and salt. Puree.
3. Reserve about 1 tbsp (15 mL) puree and stuff remaining into slits in fish. Combine reserved puree with olive oil and rub over fish.
4. Place fish on a large foil-lined baking sheet and bake in a preheated 425°F (220°C) oven for 10 minutes per inch (2.5 cm) of thickness. (If fish is 3 inches/7.5 cm thick, cook for about 30 minutes.) Garnish with lemon and cilantro sprigs.

Roasted Red Snapper with Salsa

Instead of cilantro puree, spread 2 cups (500 mL) of your favourite tomato salsa over fish and inside cavity.

COOKING FISH

The rule for cooking fish devised by the Canadian Fisheries Institute is still the norm. Cook fish at medium-high heat for 10 minutes per inch of thickness. If you are cooking frozen fish, double the cooking time.

There are two exceptions to this rule—tuna (which should be cooked rare) and roasted fish (which often needs an extra 5 minutes to allow the heat to penetrate).

PER SERVING

Calories	129
Protein	21 g
Fat	4 g
Saturates	1 g
Cholesterol	37 mg
Carbohydrate	2 g
Fibre	trace
Sodium	191 mg
Potassium	469 mg

Excellent: Vitamin B12
Good: Niacin;
Vitamin B6

CAPE MALAY PICKLED FISH AND ONIONS

If you love pickled foods, you will really love this South African favourite. Everyone prepares it a little differently, but this is a delicious version. Although many cooks fry the fish, I like to bake it.

In South Africa a fish called kingclip is typically used in this dish, but I prefer grouper or orange roughy. Serve it with seed bread (page 441).

Makes 8 servings

2 lb (1 kg) grouper fillet or orange roughy, skin removed
¹⁄₄ tsp (1 mL) salt
¹⁄₄ tsp (1 mL) pepper
2 tbsp (25 mL) olive oil

Pickling Solution

1 ¹⁄₂ cups (375 mL) white wine vinegar or cider vinegar
1 ¹⁄₂ cups (375 mL) water
¹⁄₃ cup (75 mL) granulated sugar
3 tbsp (45 mL) apricot jam
1 tbsp (15 mL) curry paste or powder
1 tsp (5 mL) salt
1 bay leaf
2 onions, sliced
2 tbsp (25 mL) raisins

PER SERVING	
Calories	183
Protein	22 g
Fat	5 g
Saturates	1 g
Cholesterol	42 mg
Carbohydrate	11 g
Fibre	1 g
Sodium	300 mg
Potassium	486 mg

Excellent: Vitamin B12
Good: Niacin; Vitamin B6

1. Pat fish dry and cut into 2-oz (60 g) pieces. Season with salt and pepper and rub with oil. Place on a baking sheet lined with parchment paper and roast on lower rack in a preheated 450°F (230°C) oven for 5 to 7 minutes for orange roughy or 12 to 15 minutes for grouper, depending on thickness. Do not overcook. Place fish in a dish in a single layer.

2. To prepare pickling solution, in a large saucepan, combine vinegar, water, sugar, jam, curry paste, salt and bay leaf. Bring to a boil and add onions. Cook gently for 10 to 15 minutes, or until onions are tender but still a little crispy. Add raisins. Cool for about 15 minutes. Taste and adjust seasonings if necessary.

3. Pour onion mixture over fish and refrigerate overnight.

GEFILTE FISH LOAF

Gefilte fish is a traditional Jewish holiday dish that is generally served as part of the Passover Seder dinner and on Rosh Hashanah. Every Jewish cook has a version, varying the types and quantities of fish used, how it is cooked, whether it is sweet or salty, peppery or mild. Traditionally the bones, heads and tails of the fish are placed on the bottom of the pot with onions and sliced carrots as a base, and the fish mixture is shaped into balls which are then poached, but a method that is becoming more popular is simply to cook the mixture in a loaf pan.

Most fish stores will prepare the fish mix for you, but be sure to order it ahead. Use the freshest fish possible. Everyone has their own favourite combination, but this is a mixture I like.

Gefilte fish is usually served cold, so I make it at least a day ahead. Serve it in slices on a lettuce leaf with cherry tomatoes and red horseradish.

Makes 16 servings

3 lb (1.5 kg) ground fish (1 ½ lb/750 g whitefish, 1 lb/500 g
    pickerel, 8 oz/250 g salmon)
3 eggs
½ cup (125 mL) cold water
½ cup (125 mL) matzo meal (page 88)
1 small onion, grated (about ¼ to ⅓ cup/50 to 75 mL)
1 carrot, finely chopped (about ½ cup/125 mL)
1 tbsp (15 mL) granulated sugar
4 tsp (20 mL) salt
1 tsp (5 mL) pepper

1. In a large bowl, combine fish, eggs, water, matzo meal, onion, carrot, sugar, salt and pepper. Combine gently. (Use your hands or a large spoon or spatula.)
2. Spoon mixture into a 9- x 5-inch (2 L) loaf pan lined with parchment paper. Smooth top and cover with foil.
3. Place a roasting pan in a preheated 350°F (180°C) oven and fill with hot or boiling water until pan is about half full. Gently place loaf pan in water bath. Bake loaf for 1 hour. Uncover pan and bake for 30 minutes longer.
4. Cool fish and refrigerate for a few hours or overnight. Remove from pan and slice.

HOMEMADE RED HORSERADISH
Peel a 6-inch (15 cm) piece horseradish root, cut it into pieces and chop it finely in a food processor with a small, peeled raw red beet. Add a few tablespoons of white vinegar and puree.

PER SERVING

Calories	139
Protein	18 g
Fat	5 g
Saturates	1 g
Cholesterol	93 mg
Carbohydrate	4 g
Fibre	trace
Sodium	643 mg
Potassium	326 mg

Excellent: Niacin; Vitamin B12
Good: Thiamine; Vitamin B6

OLIVES

OLIVES

Although olives are high in fat and sodium, they are also high in flavour, so a little goes a long way. Instead of putting out bowls of olives for nibbling, use small quantities as a seasoning in salads and sauces. Black olives are ripe olives; green olives are unripe.

Generally, the best olives are unpitted. Cut the meat off the pit with a sharp knife, or whack the olives on a cutting board with the flat side of a knife or meat pounder; in most cases the pits will pop out.

PER SERVING

Calories	202
Protein	27 g
Fat	10 g
Saturates	2 g
Cholesterol	43 mg
Carbohydrate	1 g
Fibre	trace
Sodium	238 mg
Potassium	326 mg

Excellent: Vitamin A; Niacin; Vitamin B6; Vitamin B12
Good: Thiamine; Riboflavin

SEARED TUNA WITH OLIVE AND TOMATO SALSA

I first had something like this on a trip to Spain, and I have been trying to recreate it ever since. I have never been able to duplicate the dish exactly, but all the experiments are pretty great.

Tuna steaks taste best when they are cooked rare, so buy very fresh fish and be careful not to overcook it, as the steaks dry out quickly.

Makes 8 servings

2 lb (1 kg) tuna fillet, about 1 inch (2.5 cm) thick, skin removed
2 tbsp (25 mL) olive oil, divided
1/2 tsp (2 mL) salt
1/2 tsp (2 mL) pepper
1 tbsp (15 mL) chopped fresh thyme, or 1/2 tsp (2 mL) dried
2 plum tomatoes, seeded and diced
2 tbsp (25 mL) pitted black olives, chopped
2 tbsp (25 mL) pitted green olives, chopped
Pinch hot red pepper flakes
2 tbsp (25 mL) sherry vinegar
1 tbsp (15 mL) chopped fresh parsley

1. Pat tuna dry and rub with 1 tbsp (15 mL) olive oil. Combine salt, pepper and thyme and press into tuna.
2. Heat a large, lightly oiled non-stick skillet on high heat. Add tuna and cook for 2 minutes per side. Remove to a carving board. Be sure to time this carefully as tuna overcooks easily.
3. Add remaining 1 tbsp (15 mL) oil to skillet. Add tomatoes, olives, hot pepper flakes, vinegar and parsley. Cook for 2 minutes.
4. Slice tuna and spoon olive mixture over top.

GRILLED TUNA WITH JAPANESE NOODLE SALAD

Fresh tuna has become very popular in the past couple of years. It is usually served rare, and it tastes and looks very meaty.

Although this recipe has a long list of ingredients, it is easy to make. Because the tuna is served rare, make sure your fish is very fresh. Be careful not to overcook it if you want that rare centre, as it seems to go from rare to well done in a blink.

You can prepare the tuna on its own and serve it separately, and the noodle salad can also be served alone. Buy the noodles in a health food store or Asian market.

Makes 6 servings

1 lb (500 g) tuna fillet, about 1 inch (2.5 cm) thick, skin removed
1 tbsp (15 mL) dark sesame oil
1 tbsp (15 mL) pepper
$^1/_2$ tsp (2 mL) salt
$^1/_2$ tsp (2 mL) vegetable oil

Japanese Noodle Salad

$^1/_2$ lb (250 g) whole wheat or buckwheat Japanese noodles or
      regular whole wheat noodles
1 large carrot, cut in thin strips
1 zucchini, cut in thin strips
1 sweet red pepper, seeded and cut in thin strips
1 sweet yellow pepper, seeded and cut in thin strips
2 oz (60 g) snow peas, sliced thinly on diagonal
3 green onions, cut in thin strips
1 small clove garlic, minced
1 tbsp (15 mL) minced fresh ginger root
1 tbsp (15 mL) rice wine
1 tbsp (15 mL) soy sauce
1 tbsp (15 mL) rice vinegar or cider vinegar
1 tbsp (15 mL) dark sesame oil
1 tbsp (15 mL) lemon juice
$^1/_2$ tsp (2 mL) hot red pepper sauce
$^1/_3$ cup (75 mL) chopped fresh cilantro or parsley
2 tbsp (25 mL) chopped fresh mint
2 tbsp (25 mL) shredded fresh basil

PER SERVING	
Calories	324
Protein	25 g
Fat	9 g
Saturates	2 g
Cholesterol	29 mg
Carbohydrate	37 g
Fibre	7 g
Sodium	380 mg
Potassium	513 mg

Excellent: Vitamin A; Vitamin C; Thiamine; Niacin; Vitamin B6; Vitamin B12
Good: Riboflavin; Iron

1. Pat tuna dry. Rub with sesame oil, pepper and salt.

2. Heat oil in a non-stick skillet or grill pan on high heat. Sear tuna for 2 minutes per side. Allow to rest for 10 minutes. Slice thinly on diagonal (fish should be rare).

3. Meanwhile, to prepare salad, cook noodles in a large pot of boiling water according to package directions. Rinse with cold water and drain well.

4. Bring a large pot of water to a boil. Add carrot, zucchini and sweet peppers and cook for 2 minutes. Lift out and chill under cold water. Pat dry.

5. Boil snow peas and green onions for 10 seconds, or just until brightened. Chill under cold water and pat dry.

6. In a small bowl, combine garlic, ginger, rice wine, soy sauce, rice vinegar, sesame oil, lemon juice and hot pepper sauce.

7. Toss noodles with vegetables, dressing, cilantro, mint and basil. To serve, arrange noodle salad on plates and top with slices of seared tuna.

FISH

Good fish smells clean and fresh, never "fishy." If the fish is whole, the eyes should be clear and protruding, the gills red, and the skin moist and smooth. The flesh should feel firm when you press it.

Remove fish from its plastic wrapping as soon as you get it home. Place it in a glass or stainless-steel dish, cover loosely and keep in the coldest part of the refrigerator over a pan of ice and water. Cook the fish as soon as possible—within a day or two.

I buy fresh fish if possible, but if you buy frozen fish, defrost it in the refrigerator or, tightly wrapped, in a bowl of cold water. Defrosting fish at room temperature destroys the texture, causes the fish to become dry, and can encourage the growth of bacteria. Never refreeze thawed fish.

Seafood Watch

Whether you are cooking fish at home or eating it in restaurants, it can be hard to remember which fish are safe and ecologically sound choices. For example, at the time this book is being written, imported swordfish is to be avoided, but line-caught U.S. swordfish is a good choice. Chilean sea bass, once a favourite of restaurants and home cooks, is now endangered.

One of the best resources for a consumer is the Seafood Watch site sponsored by the Monterey Bay Aquarium (www.mbayaq.org/cr/seafoodwatch.asp), which provides the latest information about the merits of farmed vs. wild fish, sustainability, which seafood to buy and why, and why seafood choices matter.

ASIAN TUNA OR SWORDFISH BURGERS

Many people want to eat more fish, but they want it to taste more like meat. Chopped tuna and swordfish (page 217) make great fish burgers because of their firm, meaty texture.

Serve these in the buns with grilled red onion slices.

Makes 6 servings

2 tsp (10 mL) olive oil
3 green onions, chopped
1 tbsp (15 mL) finely chopped fresh ginger root
1 clove garlic, finely chopped
1 lb (500 g) boneless, skinless tuna or swordfish
2 egg whites, or 1 whole egg
1/2 cup (125 mL) fresh whole wheat or regular breadcrumbs
1/2 tsp (2 mL) salt
1/4 tsp (1 mL) pepper
2 tbsp (25 mL) hoisin sauce
1 tbsp (15 mL) soy sauce
1 tsp (5 mL) dark sesame oil
6 whole wheat or regular sesame seed buns

1. Heat olive oil in a non-stick skillet on medium heat. Add green onions, ginger and garlic and cook gently for a few minutes, or until fragrant.
2. Cut fish into chunks and pat dry. Chop coarsely in a food processor. Add egg whites and breadcrumbs and chop until just combined. Blend in cooled garlic mixture, salt and pepper. Shape into 6 patties about 1/2 inch (1 cm) thick.
3. To prepare glaze, in a small bowl, combine hoisin sauce, soy sauce and sesame oil.
4. Grill burgers for a couple of minutes. Turn and brush with glaze. Turn and brush once more, cooking burgers for a total of about 3 to 4 minutes per side, or until cooked through but still juicy. Serve in buns.

Lemon Rosemary Fish Burgers

Omit ginger and glaze. Add 1 tbsp (15 mL) lemon juice and 1 tsp 5 mL) chopped fresh rosemary (or pinch dried) to burgers. Serve burgers in crusty Italian buns or pitas with barbecued eggplant and red peppers.

PER SERVING	
Calories	326
Protein	25 g
Fat	10 g
Saturates	2 g
Cholesterol	29 mg
Carbohydrate	32 g
Fibre	3 g
Sodium	730 mg
Potassium	462 mg

Excellent: Vitamin A; Thiamine; Niacin; Vitamin B12
Good: Riboflavin; Vitamin B6; Iron

PINE NUTS

Pine nuts are used in Italian and Middle Eastern cooking, but they are also very common in Chinese dishes. They are high in fat, so toast them before using. The flavour will be stronger, and you won't need to use as many. Keep pine nuts in the freezer if you are not using them right away.

To toast pine nuts, spread them on a baking sheet and bake in a preheated 350°F (180°C) oven for 3 to 5 minutes, or until lightly browned.

PER SERVING

Calories	204
Protein	23 g
Fat	9 g
Saturates	2 g
Cholesterol	41 mg
Carbohydrate	8 g
Fibre	1 g
Sodium	446 mg
Potassium	400 mg

Excellent: Niacin; Vitamin B12
Good: Vitamin B6

SWORDFISH SICILIAN

This is also a great way to cook tuna steaks, veal or lamb chops.

Makes 6 servings

1 tbsp (15 mL) olive oil, divided
1 large onion, chopped
1 clove garlic, finely chopped
1 cup (250 mL) fresh whole wheat or regular breadcrumbs
2 tbsp (25 mL) pine nuts, toasted
2 tbsp (25 mL) currants (soaked in boiling water for 5 minutes if hard)
2 tbsp (25 mL) chopped fresh parsley
2 tbsp (25 mL) grated Parmesan cheese
2 tbsp (25 mL) capers
6 swordfish steaks (about 4 oz/125 g each), 3/4 inch (2 cm) thick
1/2 tsp (2 mL) salt
1/4 tsp (1 mL) pepper

1. Heat 1 1/2 tsp (7 mL) oil in a large non-stick skillet on medium heat. Add onion and garlic and cook gently until tender, about 5 minutes. If onion begins to stick, add a few spoonfuls of water to skillet and cook until water evaporates.
2. Combine onion mixture, breadcrumbs, pine nuts, currants, parsley, Parmesan and capers.
3. Pat swordfish dry and brush with remaining 1 1/2 tsp (7 mL) oil. Sprinkle with salt and pepper. Grill for 2 minutes per side. Transfer fish to a baking sheet. Pat breadcrumb mixture evenly over top.
4. Just before serving, broil fish for 2 to 3 minutes, or until crisp and golden. Watch closely to make sure topping doesn't burn.

CEDAR-PLANKED SALMON

This is fun and delicious. Get a few planks of untreated cedar from the supermarket or a lumber yard—you can use the same board a few times until it gets too charred. You may also want to save one board just for serving; lay the cooked salmon on the board and garnish with fresh herbs.

If you do not want to barbecue this, place the soaked plank on a rimmed baking sheet, lay the marinated fish on top and cover loosely with foil. Roast in a preheated 450°F (230°C) oven for about 20 to 30 minutes, or longer, until fish barely flakes. Remove foil for the last 5 minutes of cooking time. The flavour will not be as smoky, but it will still be very good.

You can also use this marinade and simply roast, grill or barbecue the fish. Use leftover fish in sandwiches or salads, or blend with a little yogurt cheese, mayonnaise or cream cheese to make a smoky spread.

Makes 6 to 8 servings

2 lb (1 kg) salmon fillet, with skin, about 1 inch (2.5 cm) thick
1 clove garlic, minced
1 tbsp (15 mL) minced fresh ginger root
3 tbsp (45 mL) brown sugar
1 tsp (5 mL) ground cumin
1 tsp (5 mL) salt
½ tsp (2 mL) pepper
2 tsp (10 mL) dark sesame oil

1. Soak a 12- x 8-inch (30 x 20 cm) cedar plank in a tub of cold water for a few hours.
2. Pat fish dry. With salmon skin side down, score fish in serving-sized pieces, but do not cut through skin.
3. Combine garlic, ginger, sugar, cumin, salt, pepper and sesame oil. Rub into fish. Allow salmon to marinate for 10 to 20 minutes.
4. Place salmon on soaked plank. Place plank on barbecue. Close lid or cover with foil and barbecue for 15 to 25 minutes, or until salmon is cooked through. Remove cover for last 5 minutes of cooking. Do not turn fish during cooking.
5. Lift salmon off plank and serve without skin.

PER SERVING	
Calories	287
Protein	28 g
Fat	17 g
Saturates	3 g
Cholesterol	78 mg
Carbohydrate	6 g
Fibre	trace
Sodium	364 mg
Potassium	33 mg

Excellent: Thiamine; Niacin; Vitamin B6; Vitamin B12
Good: Folate

SESAME-CRUSTED SALMON ON GREENS

This is one of my most popular recipes. I usually serve it with steamed basmati rice, quinoa or couscous.

Makes 6 servings

6 salmon fillets (about 4 oz/125 g each), skin removed
1 tbsp (15 mL) honey
1 tbsp (15 mL) soy sauce
1 tsp (5 mL) honey-style mustard
1 tbsp (15 mL) sesame seeds

Orange Ginger Dressing

1 clove garlic, minced
1 tsp (5 mL) minced fresh ginger root
3 tbsp (45 mL) orange juice
2 tbsp (25 mL) soy sauce
2 tbsp (25 mL) rice vinegar or balsamic vinegar
2 tsp (10 mL) dark sesame oil
2 tsp (10 mL) honey
$1/4$ tsp (1 mL) hot red pepper sauce

Salad

12 cups (3 L) mixed greens
1 lb (500 g) cooked asparagus or green beans, cut in pieces
1 sweet red pepper, seeded and cut in strips
1 orange, peeled and sectioned
2 tbsp (25 mL) chopped fresh cilantro or parsley
2 tbsp (25 mL) chopped fresh chives or green onions

PER SERVING	
Calories	242
Protein	25 g
Fat	10 g
Saturates	1 g
Cholesterol	57 mg
Carbohydrate	16 g
Fibre	3 g
Sodium	496 mg
Potassium	1049 mg

Excellent: Vitamin A; Vitamin C; Thiamine; Niacin; Riboflavin; Vitamin B6; Folate; Vitamin B12
Good: Iron

1. Pat salmon dry. In a small bowl, combine honey, soy sauce and mustard. Rub into salmon. Sprinkle with sesame seeds.
2. Heat a lightly oiled non-stick ovenproof skillet on high heat. Add salmon and cook for 1 minute per side. Transfer to a preheated 425°F (220°C) oven. Roast for 7 to 8 minutes, or until just cooked.
3. Meanwhile, to prepare dressing, whisk together garlic, ginger, orange juice, soy sauce, vinegar, sesame oil, honey and hot pepper sauce. Taste and adjust seasonings if necessary.
4. Toss greens, asparagus, red pepper, orange, cilantro and chives with dressing. Serve salad topped with salmon.

STEAMED SALMON WITH KOREAN DRESSING

This is an adaptation of a recipe I learned from Madhur Jaffrey when I was taking cooking classes at Darina Allen's school at Ballymaloe near Cork, Ireland. Madhur Jaffrey vacationed there while she taught, and I vacationed there while I learned. Jaffrey is an accomplished actress, which enhances her teaching ability, and she casts a magical spell over her students. Eventually I convinced her that Toronto was also a great place for a vacation, and when she taught at my school the students were as spellbound as I was.

Although you can oven-steam this salmon (page 205), it is easy to put together a makeshift steaming unit as described.

This dish can also be made with a black bean sauce (page 205). It is delicious served hot or cold.

Makes 4 servings

4 oz (125 g) rice vermicelli or regular angelhair pasta
3/4 lb (375 g) fresh baby spinach (about 6 cups/1.5 L packed)
1 tbsp (15 mL) finely chopped fresh ginger root
3 green onions, chopped
4 salmon fillets (about 4 oz/125 g each), skin removed
1 lemon, cut in 8 slices
1/4 tsp (1 mL) pepper

Korean Dressing

1 1/2 tbsp (20 mL) soy sauce
2 tbsp (25 mL) water
2 tsp (10 mL) dark sesame oil
1 clove garlic, minced
1 tsp (5 mL) minced fresh ginger root
2 tsp (10 mL) granulated sugar
Pinch hot red pepper flakes
1/4 cup (50 mL) chopped fresh chives
1/4 cup (50 mL) chopped fresh cilantro or parsley
1 tbsp (15 mL) black sesame seeds (page 384), optional

1. To assemble a steaming unit, fit a rack or criss-crossed pairs of chopsticks in bottom of a wok or large deep skillet (rack should sit about 1 inch/2.5 cm from bottom). Find a shallow glass or ceramic ovenproof baking dish that fits on rack.

SPINACH

Spinach has enjoyed a revival now that you can buy prewashed baby spinach. It is not as strong-tasting as regular spinach, the leaves and stems are never tough, and you don't have to wash or trim it.

To clean mature spinach, fill a sink with cold water and swish the spinach around in it for a minute. Then just let it soak for a few minutes. The sand will sink to the bottom and the leaves will rise to the top. Lift out the leaves gently; repeat if necessary. Dry the spinach well.

PER SERVING	
Calories	311
Protein	26 g
Fat	9 g
Saturates	1 g
Cholesterol	57 mg
Carbohydrate	31 g
Fibre	3 g
Sodium	419 mg
Potassium	1021 mg

Excellent: Vitamin A; Thiamine; Niacin; Riboflavin; Iron; Vitamin B6; Folate; Vitamin B12

2. If you are using rice vermicelli, cover with warm water and allow to stand for 15 minutes. If you are using angelhair pasta, cook in boiling water until just tender. Drain well and rinse with cold water.

3. Arrange spinach leaves over bottom of baking dish. Place vermicelli on spinach. Sprinkle with half the chopped ginger and green onions. Pat fish dry and arrange on spinach in a single layer. Sprinkle with remaining ginger and green onions. Arrange 2 lemon slices on each fillet. Sprinkle with pepper.

4. Add just enough water to wok or skillet to reach rack. Bring water to a boil on medium-high heat.

5. Set baking dish containing fish on rack and cover wok with lid or foil. Cook for 8 to 10 minutes if fish is about 1 inch (2.5 cm) thick.

6. Meanwhile, prepare dressing by combining soy sauce, water, sesame oil, garlic, minced ginger, sugar and hot pepper flakes.

7. When salmon is ready, pour dressing over top and sprinkle with chives, cilantro and sesame seeds.

HOISIN-GLAZED SALMON

Hoisin sauce adds a sweet, mysterious flavour to dishes. You can use halibut or tuna in this recipe (reduce the cooking time slightly), as well as boneless, skinless chicken breasts and thinly cut lamb chops.

This dish is good cold and perfect for picnics; leftovers can be added to rice or couscous salads.

PER SERVING	
Calories	132
Protein	22 g
Fat	4 g
Saturates	1 g
Cholesterol	47 mg
Carbohydrate	3 g
Fibre	0 g
Sodium	359 mg
Potassium	296 mg
Excellent: Niacin	
Good: Vitamin B6	

Makes 4 servings

2 tbsp (25 mL) hoisin sauce
1 tbsp (15 mL) soy sauce
1 tsp (5 mL) dark sesame oil
1/4 tsp (1 mL) pepper
4 salmon fillets (about 4 oz/125 g each), 1 inch (2.5 cm) thick,
    skin removed

1. In a small bowl, combine hoisin sauce, soy sauce, sesame oil and pepper.

2. Pat fish dry and coat with sauce. Grill fish for about 5 minutes per side. (You can also bake fish in a preheated 425°F/220°C oven for 10 to 12 minutes.)

TANDOORI SALMON

This salmon is very tender and flavourful. Serve leftovers in a wrap along with rice and raita (page 118), or break up the fish and add to salads.

You can also use shrimp or boneless, skinless chicken breasts.

Makes 6 servings

6 salmon fillets (about 4 oz/125 g each), skin removed
1/3 cup (75 mL) yogurt cheese (page 391) or thick unflavoured
       low-fat yogurt
1 tbsp (15 mL) finely chopped fresh ginger root
1 clove garlic, minced
1 jalapeño, seeded and finely chopped
1 tbsp (15 mL) ground cumin
1 tbsp (15 mL) paprika
1 tsp (5 mL) pepper
1/2 tsp (2 mL) salt
1/4 tsp (1 mL) ground cloves
1/4 tsp (1 mL) ground cardamom

1. Pat salmon dry and place in a shallow baking dish.
2. In a small bowl, combine yogurt cheese, ginger, garlic, jalapeño, cumin, paprika, pepper, salt, cloves and cardamom.
3. Spoon yogurt mixture over salmon and gently rub into fish. Marinate in refrigerator for 20 minutes or up to 2 hours.
4. Place salmon on a baking sheet lined with parchment paper. Roast in a preheated 450°F (230°C) oven for 10 to 12 minutes (for fillets that are just under 1 inch/2.5 cm thick), or until salmon is just cooked through.

PER SERVING	
Calories	204
Protein	21 g
Fat	12 g
Saturates	3 g
Cholesterol	59 mg
Carbohydrate	2 g
Fibre	0 g
Sodium	167 mg
Potassium	55 mg
Excellent: Thiamine; Niacin; Vitamin B6; Vitamin B12	
Good: Folate	

QUICK SALMON DINNER

This is a quick and colourful dinner for one or two.

Season one or two salmon fillets with salt and pepper and place on a parchment-lined baking sheet. Toss 1 to 2 cups (250 mL to 500 mL) cherry tomatoes with salt, pepper and a little olive oil. Toss 1 to 2 cups (250 to 500 mL) diced squash with salt, pepper, olive oil and 1 tsp (5 mL) chopped fresh thyme or rosemary (or 1/4 tsp dried).

Place tomatoes and squash alongside salmon and roast in a preheated 425°F (220°C) oven for 12 to 15 minutes, or until salmon is just cooked, tomatoes have split and squash is tender.

ROASTED SALMON WITH LENTILS

This is my rendition of a popular French bistro dish. I like to use tiny Puy lentils in this; they are cleaner tasting and hold their shape better than regular green lentils.

Makes 6 servings

1 1/2 cups (375 mL) dried green lentils
4 tsp (20 mL) olive oil, divided
1 onion, chopped
2 cloves garlic, finely chopped
1 tsp (5 mL) ground cumin
1/4 tsp (1 mL) hot red pepper flakes
1 carrot, finely diced
1 stalk celery, finely diced
1 cup (250 mL) canned plum tomatoes, with juices, pureed
1/4 cup (50 mL) chopped fresh parsley
1/2 tsp (2 mL) pepper
Salt to taste
1 1/2 lb (750 g) salmon fillet, cut in 6 pieces, skin removed
1 tsp (5 mL) chopped fresh rosemary, or 1/4 tsp (1 mL) dried

1. Place lentils in a large pot and cover generously with water. Bring to a boil and cook gently for 25 to 35 minutes, or just until tender. Rinse and drain well.
2. Meanwhile, heat 1 tbsp (15 mL) oil in large, deep non-stick skillet on medium heat. Add onion and garlic and cook gently for 5 minutes. Add cumin and hot pepper flakes. Cook for 30 seconds.
3. Add carrot, celery and tomatoes to skillet. Cook for 8 to 10 minutes, or until carrots are just tender and liquid from tomatoes has reduced.
4. Add drained lentils, parsley and pepper to skillet. Taste and adjust seasonings, adding salt if necessary. Keep warm.
5. Heat remaining 1 tsp (5 mL) oil in a separate non-stick skillet on medium-high heat. Pat salmon dry and sprinkle with rosemary. Cook for 1 to 2 minutes per side, or until slightly browned and crusty.
6. Transfer salmon to a baking sheet lined with parchment paper (or leave in skillet if it is ovenproof). Bake in a preheated 400°F (200°C) oven for 7 to 9 minutes, or until just cooked through. Serve salmon on bed of lentils.

PER SERVING	
Calories	361
Protein	34 g
Fat	10 g
Saturates	2 g
Cholesterol	57 mg
Carbohydrate	34 g
Fibre	8 g
Sodium	129 mg
Potassium	1208 mg

Excellent: Vitamin A; Thiamine; Niacin; Riboflavin; Iron; Vitamin B6; Folate; Vitamin B12

HALIBUT WITH COUSCOUS CRUST AND TOMATO OLIVE VINAIGRETTE

The little grains of couscous add great texture to this dish, and the vinaigrette keeps the fish moist (the vinaigrette can also be used on salads). Black cod and salmon are also delicious cooked this way.

Makes 6 servings

3/4 cup (175 mL) couscous
3/4 cup (175 mL) boiling water or
    homemade chicken stock (page 109)
1 tsp (5 mL) ground cumin
1/2 tsp (2 mL) salt
1/2 cup (125 mL) all-purpose flour
1 egg, beaten
6 halibut fillets (about 4 oz/125 g each), 1 inch (2.5 cm) thick,
    skin removed

Tomato Olive Vinaigrette

2 tbsp (25 mL) red wine vinegar
2 tbsp (25 mL) lemon juice
1 clove garlic, minced
1/2 tsp (2 mL) pepper
1/4 cup (50 mL) tomato juice or V-8 juice
2 tbsp (25 mL) olive oil
2 tbsp (25 mL) chopped sun-dried tomatoes
2 tbsp (25 mL) shredded fresh basil or chopped parsley
Salt to taste

1 tbsp (15 mL) olive oil
10 cups (2.5 L) mixed salad greens

1. Place couscous in a shallow baking dish. Combine boiling water with cumin and salt and pour over couscous. Cover tightly and allow to rest for 15 minutes. Fluff with a fork.

2. Meanwhile, place flour in a shallow dish. Place beaten egg in a second shallow dish.

3. Pat fish dry. Dip fish into flour and shake off excess. Dip into egg and allow excess to drip off. Pat couscous into fish to coat all over. Refrigerate until ready to cook.

4. To prepare vinaigrette, combine vinegar, lemon juice, garlic and

---

SUN-DRIED TOMATOES

To make your own "sun"-dried tomatoes, halve or slice fresh Italian plum tomatoes and gently squeeze out the juice and seeds. Place tomatoes in a single layer on a rack over a baking sheet. Bake in a 200°F (100°C) oven for 6 to 24 hours, or until dried. Freeze.

PER SERVING

Calories	344
Protein	30 g
Fat	11 g
Saturates	2 g
Cholesterol	67 mg
Carbohydrate	30 g
Fibre	3 g
Sodium	373 mg
Potassium	973 mg

Excellent: Vitamin A; Niacin; Vitamin B6; Vitamin B12; Folate
Good: Thiamine; Riboflavin; Vitamin C; Iron

pepper. Whisk in tomato juice and oil. Stir in sun-dried tomatoes, basil and salt. Taste and adjust seasonings if necessary.

5. Heat 1 tbsp (15 mL) oil in a large, non-stick ovenproof skillet on medium-high heat. Add fish and cook for 1 minute. Turn gently and cook for 1 minute longer. Transfer to a preheated 425°F (220°C) oven and bake for 10 minutes, or until cooked through.

6. Serve fish on salad greens and drizzle with vinaigrette.

ROASTED HALIBUT WITH BALSAMIC VINEGAR

You can cook individual fillets or steaks using this recipe, but a whole piece is juicier and looks fabulous.

Instead of halibut, you could substitute cod or salmon.

Makes 6 to 8 servings

2 tbsp (25 mL) balsamic vinegar
2 tbsp (25 mL) brown sugar
1 tbsp (15 mL) olive oil
1 clove garlic, minced
1 tbsp (15 mL) chopped fresh rosemary, or 1/2 tsp (2 mL) dried
1/2 tsp (2 mL) pepper
2 lb (1 kg) halibut, cod, or salmon, in 1 piece, 2 inches (5 cm) thick, skin removed
1/2 tsp (2 mL) salt

PER SERVING	
Calories	207
Protein	32 g
Fat	6 g
Saturates	1 g
Cholesterol	48 mg
Carbohydrate	6 g
Fibre	trace
Sodium	280 mg
Potassium	707 mg
Excellent: Niacin; Vitamin B6; Vitamin B12	

1. In a small bowl, combine vinegar, brown sugar, oil, garlic, rosemary and pepper.

2. Pat fish dry, place in a shallow dish and gently rub with marinade. Marinate for 30 minutes or up to 2 hours in refrigerator.

3. Place fish on a baking sheet lined with parchment paper. Sprinkle with salt. Roast in a preheated 425°F (220°C) oven for 30 to 40 minutes, depending on thickness of the fish. (When it is cooked, it should just flake apart when prodded.) Transfer fish to a serving platter with a large spatula (the bottom of a removable-bottomed tart pan will work if you do not have a large enough spatula).

CHREIME (FISH IN SPICY CHERRY TOMATO SAUCE)

As soon as I tasted this dish in Israel, I knew it would become a favourite. I tasted many different versions and this is mine. You can cook the fish directly in the tomatoes instead of roasting it and/or serve the fish on top of asparagus or sauteed sweet peppers instead of the spinach.

This is great hot or cold. It is also delicious made with salmon.

Makes 6 to 8 servings
2 tsp (10 mL) olive oil
2 tsp (10 mL) chopped fresh thyme, or ½ tsp (2 mL) dried
½ tsp (2 mL) salt
¼ tsp (1 mL) pepper
2 lb (1 kg) thick white-fleshed fish fillets (e.g., halibut or cod),
    skin removed

Spicy Cherry Tomato Sauce
2 tbsp (25 mL) olive oil
6 cloves garlic, chopped
1 tsp (5 mL) ground cumin
1 tsp (5 mL) sweet smoked paprika
¾ tsp (4 mL) salt, divided
¼ tsp (1 mL) hot red pepper flakes
4 cups (1 L) cherry tomatoes

¾ lb (375 g) fresh baby spinach (about 6 cups/1.5 L packed)
1 tbsp (15 mL) dark sesame oil
2 tbsp (25 mL) chopped fresh cilantro

1. Combine olive oil, thyme, salt and pepper. Pat fish dry and rub marinade into fish. Marinate in refrigerator until ready to cook.
2. To prepare sauce, heat olive oil in a large, deep non-stick skillet on medium heat. Add garlic and cook gently for 2 to 3 minutes, or until fragrant but not brown. Add cumin, paprika, ½ tsp (2 mL) salt and hot pepper flakes and cook for 1 minute.
3. Add tomatoes and ¼ cup (50 mL) water. Bring to a boil. Cook for 8 to 10 minutes, or until tomatoes start to split.
4. Just before serving, place fish on a baking sheet lined with

PAPRIKA

Paprika is a powder made from a variety of mild pepper. Spanish smoked paprika can be hot or sweet, and it has a delicious smoky flavour.

PER SERVING

Calories	279
Protein	34 g
Fat	12 g
Saturates	2 g
Cholesterol	48 mg
Carbohydrate	8 g
Fibre	3 g
Sodium	616 mg
Potassium	1177 mg

Excellent: Vitamin A; Niacin; Vitamin B6; Vitamin B12; Folate; Iron
Good: Thiamine; Riboflavin; Vitamin C

parchment paper and roast in a preheated 400°F (200°C) oven for 15 minutes, or until just cooked.

5. Meanwhile, combine spinach, sesame oil and remaining ¼ tsp (1 mL) salt. Place in a large skillet and cook (without any liquid) until spinach just wilts, turning over with tongs constantly.

6. To serve, place some spinach on each plate. Top with a piece of fish. Spoon cherry tomatoes and sauce over top. Sprinkle with cilantro.

OVEN-STEAMED SEAFOOD DINNER

The Kingfisher Spa in Courtenay, British Columbia, serves delicious spa-style food. I had something like this there and it was beautifully presented in individual Chinese steamer baskets. At home, I improvise by steaming it in the oven.

Makes 4 servings

3 cups (750 mL) fresh baby spinach
½ lb (250 g) salmon fillet, cut in four pieces, skin removed
½ lb (250 g) halibut fillet, cut in four pieces, skin removed
8 large shrimp, cleaned
8 scallops, trimmed
8 mussels, cleaned
8 spears asparagus, trimmed
8 green beans, trimmed
16 baby carrots
2 tbsp (25 mL) sweet Thai chili sauce or red pepper jelly
1 tbsp (15 mL) soy sauce
1 tbsp (15 mL) water
1 tbsp (15 mL) lemon juice

1. Line a 13- x 9-inch (3.5 L) baking dish with spinach. Pat fish and shellfish dry and arrange in a single layer on top. Arrange asparagus, beans and carrots on top of fish.

2. Combine sweet chili sauce, soy sauce, water and lemon juice. Spoon over fish and vegetables. Cover tightly with foil.

3. Bake in a preheated 425°F (220°C) oven for 20 to 25 minutes, or until fish is cooked through and vegetables are tender-crisp.

PER SERVING

Calories	330
Protein	49 g
Fat	10 g
Saturates	2 g
Cholesterol	204 mg
Carbohydrate	10 g
Fibre	3 g
Sodium	628 mg
Potassium	1151 mg

Excellent: Vitamin A; Thiamine; Niacin; Vitamin B6; Vitamin B12; Folate; Iron
Good: Riboflavin; Vitamin C

RISOTTO WITH SEAFOOD AND PEPPERS

Although I usually like to prepare things in advance, risotto really should be made just before serving. So invite people that you feel comfortable having in your kitchen, and serve appetizers while they help you stir.

I like to serve risotto as the first sit-down course so that I don't have to leave people sitting at the table while I make it.

When I make risotto I always make lots, but there still never seems to be any left over! If you do have leftover risotto, it can be reheated in small portions in the microwave. Better still, shape into patties and make risotto cakes (page 354).

Makes 6 to 8 servings

3 tbsp (45 mL) olive oil, divided
3 cloves garlic, finely chopped
¼ tsp (1 mL) hot red pepper flakes
1 sweet red pepper, seeded and diced
1 sweet yellow pepper, seeded and diced
½ lb (250 g) cleaned shrimp, diced
½ lb (250 g) scallops, trimmed and diced
¼ cup (50 mL) chopped fresh parsley
¼ cup (50 mL) shredded fresh basil
4 cups (1 L) homemade chicken stock (page 109) or
        low-sodium commercial broth
½ cup (125 mL) dry white wine
1 onion, chopped
1½ cups (375 mL) short-grain Italian rice
Salt and pepper to taste

1. Heat 1 tbsp (15 mL) oil in a large non-stick skillet on medium heat. Add garlic and hot pepper flakes and cook until fragrant but not brown, about 30 seconds. Add red and yellow peppers and cook until wilted, about 10 minutes.

2. Add shrimp and scallops and stir well. Cook just until cooked through, about 2 to 3 minutes. Stir in parsley and basil. (Recipe can be prepared ahead to this point.)

3. About 20 minutes before serving, combine stock and wine in a saucepan. Bring to a boil and keep at a simmer.

4. Heat remaining 2 tbsp (25 mL) oil in a large saucepan on medium

PER SERVING	
Calories	365
Protein	21 g
Fat	9 g
Saturates	1 g
Cholesterol	71 mg
Carbohydrate	47 g
Fibre	2 g
Sodium	142 mg
Potassium	481 mg
Excellent: Vitamin C; Niacin; Vitamin B12	
Good: Vitamin A	

heat. Add onion and cook gently for about 5 minutes, or until tender and fragrant.

5. Stir in rice and coat well. Add 1 cup (250 mL) stock and cook over medium to medium-high heat, stirring constantly, until liquid evaporates or has been absorbed. When pan is dry, add stock about 1/2 cup (125 mL) at a time, stirring constantly, until rice is barely tender (you may use more or less stock than called for). This should take about 15 minutes. (Rice will cook a bit more after you add seafood.)

6. Stir seafood into rice. Cook for 4 minutes. Taste and season with salt and pepper if necessary. Serve immediately.

WARM SEA SCALLOPS WRAPPED IN PROSCIUTTO ON GREENS

This makes a very elegant appetizer or main course lunch. The first time I made it I had a glass of wine and overcooked the scallops. Another law of entertaining—don't drink wine until after you've cooked the scallops!

Makes 6 servings

12 large scallops, trimmed
6 thin slices prosciutto ham, sliced in half lengthwise
1/4 tsp (1 mL) pepper
1 tbsp (15 mL) olive oil
3 tbsp (45 mL) balsamic vinegar
1 tbsp (15 mL) lemon juice
1 tbsp (15 mL) shredded fresh sage
1/4 lb (125 g) fresh baby spinach (about 2 cups/500 mL)

1. Pat scallops dry and wrap with strips of prosciutto. Secure with a skewer. Season with pepper.
2. Heat oil in a large nonstick skillet on medium-high heat. Add scallops and sear for a few minutes per side until barely cooked through.
3. Add vinegar and lemon juice to skillet and bring to a boil. Add sage. (If liquid evaporates too quickly, add 1/4 cup/50 mL water.)
4. Spoon scallops and juices over spinach.

PER SERVING	
Calories	87
Protein	10 g
Fat	4 g
Saturates	1 g
Cholesterol	20 mg
Carbohydrate	3 g
Fibre	1 g
Sodium	321 mg
Potassium	294 mg
Excellent: Vitamin B12	
Good: Folate	

SPICY THAI SHRIMP

This is a version of a recipe I learned when I attended classes at the fabulous cooking school at the Oriental Hotel in Bangkok. Spearing the shrimp from head to tail keeps them straight and prevents them from rolling around on the skewers when you turn them. (This method also works well with chicken fingers and salmon strips.)

The shrimp looks pretty served on a platter lined with banana leaves or cilantro.

Leftovers can be frozen. Chop them up and use in a salad, stir-fry or as a filling for wraps with rice and peanut sauce or even in sushi rolls (page 54).

Makes 6 servings

2 lb (1 kg) extra-large shrimp (about 32), cleaned
3 cloves garlic, peeled
1 1-inch (2.5 cm) piece fresh ginger root, peeled
1 hot pepper, seeded
1/4 cup (50 mL) fresh cilantro leaves, stems and roots
2 tbsp (25 mL) hoisin sauce
1 tbsp (15 mL) Thai fish sauce or soy sauce
1 tbsp (15 mL) lime juice or lemon juice
1 tbsp (15 mL) honey
1 tbsp (15 mL) rice vinegar
1 tsp (5 mL) dark sesame oil
1/2 cup (125 mL) sweet Thai chili sauce

1. Pat shrimp dry and place in a large bowl.
2. In a food processor, combine garlic, ginger, hot pepper and cilantro and blend into a paste. Blend in hoisin sauce, fish sauce, lime juice, honey, vinegar and sesame oil.
3. Combine marinade with shrimp and marinate for at least 30 minutes in refrigerator.
4. If you are using wooden skewers, soak in cold water for 30 minutes before using.
5. Thread shrimp on skewers from head to tail so shrimp are relatively straight. (Make sure shrimp is pushed right to points of skewers so wooden tips don't burn.)
6. Grill shrimp for a few minutes on each side or until pink and opaque. Place sweet Thai chili sauce in a small bowl in middle of serving platter. Arrange shrimp around sauce.

FRESH VS. FROZEN SHRIMP

Shrimp is highly perishable, so most "fresh" shrimp that you see in stores has been previously frozen.

I usually buy a 4-lb (2 kg) block of raw shrimp frozen in the shell. The shells provide protection from freezer burn and shrimp cooked in the shell is more flavourful. Then I defrost and clean them as I need them. Hold part of the chunk under cold water until it breaks off and then return the rest to the freezer, well wrapped. Defrost the shrimp you are using in the refrigerator, or in a sink or bowl of cold water.

I don't usually buy frozen cooked shrimp, as it is usually very wet and soggy when defrosted.

PER SERVING

Calories	156
Protein	25 g
Fat	2 g
Saturates	0 g
Cholesterol	229 mg
Carbohydrate	8 g
Fibre	1 g
Sodium	582 mg
Potassium	389 mg

Excellent: Vitamin A; Niacin; Vitamin B12
Good: Vitamin C

CLEANING SHRIMP

To clean and shell shrimp, peel the shells off with your fingers and then wiggle the tail part off gently. Run a knife about ¹/₄ inch (5 mm) deep along the top of the shrimp. If the intestinal tract is black and full of sand, remove and discard it. Pat the shrimp dry.

GRILLED BUTTERFLIED SHRIMP WITH SALSA VERDE

Like meat or chicken cooked on the bone, shrimp cooked in the shells will be more juicy and flavourful. But they are a bit messy to eat, so save this for casual dining with close friends! (You could also remove the shells before or after cooking.)

Salsa verde is a classic Italian green sauce that adds a lot of flavour to boiled or grilled meat or seafood.

Makes 6 servings

Salsa Verde

2 cups (500 mL) packed fresh parsley leaves
2 anchovies, rinsed
1 tbsp (15 mL) capers
1 clove garlic, peeled
1 tsp (5 mL) Dijon mustard
2 tbsp (25 mL) red wine vinegar
3 tbsp (45 mL) olive oil
Salt to taste

Shrimp

2 lb (1 kg) extra-large shrimp (16/20 per pound)
1 tbsp (15 mL) chopped fresh rosemary, or ¹/₂ tsp (2 mL) dried
¹/₂ tsp (2 mL) salt
¹/₄ tsp (1 mL) hot red pepper flakes
2 cloves garlic, minced
6 cups (1.5 L) baby arugula or other mixed greens

PER SERVING	
Calories	195
Protein	26 g
Fat	9 g
Saturates	1 g
Cholesterol	225 mg
Carbohydrate	3 g
Fibre	1 g
Sodium	561 mg
Potassium	413 mg

Excellent: Niacin; Vitamin B12; Vitamin C; Folate; Iron
Good: Vitamin A

1. Place parsley, anchovies, capers and garlic in a food processor and chop until fine. Add mustard, vinegar and oil. Blend into a rough paste by chopping on/off. Taste and add salt only if necessary. Mixture will be quite pasty. Thin with a bit of water if you wish.
2. With a sharp knife or pair of scissors, cut along back of shrimp and open up to butterfly. Remove intestinal tract (sometimes called the vein) if it is full of dirt or sand.
3. Toss shrimp with rosemary, salt, hot pepper flakes and minced garlic. Rub in and marinate until ready to cook.
4. Grill shrimp for about 2 minutes per side or until opaque, red and slightly curled. Do not overcook! Toss immediately with salsa verde. Serve on a bed of arugula.

MUSSELS PROVENÇALE

People eat mussels in restaurants all the time, but don't often think to cook them at home. Yet they are easy to prepare. If you are serving them for dinner, count on 1 lb (500 g) per person; if you are serving them as an appetizer, serve ½ lb (250 g) per person. Set bowls on the table for the empty shells.

You can serve the mussels and sauce on pasta or rice. You can also remove the mussels from their shells and serve the sauce, juices and shelled mussels as a soup.

Makes 8 servings as an appetizer; 4 as a main course

4 lb (2 kg) mussels (about 90 to 100)
1 tbsp (15 mL) olive oil
1 shallot, chopped
4 cloves garlic, chopped
1 28-oz (796 mL) can plum tomatoes, drained and chopped (about
    1 ½ cups/375 mL), or 1 ½ lb (750 g) fresh tomatoes, peeled,
    seeded and diced
1 cup (250 mL) dry white wine, stock or water
1 tbsp (15 mL) chopped fresh tarragon, or 1 tsp (5 mL) dried
¼ tsp (1 mL) salt
Pinch pepper
3 tbsp (45 mL) chopped fresh parsley
2 whole wheat or regular baguette, sliced

1. Clean mussels and discard any that have broken shells or that do not close when lightly tapped.
2. Heat oil in a large Dutch oven or wok on medium-high heat. Add shallot and garlic. Cook for a few minutes until fragrant and tender, but do not brown. Add tomatoes and bring to a boil.
3. Add mussels and turn to coat well. Add wine and bring to a boil. Sprinkle with tarragon, salt and pepper.
4. Cover and cook mussels for 5 minutes, or until mussels open. Discard any that do not open after another minute of cooking.
5. Transfer mussels to large bowls. Sprinkle with parsley and serve with lots of bread to soak up juices.

PER APPETIZER SERVING	
Calories	300
Protein	17 g
Fat	6 g
Saturates	1 g
Cholesterol	18 mg
Carbohydrate	45 g
Fibre	6 g
Sodium	729 mg
Potassium	462 mg

Excellent: Niacin; Vitamin B12; Iron
Good: Thiamine; Folate

MUSSELS

Cultivated mussels are milder in flavour than wild ones. They are usually a little more expensive, but they are much easier to clean (and often easier to find).

To clean wild mussels, scrub them well and remove the beards. To clean culti-vated mussels, simply wash and remove the beards (if there are any). When you are cleaning the mussels, discard any that do not close tightly when touched, any with broken shells and any that are very heavy (they may be full of sand). When the mussels are cooked, discard any that have not opened.

PER SERVING	
Calories	143
Protein	12 g
Fat	5 g
Saturates	1 g
Cholesterol	25 mg
Carbohydrate	12 g
Fibre	2 g
Sodium	319 mg
Potassium	308 mg

Excellent: **Vitamin C; Iron; Folate; Vitamin B12**
Good: **Vitamin A; Thiamine; Niacin**

MUSSELS WITH BLACK BEAN SAUCE

This recipe serves six to eight people as a main course, or eight to ten as an appetizer (or serve the cooked, shelled mussels on tooth-picks as hors d'oeuvres). Serve over pasta or rice or just with lots of crusty bread. Put a few extra bowls on the table to collect the empty shells, and provide spoons for the juices.

Makes 6 to 8 servings

4 lb (2 kg) mussels (about 90 to 100)
2 tsp (10 mL) vegetable oil
3 green onions, chopped
1 tbsp (15 mL) finely chopped fresh ginger root
3 cloves garlic, finely chopped
1/2 tsp (2 mL) hot Asian chili paste
2 tbsp (25 mL) fermented black beans, rinsed and chopped
1 tsp (5 mL) grated lemon peel
2 leeks or small onions, trimmed and thinly sliced
2 sweet red peppers, seeded and thinly sliced
1/2 cup (125 mL) homemade chicken stock (page 109), fish stock,
     dry white wine or water
1/2 cup (125 mL) water
2 tbsp (25 mL) rice vinegar or cider vinegar
1 tbsp (15 mL) soy sauce
2 tsp (10 mL) dark sesame oil
1/4 cup (50 mL) chopped fresh cilantro or parsley

1. Clean mussels and discard any that have broken shells or that do not close when lightly tapped.
2. Heat vegetable oil in a wok or Dutch oven on medium-high heat. Add green onions, ginger, garlic, chili paste, black beans and lemon peel. Stir-fry for 30 seconds, or until very fragrant.
3. Add leeks and red peppers and cook for 2 minutes, or until vegeta-bles are slightly wilted.
4. Add stock, water, vinegar, soy sauce and sesame oil. Stir well and bring to a boil.
5. Add mussels and return to a boil. Cover and cook for 5 to 7 minutes, or until mussels have opened and are thoroughly cooked (discard any mussels that do not open). Stir well. Sprinkle with cilantro.

Red Curry Chicken
Sweet Chili Chicken
Thai Mango Chicken with Vegetables
Thai Chicken and Noodle Stir-fry
Stir-fried Chicken and Vegetables
Grilled Peruvian Chicken
Grilled Chicken and Tahina Pita Sandwiches
Chicken Fajitas
Chicken Tagine with Green Olives and Preserved Lemons
Chicken Tagine with Dried Fruits
Coq au Vin
Asian Chicken Chili
Chicken with Forty Cloves of Garlic
Chicken Pot Pie
Breaded Chicken Fingers
Chicken Adobo
Chicken "Meatloaf"
Flattened Chicken Breasts with Roasted
    Garlic Couscous
Twist and Shout Chicken Drumsticks
Breaded Chicken Cutlets with Tomato Sauce
Roast Chicken with Bulgur Stuffing
Musakhan (Roast Chicken with Onions and
    Pine Nuts on Pita)

Barbecued Chicken Fingers
Chicken Jambalaya
Chicken Breasts with Black Bean Sauce
Roast Cornish Hens with Herbs
Indian-flavoured Grilled Chicken Thighs
Turkey Burgers with Old-fashioned Coleslaw
Turkey and Sweet Potato Shepherd's Pie
Rolled Turkey Breast with Gravy
Roast Turkey Breast with Rosemary and Garlic
Old-fashioned Whole Roast Turkey
Bread Stuffing with Herbs

HEART

SMART

POULTRY

RED CURRY CHICKEN

You can also make this using six to eight skinless chicken breasts. Serve over couscous or rice noodles instead of rice. Leftover chicken can be used with rice to fill wraps, or you can dice the chicken and vegetables, add stock and serve as a soup. If you don't like things too spicy, use half the curry paste.

Makes 6 servings

1 4-lb (2 kg) chicken, cut in 8 pieces, skin removed
2 tsp (10 mL) vegetable oil
2 tbsp (25 mL) red Thai curry paste
1 large onion, thickly sliced
2 carrots, thickly sliced
2 cloves garlic, chopped
2 potatoes (about 1 lb/500 g),
    peeled and cut in 2-inch (5 cm) chunks
1 sweet red pepper, seeded and cut in chunks
3 whole jalapeños
½ lb (250 g) mushrooms, trimmed
1 stalk lemongrass, cut in 2-inch (5 cm) pieces, smashed
2 cups (500 mL) homemade chicken stock (page 109) or water
2 tbsp (25 mL) Thai fish sauce or soy sauce
½ cup (125 mL) tomato puree, tomato sauce or
    light coconut milk
6 cups (1.5 L) cooked brown or white rice, hot
¼ cup (50 mL) chopped fresh cilantro

1. Trim fat from chicken pieces and pat chicken dry. Heat oil in a large, deep non-stick skillet or Dutch oven on medium-high heat. Brown chicken pieces for about 5 minutes per side. Remove chicken from skillet.

2. Discard all but a thin film of oil from skillet. Add curry paste and cook for 30 to 60 seconds, or until fragrant. Add onion, carrots, garlic, potatoes, red pepper, jalapeños, mushrooms and lemongrass. Cook for about 1 minute. If vegetables begin to stick, add ¼ cup (50 mL) stock now.

3. Add stock and fish sauce to skillet. Bring to a boil. Add chicken pieces. Reduce heat, cover and simmer for 30 minutes, or until chicken is cooked through.

4. Remove chicken and vegetables from skillet (discarding jalapeños and lemongrass), cover and keep warm. Return skillet with stock to

THAI CURRY PASTES

Thai curry has a very different taste from West Indian or East Indian curry. Red and green Thai curry pastes are now easy to find in supermarkets and specialty stores. Red curry is more spice based and green curry is more herb based. Different brands vary in heat.

PER SERVING

Calories	583
Protein	42 g
Fat	10 g
Saturates	2 g
Cholesterol	103 mg
Carbohydrate	79 g
Fibre	6 g
Sodium	603 mg
Potassium	910 mg

Excellent: Vitamin A; Thiamine; Niacin; Vitamin B6; Vitamin B12; Vitamin C
Good: Riboflavin; Folate; Iron

EAST INDIAN CURRY POWDERS AND PASTES

There are many different blends of curry powder, but you can also make your own. Combine 2 tbsp (25 mL) ground coriander, 1 tsp (5 mL) ground cumin, 1 tsp (5 mL) turmeric, 1 tsp (5 mL) ground cardamom, 1/2 tsp (2 mL) ground cinnamon, 1/4 tsp (1 mL) ground cloves, 1/4 tsp (1 mL) salt and about 1 tsp (5 mL) cayenne (more or less to taste).

I now prefer to use Indian curry paste instead of curry powder, because the spices have been roasted in oil and do not add a dry, raw taste to dishes. Patak's Madras curry paste is a good all-purpose product.

PER SERVING

Calories	276
Protein	39 g
Fat	8 g
Saturates	1 g
Cholesterol	95 mg
Carbohydrate	11 g
Fibre	2 g
Sodium	716 mg
Potassium	790 mg

Excellent: Vitamin A; Niacin; Vitamin B6; Folate
Good: Riboflavin; Vitamin B12; Iron

heat. Bring to a boil and cook, uncovered, for about 10 minutes, or until 1 to 1 1/2 cups (250 to 375 mL) stock remains. Add tomato puree and cook, uncovered, for 5 minutes, or until thickened.

5. Place rice on a large platter. Make an indentation for chicken. Place chicken, vegetables and sauce on rice. Sprinkle with cilantro.

Red Curry Lamb

Instead of chicken, use 2 lb (1 kg) stewing lamb cut in 2-inch (5 cm) chunks. Cook for 1 to 1 1/2 hours, or until lamb is very tender.

SWEET CHILI CHICKEN

This is one of the best fast recipes I know. Leave out the spinach if your kids refuse to eat anything green.

Sweet Thai chili sauce can be found in Asian stores and some grocery stores. Although it is slightly hot, it can be used on its own as a dip for dumplings or spring rolls. If you can't find it, use red pepper jelly; do not substitute the really hot Asian chili paste!

Makes 4 servings

1 lb (500 g) boneless, skinless chicken breasts
3 tbsp (45 mL) hoisin sauce
3 tbsp (45 mL) sweet Thai chili sauce
2 tbsp (25 mL) soy sauce
1 tbsp (15 mL) vegetable oil
1 tbsp (15 mL) chopped fresh ginger root
2 green onions, chopped
2 cloves garlic, finely chopped
2 cups (500 mL) fresh baby spinach
2 tbsp (25 mL) chopped fresh cilantro

1. Pat chicken dry and cut into cubes.
2. To prepare sauce, combine hoisin, sweet chili sauce and soy sauce.
3. Heat oil in a large, deep non-stick skillet or wok on medium-high heat. Add ginger, green onions and garlic and stir-fry for 30 seconds, or until fragrant. Add chicken and stir-fry for 2 minutes, or until browned.
4. Add sauce and combine well. Cook for 3 to 4 minutes, or until chicken is barely cooked through. Add spinach and cook for 1 minute longer. Sprinkle with cilantro.

THAI MANGO CHICKEN WITH VEGETABLES

Look for the smaller yellow Alfonso mangoes. They have a less fibrous texture than other mangoes and are very sweet.

Makes 4 servings

1 lb (500 g) boneless, skinless chicken breasts
1/4 cup (50 mL) hoisin sauce
2 tbsp (25 mL) peanut butter
1/4 cup (50 mL) light coconut milk
1 1/4 cups (300 mL) homemade chicken stock (page 109) or water
2 tbsp (25 mL) cornstarch
1 tbsp (15 mL) vegetable oil
1 tbsp (15 mL) green Thai curry paste (page 238)
1 sweet red pepper, seeded and cut in chunks
1 cup (250 mL) broccoli florets
1/4 lb (125 g) mushrooms, trimmed and halved
1 mango, peeled and diced
2 tbsp (25 mL) chopped fresh cilantro

1. Pat chicken dry and cut into strips.
2. Blend or whisk hoisin sauce and peanut butter until smooth. Whisk in coconut milk, stock and cornstarch.
3. Heat oil in a large, deep non-stick skillet on medium-high heat. Add curry paste and cook for 10 seconds. Add chicken and stir-fry for 1 minute, or until chicken loses its raw appearance.
4. Add red pepper, broccoli and mushrooms to skillet and stir-fry for about 4 minutes.
5. Add mango to skillet. Stir up reserved sauce. Add sauce to skillet, bring to a boil and cook for 1 minute, or until thick. Sprinkle with cilantro.

PER SERVING	
Calories	364
Protein	36 g
Fat	13 g
Saturates	3 g
Cholesterol	79 mg
Carbohydrate	27 g
Fibre	4 g
Sodium	506 mg
Potassium	809 mg

Excellent: Vitamin A; Niacin; Vitamin B6; Vitamin C
Good: Thiamine; Riboflavin; Vitamin B12; Folate; Iron

THAI CHICKEN AND NOODLE STIR-FRY

Be sure to remove the whole chiles after cooking, or warn guests not to eat them—unless they have iron stomachs! Or omit the chiles and add 1 tsp (5 mL) hot Asian chili paste with the onions.

Thai basil, also known as holy basil, has more of an anise taste than other types of basil, and its stems are purply green. Look for it in Thai and Asian markets, but if you can't find it, just use regular basil.

Makes 4 to 6 servings

3/4 lb (375 g) whole wheat or regular linguine
1 lb (500 g) boneless, skinless chicken breasts
1 tbsp (15 mL) vegetable oil
1 onion, thinly sliced
1 tbsp (15 mL) chopped fresh ginger root
2 cloves garlic, finely chopped
1 tsp (5 mL) curry powder or red Thai curry paste (page 238)
1/2 cup (125 mL) tomato juice
1/3 cup (75 mL) homemade chicken stock (page 109) or water
1/3 cup (75 mL) light coconut milk or tomato juice
1 tbsp (15 mL) Thai fish sauce or soy sauce
12 small hot green chiles
Handful fresh Thai basil or regular basil
Salt and pepper to taste

PER SERVING	
Calories	509
Protein	39 g
Fat	8 g
Saturates	1 g
Cholesterol	66 mg
Carbohydrate	69 g
Fibre	4 g
Sodium	576 mg
Potassium	572 mg
Excellent: Niacin;	
Vitamin B6	
Good: Vitamin B12;	
Folate; Iron	

1. Bring a large pot of water to a boil. Add linguine and cook until tender. Drain. If not using right away, rinse with cold water.
2. Pat chicken dry and cut into 1 1/2-inch (4 cm) chunks.
3. Heat oil in a large, deep non-stick skillet or wok on medium-high heat. Add chicken and stir-fry for 1 minute, or just until it loses its raw appearance.
4. Add onion, ginger and garlic to skillet and stir-fry for 30 to 60 seconds, or until fragrant.
5. Stir in curry powder, tomato juice, stock, coconut milk and fish sauce. Bring to a boil.
6. Add chiles and basil and cook for 3 minutes.
7. Add noodles and combine well until noodles are thoroughly heated. Taste and add salt and pepper if necessary.

STIR-FRIED CHICKEN AND VEGETABLES

Kids love taking my university survival course—as soon as they realize that if you know how to cook, you become the most popular kid on campus, and invitations to dinner at your place become really hot tickets!

Serve this with steamed rice.

Makes 4 to 5 servings

1 tbsp (15 mL) soy sauce
2 tbsp (25 mL) cornstarch, divided
1 lb (500 g) boneless, skinless chicken breasts
2/3 cup (150 mL) homemade chicken stock (page 109) or water
2 tbsp (25 mL) hoisin sauce
1 tbsp (15 mL) rice wine
2 tsp (10 mL) dark sesame oil
1 tbsp (15 mL) vegetable oil
1 tbsp (15 mL) finely chopped fresh ginger root
3 green onions, chopped
2 cloves garlic, finely chopped
1 tsp (5 mL) hot Asian chili paste
1 sweet red pepper, seeded and cut in strips
1 carrot, thinly sliced
1 bunch broccoli, cut in 1-inch (2.5 cm) pieces
2 tbsp (25 mL) chopped fresh cilantro or green onions

1. In a large bowl, combine soy sauce and 1 tbsp (15 mL) cornstarch.
2. Pat chicken dry and cut into 1-inch (2.5 cm) chunks. Add chicken to soy sauce mixture and combine well.
3. In a separate bowl, combine stock, hoisin sauce, rice wine, sesame oil and remaining 1 tbsp (15 mL) cornstarch.
4. Heat vegetable oil in a large, deep non-stick skillet on medium-high heat. Add ginger, green onions, garlic and hot chili paste. Cook for 30 seconds.
5. Add chicken to skillet and cook for a couple of minutes until lightly browned. Add red pepper, carrot, broccoli and 1/4 cup (50 mL) water. Cover and cook for 3 to 5 minutes, or until chicken is just cooked through and broccoli is bright green.
6. Stir reserved sauce well and add to chicken/vegetable mixture. Bring to a boil, stirring constantly. Taste and adjust seasonings if necessary. Serve sprinkled with cilantro.

RICE COOKERS
If you serve rice more than twice a week, you might want to invest in an electric rice cooker. The cooker turns off automatically and keeps the rice hot. I like the 10-cup (2.5 L) size (Japanese cups are smaller than North American cups, so it is not as big as it sounds). Follow the manufacturer's directions.

PER SERVING

Calories	278
Protein	32 g
Fat	8 g
Saturates	1 g
Cholesterol	66 mg
Carbohydrate	19 g
Fibre	4 g
Sodium	501 mg
Potassium	823 mg

Excellent: Vitamin A; Vitamin C; Niacin; Vitamin B6; Folate
Good: Riboflavin; Iron; Vitamin B12

STEAMING RICE

To steam rice on the stove, rinse 1 1/2 cups (375 mL) rice in a strainer until water runs clear. Drain well. Place in a medium saucepan with 2 1/4 cups (550 mL) cold water. Bring to a boil, reduce heat to medium and cook, uncovered, until surface water disappears and crater-like holes appear on surface of rice, about 5 to 8 minutes. Cover tightly, reduce heat to very low and cook for 15 minutes. Remove from heat and allow to rest, without lifting lid, for 10 to 30 minutes before serving. (For brown rice, increase water by 1/4 cup/50 mL and cook for 30 minutes instead of 15 minutes.)

Makes about 3 cups (750 mL).

PER SERVING

Calories	225
Protein	29 g
Fat	10 g
Saturates	2 g
Cholesterol	86 mg
Carbohydrate	4 g
Fibre	trace
Sodium	203 mg
Potassium	300 mg

Excellent: Niacin; Vitamin B6
Good: Vitamin B12

GRILLED PERUVIAN CHICKEN

According to my good friend Mitchell Davis, cookbook author and director of publications for the James Beard Foundation, small inexpensive Peruvian restaurants are all the rage in New York City. Here's his take on the irresistible grilled chicken they serve. (You can also roast this on a parchment-lined baking sheet in a 400°F/200°C oven for 35 to 40 minutes, or until cooked through.)

You can make this with all white meat or all dark meat.

Makes 10 servings

2 chickens, cut in quarters (8 pieces), skin removed
2 lemons, halved
2 heads garlic, halved
2 tsp (10 mL) ground cumin
2 tsp (10 mL) paprika (preferably smoked)
3/4 tsp (4 mL) ground cinnamon
3/4 tsp (4 mL) pepper
1/2 tsp (2 mL) salt
1/2 tsp (2 mL) cayenne
2 tbsp (25 mL) olive oil
2 tbsp (25 mL) chopped fresh cilantro

1. Pat chicken pieces dry and place in a large bowl. Squeeze juice from lemon halves all over chicken. Add lemon halves to bowl. Rub chicken with cut sides of garlic heads and add garlic to bowl.
2. To make paste, in a small bowl, combine cumin, paprika, cinnamon, pepper, salt, cayenne and oil.
3. Rub paste into chicken pieces and sprinkle with cilantro. Marinate chicken for 1 hour or up to overnight in refrigerator.
4. Grill chicken for about 5 minutes per side. Reduce heat to low, cover and cook for 15 to 20 minutes longer, or until chicken is cooked through. If you cannot reduce grilling heat low enough, simply transfer to a preheated 350°F (180°C) oven and roast. Chicken should be cooked until internal temperature reaches 165°F (74°C) when measured with a meat thermometer.

Peruvian Roast Chicken

Rub paste over a whole chicken (you may have enough paste for two chickens). Place lemons and garlic in cavity and roast chicken in a preheated 400°F (200°C) oven for 50 to 60 minutes, or until a meat thermometer reads 165°F (74°C).

GRILLED CHICKEN AND TAHINA PITA SANDWICHES

This tahina sauce, which has an amazing sesame flavour, can also be used as a salad dressing, sandwich spread, dip or drizzle over roasted vegetables. These sandwiches can also be served with Middle Eastern Dressing.

Makes 4 sandwiches

4 boneless, skinless single chicken breasts (about 4 oz/125 g each)
1 tbsp (15 mL) olive oil
$^1/_2$ tsp (2 mL) salt
$^1/_2$ tsp (2 mL) dried oregano
$^1/_2$ tsp (2 mL) dried thyme

Tahina Sauce

3 tbsp (45 mL) tahina (page 40)
2 cloves garlic, minced
2 tbsp (25 mL) lemon juice
Dash hot red pepper sauce
$^1/_2$ cup (125 mL) unflavoured low-fat yogurt
Salt to taste

4 4-inch (10 cm) whole wheat or regular pita breads
1 tomato, seeded and sliced
$^1/_2$ English cucumber, thinly sliced
1 tbsp (15 mL) chopped fresh cilantro
1 tbsp (15 mL) chopped fresh parsley

1. Remove filets from chicken breasts (page 257) and reserve for another use such as chicken fingers or stir-fries. Pat chicken breasts dry. Place in a heavy plastic bag, one at a time, and pound until about $^1/_2$ inch (1 cm) thick.
2. In a large bowl, combine chicken, oil, salt, oregano and thyme.
3. Grill chicken for 4 to 6 minutes per side, depending on thickness, until just cooked through. Cut chicken into chunks or strips.
4. To prepare sauce, blend tahina, garlic, lemon juice, hot pepper sauce and yogurt. Taste and adjust seasonings, adding salt if necessary. Mixture should be creamy in texture. Thin with water if necessary.
5. Open pita breads and fill with chicken. Drizzle with sauce. Add tomato and cucumber. Sprinkle with cilantro and parsley.

MIDDLE EASTERN DRESSING

Combine 1 minced clove garlic, $^3/_4$ tsp (4 mL) ground cumin, $^3/_4$ tsp (4 mL) paprika, $^1/_4$ tsp (1 mL) cayenne, 1/2 cup (125 mL) yogurt cheese (page 391) or thick yogurt and 1 tbsp (15 mL) lemon juice. Stir in 2 tbsp (25 mL) chopped fresh cilantro or parsley and 2 tbsp (25 mL) mayonnaise (optional).

Makes about $^1/_2$ cup (125 mL).

PER SERVING

Calories	316
Protein	30 g
Fat	12 g
Saturates	2 g
Cholesterol	62 mg
Carbohydrate	23 g
Fibre	2 g
Sodium	521 mg
Potassium	565 mg

Excellent: Thiamine; Niacin; Vitamin B6
Good: Riboflavin; Vitamin B12; Folate; Iron

CHICKEN FAJITAS

This Eastern-flavoured adaptation of fajitas is perfect for a Super Bowl or World Series party instead of chili or whatever you had last year! You can use pita breads and fill the pockets with the chicken, vegetables and lettuce. Add vegetables such as red pepper strips if you wish.

Makes 8 servings

8 small boneless, skinless single chicken breasts
    (about 3 oz/90 g each)
1 tbsp (15 mL) hoisin sauce
1 tbsp (15 mL) honey
1 tbsp (15 mL) dark sesame oil
1 tbsp (15 mL) minced fresh ginger root
1 tsp (5 mL) hot Asian chili paste
2 cloves garlic, minced
1 lb (500 g) Asian eggplant or zucchini (about 4),
    cut lengthwise in 1/4-inch (5 mm) slices
2 large onions, sliced
8 10-inch (25 cm) whole wheat or regular flour tortillas
1/3 cup (75 mL) hoisin sauce
2 cups (500 mL) shredded lettuce
1/4 cup (50 mL) chopped fresh cilantro or parsley

1. Pat chicken dry. Combine 1 tbsp (15 mL) hoisin sauce, honey, sesame oil, ginger, chili paste and garlic. Combine half of sauce with chicken and marinate in refrigerator until ready to cook.

2. Brush remaining marinade on eggplant and onion slices. Grill eggplant and onions for a few minutes on each side until browned and cooked through.

3. Grill chicken for 3 to 4 minutes per side, or until browned and cooked through, but do not overcook. Cut vegetables and chicken into 2-inch (5 cm) pieces and toss together if you wish, or leave in large pieces.

4. To warm tortillas, wrap in foil and place in a preheated 350°F (180°C) oven for 5 to 10 minutes, or until warm.

5. To assemble, spread a spoonful of hoisin sauce over middle of each tortilla. Place chicken and vegetable mixture in centre. Top with lettuce and cilantro. Fold up bottom, fold in sides and continue to roll up to enclose filling.

PER SERVING

Calories	340
Protein	26 g
Fat	7 g
Saturates	1 g
Cholesterol	53 mg
Carbohydrate	41 g
Fibre	4 g
Sodium	444 mg
Potassium	497 mg

Excellent: Niacin; Vitamin B6

CHICKEN TAGINE WITH GREEN OLIVES AND PRESERVED LEMONS

We all really love this recipe. A tagine is a Moroccan cooking vessel with a funnel-like top traditionally used for cooking but now mostly used as a serving dish.

Makes 6 servings

1 3-lb (1.5 kg) chicken, cut in 8 to 10 pieces, skin removed
1 tsp (5 mL) salt
1 tsp (5 mL) pepper
1 tsp (5 mL) paprika
1/4 tsp (1 mL) saffron threads, crushed
1/4 tsp (1 mL) cayenne
1 tbsp (15 mL) olive oil
2 large onions, sliced
3 cloves garlic, finely chopped
1/4 tsp (1 mL) hot red pepper flakes
1 cup (250 mL) pitted green olives
1 cup (250 mL) pitted black olives
1 preserved lemon, thinly sliced, or
     1 tbsp (15 mL) grated lemon peel
1/3 cup (75 mL) chopped fresh parsley, divided
1/3 cup (75 mL) chopped fresh cilantro, divided
1 lemon, thinly sliced

1. Pat chicken pieces dry. Combine salt, pepper, paprika, saffron and cayenne and rub into chicken. Marinate for a few hours in refrigerator.
2. Heat oil in a Dutch oven on medium-high heat. Cook chicken (in batches if necessary) for about 5 to 8 minutes per side, or until browned. Remove chicken from pan.
3. Return pan to heat. Add onions and cook for 8 to 10 minutes, or until brown. Stir in garlic and hot pepper flakes.
4. Return chicken to pan in a single layer and spoon some onions over top. Sprinkle with olives, preserved lemon and half the parsley and cilantro.
5. Roast chicken in a preheated 350°F (180°C) oven for 30 to 40 minutes, or until chicken is cooked through.
6. Serve chicken sprinkled with remaining fresh parsley and cilantro and fresh lemon slices.

PRESERVED LEMONS
Preserved lemons are sold in Middle Eastern stores, but you can also make your own. Simply cut several lemons into quarters lengthwise, leaving the stem end attached. Open up lemons slightly, fill with kosher salt and pack tightly into a preserving jar. Cover with freshly squeezed lemon juice and refrigerate, covered, for 3 weeks before using. Discard the pulp and use the sliced peel.

PER SERVING

Calories	246
Protein	25 g
Fat	13 g
Saturates	3 g
Cholesterol	72 mg
Carbohydrate	8 g
Fibre	2 g
Sodium	910 mg
Potassium	330 mg

Excellent: Niacin; Vitamin B6
Good: Iron

CHICKEN TAGINE WITH DRIED FRUITS

If you can find sour dried apricots, use them instead of the sweet ones. Look for them in health food stores or Middle Eastern stores.

Makes 6 servings

1 3-lb (1.5 kg) chicken, cut in 8 pieces, skin removed
1 tsp (5 mL) salt
1/2 tsp (2 mL) ground ginger
1/2 tsp (2 mL) ground cinnamon
1/2 tsp (2 mL) pepper
Pinch saffron threads
1 tbsp (15 mL) olive oil
2 onions, sliced
2 cloves garlic, finely chopped
1 tbsp (15 mL) chopped fresh ginger root
1 lb (500 g) baby carrots
1/2 cup (125 mL) dried apricots
1/2 cup (125 mL) pitted dates, halved
1/2 cup (125 mL) pitted prunes
1 cup (250 mL) water
1 tbsp (15 mL) honey
2 cups (500 mL) cooked chickpeas, or 1 19-oz (540 mL) can chickpeas, rinsed and drained
1 tbsp (15 mL) lemon juice
2 tbsp (25 mL) sliced almonds, toasted (page 464)
2 tbsp (25 mL) chopped fresh parsley or cilantro

PER SERVING	
Calories	420
Protein	30 g
Fat	11 g
Saturates	2 g
Cholesterol	72 mg
Carbohydrate	54 g
Fibre	8 g
Sodium	639 mg
Potassium	977 mg

Excellent: Vitamin A; Niacin; Vitamin B6; Folate; Iron
Good: Thiamine; Riboflavin; Vitamin B12

1. Pat chicken dry. Combine salt, ground ginger, cinnamon, pepper and saffron. Rub into chicken.
2. Heat oil in a Dutch oven on medium-high heat. Cook chicken for 5 to 8 minutes per side, or until browned. Remove from pan.
3. Add onions, garlic and ginger root to pan and cook for 5 to 10 minutes, or until browned. Add carrots, apricots, dates, prunes, water and honey and bring to a boil.
4. Return chicken pieces to pan, cover and transfer to a preheated 350°F (180°C) oven. Bake for 20 minutes. Add chickpeas, cover and cook for 15 minutes longer, or until chicken is just cooked through.
5. Stir in lemon juice. Taste and adjust seasonings if necessary. Sprinkle with almonds and parsley.

COQ AU VIN

Coq au vin is one of those delicious comfort-food dishes that is making a big comeback. It is easy to make and can be prepared ahead and reheated, so it is great for entertaining. It is traditionally made with white and dark meat, but you can use just the breasts— do not overcook them.

If you prefer, just use brown cremini mushrooms to reduce the expense. Slice them if they are large.

This recipe can be halved.

Makes 8 to 10 servings

2 3-lb (1.5 kg) chickens, cut in 4 pieces each, skin removed
1/2 cup (125 mL) all-purpose flour
1/2 tsp (2 mL) salt
1/4 tsp (1 mL) pepper
1 tbsp (15 mL) olive oil, or 2 slices bacon,
        cut in 1-inch (2.5 cm) pieces
1/4 cup (50 mL) brandy, optional
24 pearl onions or shallots, peeled
24 cloves garlic, peeled but left whole
1 lb (500 g) wild mushrooms, trimmed
4 large carrots, sliced thickly on diagonal
1 cup (250 mL) dry red wine or stock
2 cups (500 mL) homemade beef stock (page 109) or
        chicken stock
1 bay leaf
1 tbsp (15 mL) chopped fresh thyme, or pinch dried
1 tbsp (15 mL) chopped fresh rosemary, or pinch dried
1 tbsp (15 mL) chopped fresh tarragon, or pinch dried
1/4 cup (50 mL) chopped fresh parsley

1. Pat chicken pieces dry. In a shallow dish, combine flour, salt and pepper. Coat chicken pieces with mixture, dusting off any excess. (You'll have to discard excess flour, but it is much easier to work with more than you need.)

2. Heat olive oil in a large, deep non-stick skillet or Dutch oven on medium-high heat. Cook chicken pieces, in batches if necessary, for about 5 minutes per side, or until brown. (If you are using bacon, brown bacon pieces. Remove bacon and reserve. Discard fat, but do not wash pan. Brown chicken in same pan.)

PEELING PEARL ONIONS

To peel pearl onions or shallots more easily, trim them and immerse in boiling water for 1 minute. Cool under cold water and peel.

PER SERVING

Calories	342
Protein	48 g
Fat	9 g
Saturates	2 g
Cholesterol	144 mg
Carbohydrate	15 g
Fibre	3 g
Sodium	279 mg
Potassium	869 mg

Excellent: Vitamin A; Riboflavin; Niacin; Vitamin B6; Vitamin B12; Iron
Good: Thiamine; Folate

3. Return all chicken to pan and sprinkle with brandy if using. Flambé. Once flames subside, remove chicken from pan. (Do not worry if flambé doesn't work. Alcohol will evaporate when sauce comes to a boil.)

4. Add onions, garlic, mushrooms and carrots to pan. Cook for about 8 minutes, or until brown.

5. Add wine and bring to a boil. Scrape up browned bits from bottom of pan. Add stock, bay leaf, thyme, rosemary and tarragon. Add chicken. Bring to a boil and reduce heat. Cook gently, covered, for about 45 minutes.

6. Remove chicken and vegetables to a serving platter. Cover to keep warm. Discard bay leaf. Spoon fat from surface of pan juices.

7. Bring juices to a simmer and cook, uncovered, until thickened. Pour sauce over chicken. Sprinkle with parsley.

Boeuf Bourguignon

Use stewing beef instead of chicken. Cut 2-lb (1 kg) stewing beef into chunks and cook with vegetables for 2 hours, or until beef is very tender.

FLAMBÉS

Food is flambéed for three reasons. First, flambéing burns off most of the alcohol in a dish, making it sweeter and less harsh tasting.

Another reason to flambé is to lightly singe the top of the food to seal in flavour and make a crust.

The third reason to flambé is for show.

To flambé, you can heat the alcohol in a small pot. Standing back, light a long match and hold it over the pot at the edge of the pan until the evaporating fumes ignite the alcohol. Pour the flaming alcohol over the dish and wait for the flames to die down before serving.

You can also flambé food right in the pan. Drizzle the alcohol on top of the hot food and, standing back, light it with a long match. The hot alcohol should ignite in 2 to 10 seconds. If it doesn't work, don't worry. (Don't try to flambé something more than once or twice, or the dish will taste too boozy.)

FLAMBÉ TIPS

- Turn off the smoke alarm.
- Tie back long hair.
- Never pour alcohol directly from the bottle. Pour the amount you need into a glass first, and keep the bottle away from the heat.
- The alcohol doesn't always ignite right away, so continue to stand back while you are flambéing.
- Make sure no alcohol is spilled, otherwise you may have "table flambé"!

ASIAN CHICKEN CHILI

This dish combines Eastern flavours with Western ideas. It is old-fashioned comfort food updated with international ingredients and a lighter style.

Serve it over steamed rice or couscous.

Makes 8 to 10 servings

1 tbsp (15 mL) vegetable oil
2 tbsp (25 mL) finely chopped fresh ginger root
6 green onions, chopped
3 cloves garlic, finely chopped
2 sweet red peppers, seeded and diced
2 tsp (10 mL) hot Asian chili paste, or to taste
1 lb (500 g) boneless, skinless chicken breasts, diced,
    or ground chicken
1 28-oz (796 mL) can plum tomatoes, drained and pureed
4 cups (1 L) cooked red kidney beans, or
    2 19-oz (540 mL) cans, rinsed and drained
2 tbsp (25 mL) soy sauce
1 tbsp (15 mL) rice wine
1 tsp (5 mL) dark sesame oil
1/2 cup (125 mL) chopped fresh cilantro or parsley

1. Heat vegetable oil in a large, deep non-stick skillet or wok on medium heat. Add ginger, green onions and garlic and cook gently for 30 seconds, or until fragrant. Add red peppers and chili paste and cook for a few minutes.

2. Pat chicken dry and add chicken to skillet. Cook, stirring constantly, for about 5 minutes, until chicken pieces are white on outside.

3. Add tomatoes and bring to a boil. Reduce heat and simmer gently for 30 minutes, or until mixture is quite thick and almost all juices have evaporated.

4. Stir in beans, soy sauce and rice wine. Cook for 10 minutes.

5. Stir in sesame oil and cilantro. Taste and adjust seasonings if necessary.

SESAME OIL

The sesame oil used in this book is dark, fragrant roasted sesame oil. Do not confuse it with the unflavoured golden sesame oil. Once the oil is opened, store it in the refrigerator.

Dark sesame oil is used in small quantities, as the flavour is very intense. It is usually used as a last-minute seasoning in stir-fries, salad dressings, dips, etc., but is rarely used for sauteing.

PER SERVING

Calories	229
Protein	22 g
Fat	4 g
Saturates	1 g
Cholesterol	33 mg
Carbohydrate	27 g
Fibre	10 g
Sodium	358 mg
Potassium	780 mg

Excellent: Vitamin C; Niacin; Iron; Vitamin B6; Folate
Good: Vitamin A; Thiamine

CHICKEN WITH FORTY CLOVES OF GARLIC

Some people are actually afraid of the forty cloves of garlic in this recipe (once in a large class I had to triple the amount, and students really went ballistic!). But it is as I always say—the longer garlic cooks, the milder and sweeter it becomes.

This is a good make-ahead dish, as it tastes even better after sitting in its juices overnight and being reheated. Serve the chicken over mashed potatoes with some of the juices and lots of garlic. Although it is not traditional, Goat Cheese Cream is sensational drizzled over the chicken (it is also great on baked potatoes).

Makes 6 servings

1 3-lb (1.5 kg) chicken, cut in pieces, skin removed
1 tbsp (15 mL) olive oil
40 cloves garlic, peeled but left whole
10 shallots, peeled (page 248), optional
3 tbsp (45 mL) Cognac or brandy
½ tsp (2 mL) salt
½ tsp (2 mL) pepper
¾ cup (175 mL) dry white wine or
     homemade chicken stock (page 109)
2 tbsp (25 mL) chopped fresh chives or green onions, optional

1. Pat chicken pieces dry. Heat oil in a large, deep non-stick skillet on medium-high heat. Cook chicken pieces, in batches if necessary, for about 5 minutes per side, or until brown.
2. Add garlic cloves and shallots and shake pan well to move cloves under chicken a bit. Cook for another 10 to 15 minutes, or until garlic and shallots brown lightly.
3. Discard any fat from pan. Pour in Cognac and flambé if desired (page 427).
4. Add salt, pepper and wine. Bring to a boil, cover, reduce heat and simmer gently for 30 minutes. Sprinkle with chives before serving.

PER SERVING

Calories	192
Protein	25 g
Fat	6 g
Saturates	1 g
Cholesterol	76 mg
Carbohydrate	7 g
Fibre	trace
Sodium	280 mg
Potassium	355 mg

Excellent: Niacin; Vitamin B6

CHICKEN POT PIE

Chicken pot pie is great with a biscuit or phyllo pastry crust, but I love it topped with mashed potatoes or mashed sweet potatoes (page 341).

You can also make this with leftover turkey.

Makes 8 to 10 servings

2 tbsp (25 mL) olive oil
½ lb (250 g) mushrooms, quartered
2 leeks or onions, trimmed and chopped
1 cup (250 mL) diced carrots
⅓ cup (75 mL) all-purpose flour
2 cups (500 mL) homemade chicken stock (page 109) or milk
1 tbsp (15 mL) chopped fresh thyme, or ½ tsp (2 mL) dried
½ tsp (2 mL) pepper
¼ tsp (1 mL) hot red pepper sauce
Salt to taste
4 cups (1 L) diced cooked chicken breast
½ cup (125 mL) corn kernels
1 cup (250 mL) peas
¼ cup (50 mL) diced pimento or
        roasted sweet red pepper (page 146)

Cheddar Mashed Potato Topping

2 lb (1 kg) baking potatoes, peeled and cut in 2-inch (5 cm) pieces
¾ cup (175 mL) milk, hot
¼ tsp (1 mL) pepper
Salt to taste
¾ cup (175 mL) grated light Cheddar cheese
1 tsp (5 mL) paprika

1. Heat oil in a large saucepan or Dutch oven on medium heat. Add mushrooms, leeks and carrots. Cook for a few minutes. Sprinkle with flour and cook gently for 5 minutes, but do not brown.
2. Whisk in stock and bring to a boil. Reduce heat and add thyme, pepper, hot pepper sauce and salt. Simmer gently for 10 minutes, stirring occasionally.
3. Stir in chicken, corn, peas and pimento. Taste and adjust seasonings if necessary.

PER SERVING	
Calories	333
Protein	31 g
Fat	9 g
Saturates	3 g
Cholesterol	68 mg
Carbohydrate	32 g
Fibre	3 g
Sodium	184 mg
Potassium	735 mg

Excellent: Vitamin A; Niacin; Vitamin B6
Good: Thiamine; Riboflavin; Iron; Folate; Vitamin B12

4. To make topping, cook potatoes in a large pot of boiling water until tender. Drain well and pat dry. Mash. Beat in hot milk, pepper, salt and cheese. Taste and adjust seasonings if necessary. (Add more milk if necessary so that you can spread potatoes.)

5. Spoon chicken mixture into a lightly oiled 3-qt (3 L) casserole dish. Pipe or spoon potato mixture over chicken and sprinkle with paprika.

6. Bake in a preheated 400°F (200°C) oven for 30 to 35 minutes, or until hot and bubbly.

CHICKEN

- Keep chicken refrigerated and use it quickly, or freeze it. Uncooked chicken might be contaminated with salmonella or other bacteria; defrost it in the refrigerator or in the microwave but never at room temperature, as that's when bacteria can grow most quickly.

- Prepare chicken on an easy-to-sanitize cutting board, and wash the board, counter, utensils and your hands carefully afterwards. If you are barbecuing, take care to keep the cooked chicken away from any uncooked juices or marinades.

- I usually remove the skin from chicken before cooking. I often leave the breast on the bones, however, as the bones help to keep the meat juicy when there is no skin. Save any raw skin and bones to use in chicken stock (page 109).

- Chicken and turkey should be thoroughly cooked (to at least 165°F/74°C), but if you are using skinless, boneless chicken breasts, be careful not to overcook them, as they can easily become dry and tough.

- Ground chicken is very perishable, so use it the same day you buy it or freeze it. Most storebought ground chicken is made from both light and dark meat, and it can even contain skin or fat. If you have a food processor, grind boneless, skinless chicken breasts yourself so you know that the chicken is fresh and lean (or ask your butcher to do this for you).

- One of my favourite ways to roast a chicken is on a vertical roasting rack. You slip the chicken onto the rack and place it in a roasting pan lined with foil or parchment paper. Because the rack conducts heat to the inside of the bird, the chicken cooks faster, and any fat drains off.

BREADED CHICKEN FINGERS

In my constant attempt to cook things that my children would eat when they were little, I kept trying to make chicken fingers that were not deep-fried but still delicious. This is a great version.

Instead of breadcrumbs you could use your children's favourite crackers or cereal to make the crumbs (or use half crackers or cereal and half breadcrumbs). Make the crumbs in the food processor or place the crackers or cereal in a plastic bag and crush with a rolling pin. Panko breadcrumbs (page 204) also make the chicken very crisp.

You can bake whole chicken breasts this way (just bake for about 10 minutes longer). Serve with a dipping sauce.

Makes 4 to 6 servings
1 tsp (5 mL) vegetable oil
1 lb (500 g) boneless, skinless chicken breasts
$^1/_3$ cup (75 mL) yogurt cheese (page 391) or light mayonnaise
1 tbsp (15 mL) ketchup
1 tsp (5 mL) Dijon mustard
$^1/_2$ tsp (2 mL) Worcestershire sauce
$^1/_4$ tsp (1 mL) pepper
1$^1/_2$ cups (375 mL) dry whole wheat breadcrumbs, cracker crumbs
    or crushed cereal

1. Brush a baking sheet with vegetable oil and place in a preheated 400°F (200°C) oven.
2. Pat chicken dry and cut each breast into 4 or 5 strips.
3. In a large bowl, combine yogurt cheese, ketchup, mustard, Worcestershire and pepper. Add chicken pieces and coat well.
4. Place breadcrumbs on a large plate. Roll chicken fingers in crumbs one at a time and pat in.
5. Place chicken in a single layer on hot baking sheet and bake for 15 minutes. Turn and bake for 10 to 12 minutes longer, or until crisp and cooked through.

PLUM DIPPING SAUCE
Combine $^1/_4$ cup (50 mL) plum sauce, 1 tsp (5 mL) soy sauce and $^1/_2$ tsp (2 mL) ground ginger.
    Makes about $^1/_4$ cup (50 mL).

HONEY GARLIC DIPPING SAUCE
Combine $^1/_4$ cup (50 mL) honey, 1 tbsp (15 mL) soy sauce and 1 minced clove garlic.
    Makes about $^1/_4$ cup (50 mL).

PER SERVING

Calories	279
Protein	34 g
Fat	4 g
Saturates	1 g
Cholesterol	68 mg
Carbohydrate	27 g
Fibre	3 g
Sodium	411 mg
Potassium	480 mg

Excellent: Niacin; Vitamin B6
Good: Riboflavin; Vitamin B12; Iron

CHICKEN ADOBO

This version of the famous Filipino dish is from Dely Balagtas, who works with me at the cooking school. Children like it, too (even mine!). Serve it with steamed rice and any plain vegetable.

Cooking chicken breasts with the bone in keeps them juicier and more flavourful. You can also use one whole chicken in this recipe; cut it into serving pieces and remove the skin.

Makes 4 servings

1 tbsp (15 mL) vegetable oil
1 large onion, cut in 1/4-inch (5 mm) slices
4 single chicken breasts, bone in, skin removed
3 cloves garlic, finely chopped
3 tbsp (45 mL) lemon juice or white vinegar
2 tbsp (25 mL) soy sauce
1/4 cup (50 mL) water
1/2 tsp (2 mL) pepper
1 bay leaf

PER SERVING	
Calories	198
Protein	31 g
Fat	5 g
Saturates	1 g
Cholesterol	76 mg
Carbohydrate	5 g
Fibre	1 g
Sodium	504 mg
Potassium	422 mg

Excellent: Niacin;
Vitamin B6
Good: Vitamin B12

1. Heat oil in a large, deep non-stick skillet on medium-high heat. Add onion and cook for 8 to 10 minutes, or until browned. Remove from pan.
2. Add chicken, garlic, lemon juice, soy sauce, water and pepper to skillet. Stir everything together well. Add bay leaf. Cook gently, covered, for 25 to 30 minutes.
3. Return onion to skillet. Continue to cook, uncovered, until chicken is cooked through and tender, about 5 to 10 minutes. Taste and adjust seasonings if necessary.

CHICKEN "MEATLOAF"

I love this served hot with mashed potatoes, peas and tomato sauce or ketchup, but it is also delicious cold. Try it in sandwiches with grilled onions, peppers and pesto (page 167). You can also make chicken burgers with this mixture. Or use extra-lean ground beef instead of the chicken for a traditional meatloaf.

Makes 8 servings

2 tsp (10 mL) olive oil
1 onion, chopped
2 cloves garlic, finely chopped
2 lb (1 kg) lean ground chicken breast
1 egg
2 egg whites, or 1 whole egg
1/2 cup (125 mL) ketchup
1 tbsp (15 mL) Worcestershire sauce
1 tbsp (15 mL) Dijon mustard
1 tsp (5 mL) hot Asian chili paste
1 tsp (5 mL) salt
1/2 tsp (2 mL) pepper
1 cup (250 mL) fresh whole wheat or regular breadcrumbs
2 tbsp (25 mL) chopped fresh basil or parsley
2 tbsp (25 mL) chopped fresh chives or green onion

1. Heat oil in a non-stick skillet on medium heat. Add onion and garlic and cook gently for a few minutes until fragrant but not brown. Cool.
2. In a large bowl, combine chicken, egg, egg whites, ketchup, Worcestershire, mustard, hot chili paste, salt, pepper, breadcrumbs and onion mixture. Knead everything together. Mix in basil and chives.
3. Spoon mixture into a lightly oiled or parchment-lined 9- x 5-inch (2 L) loaf pan. Cover with parchment paper or foil.
4. Bake in a preheated 350°F (180°C) oven for 1 hour. Uncover and bake for 20 minutes longer. Cool for a few minutes. Drain off any liquid accumulated in pan. Unmould and serve hot, or cool in pan and unmould before serving.

PER SERVING	
Calories	189
Protein	29 g
Fat	4 g
Saturates	1 g
Cholesterol	93 mg
Carbohydrate	9 g
Fibre	1 g
Sodium	665 mg
Potassium	443 mg
Excellent: Niacin; Vitamin B6	
Good: Vitamin B12	

FLATTENED CHICKEN BREASTS WITH ROASTED GARLIC COUSCOUS

If you don't have roasted garlic, use 1 chopped clove garlic gently cooked in 1 tbsp (15 mL) olive oil. Or stir 2 tbsp (25 mL) pesto (page 167) into the Israeli couscous instead of the garlic paste.

Makes 6 servings

6 boneless, skinless single chicken breasts (about 4 oz/125 g each)
1 tbsp (15 mL) olive oil
2 tbsp (25 mL) orange juice concentrate
1 tsp (5 mL) ground cumin
2 cloves garlic, minced
½ tsp (2 mL) salt
½ tsp (2 mL) pepper

Roasted Garlic Couscous

4 cups (1 L) homemade chicken stock (page 109) or water
½ lb (250 g) Israeli couscous (page 357) or orzo
        (about 2 cups/500 mL)
1 head roasted garlic (page 67), pureed (about 2 tbsp/25 mL)
Salt and pepper to taste

PER SERVING

Calories	392
Protein	37 g
Fat	5 g
Saturates	1 g
Cholesterol	71 mg
Carbohydrate	46 g
Fibre	3 g
Sodium	238 mg
Potassium	447 mg

Excellent: Niacin; Vitamin B6
Good: Vitamin B12; Iron

1. Remove filets (tender strips on the underside of breasts) from chicken and freeze to use in stir-fries or chicken fingers. Pat chicken dry. Place chicken breasts in a heavy plastic bag, one at a time, and pound until about ½ inch (1 cm) thick.
2. In a small bowl, combine oil, orange juice concentrate, cumin, garlic, salt and pepper. Rub mixture into chicken breasts. Marinate for 10 minutes or up to overnight in refrigerator.
3. Grill chicken for 3 to 5 minutes per side, or just until cooked through.
4. Meanwhile, to prepare couscous, in a saucepan, bring stock to a boil. Add couscous and cook for 10 minutes, or until tender.
5. Stir garlic puree into couscous. Season with salt and pepper. Place couscous in a serving dish and arrange chicken on top.

TWIST AND SHOUT CHICKEN DRUMSTICKS

My kids were enthralled when they first had Shake 'n' Bake chicken at a school potluck lunch. Because we don't use commercial mixes at home, they weren't familiar with the name; they said it sounded something like "twist and shout" chicken, and that's what we've been calling this dish ever since.

Drumsticks are often overlooked, but they are popular with children and have less fat than chicken wings. Try using them in your favourite chicken wing recipe.

You can also make this with chicken breasts.

Makes 6 servings

12 chicken drumsticks (about 3 oz/90 g each), skin removed
½ cup (125 mL) orange juice or buttermilk
2 cloves garlic, minced
1 cup (250 mL) dry whole wheat or regular breadcrumbs
2 tbsp (25 mL) cornmeal
1 tbsp (15 mL) paprika
1 tbsp (15 mL) granulated sugar
1 tsp (5 mL) chili powder
1 tsp (5 mL) salt
1 tsp (5 mL) dry mustard
½ tsp (2 mL) ground cumin
½ tsp (2 mL) cayenne, optional

1. Pat drumsticks dry and toss with orange juice and garlic. Marinate for 10 minutes. Shake off excess liquid.
2. Meanwhile, in a plastic bag, combine breadcrumbs, cornmeal, paprika, sugar, chili powder, salt, mustard, cumin and cayenne.
3. Add drumsticks to plastic bag and shake in seasoned breadcrumbs until coated. Place on a non-stick or parchment-lined baking sheet.
4. Bake in a preheated 350°F (180°C) oven for 40 to 45 minutes, or until cooked through, brown and crisp.

PER SERVING (2 DRUM-STICKS)	
Calories	197
Protein	20 g
Fat	6 g
Saturates	2 g
Cholesterol	66 mg
Carbohydrate	14 g
Fibre	2 g
Sodium	344 mg
Potassium	251 mg

Excellent: Niacin
Good: Riboflavin; Vitamin B6

BREADED CHICKEN CUTLETS WITH TOMATO SAUCE

These chicken cutlets also make wonderful sandwiches served on whole wheat buns with the tomato sauce. Or you can just serve the cutlets plain topped with a little freshly squeezed lemon juice, or slice them into strips and serve on a green or Caesar salad (page 121) or with a dip.

Makes 4 servings

4 boneless, skinless single chicken breasts (about 4 oz/125 g each)
¹/₂ cup (125 mL) whole wheat or all-purpose flour
1 tsp (5 mL) paprika
¹/₂ tsp (2 mL) ground cumin
¹/₄ tsp (1 mL) salt
Pinch pepper
1 egg
2 cups (500 mL) fresh whole wheat or panko breadcrumbs (page 204)
2 tbsp (25 mL) finely chopped fresh parsley
1 tsp (5 mL) chopped fresh thyme, or pinch dried
2 tbsp (25 mL) olive oil
1 lemon
1 recipe tomato sauce (page 151) or cherry tomato sauce (page 176)

PER SERVING	
Calories	385
Protein	34 g
Fat	15 g
Saturates	3 g
Cholesterol	113 mg
Carbohydrate	31 g
Fibre	5 g
Sodium	657 mg
Potassium	947 mg

Excellent: Niacin; Vitamin B6; Vitamin C
Good: Vitamin A; Thiamine; Riboflavin; Vitamin B12; Folate; Iron

1. Remove filets from chicken breasts (page 257) and save for chicken fingers or stir-fries. Pat chicken dry. Place in a heavy plastic bag, one at a time, and pound until ¹/₂ inch (1 crn) thick.
2. In a wide shallow dish, combine flour, paprika, cumin, salt and pepper.
3. In another shallow dish, beat egg lightly. In a third dish, combine breadcrumbs, parsley and thyme.
4. Dip chicken in flour mixture and shake off excess. Dip chicken into egg and allow excess to run off. Pat breadcrumb mixture into chicken. If not cooking right away, place chicken on a rack set over a baking sheet (so that chicken does not get soggy on bottom) and refrigerate.
5. Place chicken in a single layer on a baking sheet lined with parchment paper. Drizzle with oil. Bake in a preheated 400°F (200°C) oven for 20 to 25 minutes, depending on thickness, or until cooked through and crispy.
6. Place chicken on a platter and squeeze lemon juice over top. Serve with tomato sauce.

ROAST CHICKEN WITH BULGUR STUFFING

This bulgur stuffing can be cooked separately and served on its own as a side dish, or you can omit the stuffing altogether.

To turn the chicken easily I use True Blues (they come in pink now, too!)—thick rubber gloves that are great for washing dishes in really hot water and for rubbing the skins off peppers, peeling hot beets or potatoes, or transferring a roast to a carving board. The gloves are heat-resistant but don't touch hot pans with them, or they will melt.

Makes 6 servings

Bulgur Stuffing

2 tsp (10 mL) olive oil
2 onions, chopped
1 clove garlic, finely chopped
2 stalks celery, chopped
1/4 cup (50 mL) chopped dried apricots
2 tbsp (25 mL) raisins
1 tbsp (15 mL) pine nuts, toasted (page 219)
1 cup (250 mL) bulgur
2 cups (500 mL) homemade chicken stock (page 109) or water, hot
1/2 tsp (2 mL) salt
1/2 tsp (2 mL) pepper
1/4 cup (50 mL) chopped fresh parsley

Roast Chicken

1 3-lb (1.5 kg) chicken
1 tbsp (15 mL) soy sauce
1 tbsp (15 mL) apricot jam

1. To prepare stuffing, heat oil in a large saucepan on medium heat. Add onions and garlic and cook gently for 5 minutes. Add celery, apricots, raisins and pine nuts. Cook for 2 minutes.
2. Add bulgur, hot stock, salt and pepper and bring to a boil. Reduce heat, cover and cook on low heat for 10 minutes, or until bulgur is just tender and liquid has been absorbed. Stir in parsley and taste and adjust seasonings if necessary. Cool.
3. Pat chicken dry inside and out. Stuff with bulgur mixture and place any remaining stuffing in a lightly oiled baking dish. Truss chicken if you wish.

PER SERVING

(stuffing and chicken, no skin)

Calories	312
Protein	30 g
Fat	9 g
Saturates	2 g
Cholesterol	73 mg
Carbohydrate	29 g
Fibre	6 g
Sodium	291 mg
Potassium	549 mg

Excellent: Niacin; Vitamin B6
Good: Iron; Folate; Vitamin B12

PER SERVING

(stuffing and chicken, with skin)

Calories	406
Protein	33 g
Fat	17 g
Saturates	4 g
Cholesterol	88 mg
Carbohydrate	31 g
Fibre	6 g
Sodium	442 mg
Potassium	581 mg

Excellent: Niacin; Vitamin B6
Good: Riboflavin; Folate; Vitamin B12; Iron

4. Combine soy sauce and jam. Brush on chicken.

5. Roast chicken in a preheated 375°F (190°C) oven for 1¼ to 1½ hours, or until juices run clear and a meat thermometer inserted into stuffing reads 165°F (74°C). Check chicken after 45 minutes and if it is browning too much, reduce oven temperature to 325°F (160°C) and cover chicken lightly with a tent of foil. After chicken has cooked for 45 minutes, place dish of extra stuffing, covered, in oven to heat.

6. Carve chicken and serve with stuffing.

Lemon Roast Chicken

For a plain old-fashioned roast chicken, buy the best chicken you can find (organic or naturally raised), sprinkle it with coarse salt and a bit of pepper and place a pierced lemon in the cavity. Truss chicken if you wish. Roast in a preheated 400°F (200°C) oven for 1 to 1¼ hours for a 3- to 4-lb (1.5 to 2 kg) chicken (until a meat thermometer inserted into thigh reads 165°F/74°C).

Makes 4 to 6 servings.

MUSAKHAN (ROAST CHICKEN WITH ONIONS AND PINE NUTS ON PITA)

On a recent culinary mission to Israel, I visited an Arab high school where the kids in the culinary program cooked a version of this Middle Eastern recipe for us. It is a real winner.

This is my interpretation. The roast chicken is served over pita and topped with pine nuts and onions, and the juices soak into the pita for an amazing taste.

Ground sumac is a spice made from crushed sumac berries. It adds a tart, citrusy flavour to Middle Eastern dishes and can be found in Middle Eastern markets. If you can't find it, substitute lemon juice and lemon peel.

Makes 6 servings

2 tbsp (25 mL) lemon juice
2 tbsp (25 mL) olive oil, divided
2 tbsp (25 mL) ground sumac
1 tbsp (15 mL) sweet smoked paprika (page 228)
1/2 tsp (2 mL) salt
1/4 tsp (1 mL) ground cloves
1/4 tsp (1 mL) ground allspice
1/4 tsp (1 mL) ground cinnamon
1/4 tsp (1 mL) ground turmeric
1/4 tsp (1 mL) ground nutmeg
1 3- to 4-lb (2 kg) chicken, skin removed, cut in 8 to 10 pieces
4 large onions, thinly sliced
4 cloves garlic, finely chopped
Salt and pepper to taste
6 4-inch (10 cm) whole wheat or regular pita breads
    (or 3 larger pitas cut in half)
2 tbsp (25 mL) pine nuts
1/4 cup (50 mL) chopped fresh cilantro or parsley

1. Combine lemon juice and 1 tbsp (15 mL) oil. Stir in sumac, paprika, salt, cloves, allspice, cinnamon, turmeric and nutmeg.
2. Pat chicken dry and rub paste into chicken. Arrange chicken in a single layer on a baking sheet lined with parchment paper. Roast in a preheated 375°F (190°C) oven for 20 to 30 minutes, or until chicken is almost cooked.

PER SERVING	
Calories	331
Protein	28 g
Fat	13 g
Saturates	3 g
Cholesterol	72 mg
Carbohydrate	27 g
Fibre	4 g
Sodium	418 mg
Potassium	458 mg

Excellent: Niacin; Vitamin B6
Good: Thiamine; Vitamin B12; Iron

3. Meanwhile, heat remaining 1 tbsp (15 mL) oil in a large skillet on medium-high heat. Add onions and garlic and cook for 10 to 15 minutes, or until tender and brown. Add juices from chicken to onions. Season with salt and pepper.

4. When chicken is ready, place pita breads in a single layer on baking sheets. Place half the onions (with their juices) on pitas. Top with chicken. Top with onions and pine nuts. Roast for 10 minutes longer.

5. Sprinkle with chopped cilantro.

BARBECUED CHICKEN FINGERS

This recipe is a hit with both children and adults. It can be served warm or cold, and you can leave the chicken breasts whole instead of cutting them into fingers.

I serve these over rice as a main course, or as an appetizer with a yogurt dip for the kids and a spicy salsa dip for the adults.

Makes 4 to 6 servings

1 lb (500 g) boneless, skinless chicken breasts
2 tbsp (25 mL) honey
2 tbsp (25 mL) lemon juice
1 tbsp (15 mL) ketchup or commercial chili sauce
1/4 tsp (1 mL) ground cumin
1/2 tsp (2 mL) salt

1. Pat chicken dry and cut each breast into 4 or 5 strips.
2. In a large bowl, combine honey, lemon juice, ketchup and cumin. Add chicken and marinate in refrigerator for up to 8 hours.
3. Just before cooking, stir salt into chicken mixture. Grill chicken pieces for 5 to 7 minutes per side, depending on thickness, until just cooked through.

PER SERVING	
Calories	151
Protein	26 g
Fat	2 g
Saturates	trace
Cholesterol	70 mg
Carbohydrate	8 g
Fibre	trace
Sodium	330 mg
Potassium	239 mg
Excellent: Niacin; Vitamin B6	

CHICKEN JAMBALAYA

This is a kid-friendly one-dish meal. Add other vegetables if you like. Serve it with cornbread (page 402) and a salad. For a spicier version, add a diced jalapeño to the onions. If you are using white rice, this will cook in the oven in only 20 minutes, and you can reduce the stock to 2 cups (500 mL).

Makes 6 servings

2 tbsp (25 mL) olive oil, divided
1 onion, chopped
2 cloves garlic, finely chopped
1 sweet red pepper, seeded and diced
1 sweet green pepper, seeded and diced
2 stalks celery, sliced
1 1/2 lb (750 g) boneless, skinless chicken breasts,
        cut in 1 1/2-inch (4 cm) cubes
2 tomatoes, peeled, seeded and diced
1 1/2 cups (375 mL) long-grain brown or white rice
1/2 cup (125 mL) tomato juice or tomato puree
2 1/2 cups (625 mL) homemade chicken stock (page 109)
        or water
1/2 tsp (2 mL) hot red pepper sauce
1 tsp (5 mL) salt
1/4 tsp (1 mL) pepper
1/4 tsp (1 mL) dried thyme
1/4 tsp (1 mL) dried oregano
1/4 tsp (1 mL) cayenne, optional
1/4 lb (125 g) medium shrimp, cleaned and butterflied, optional
2 green onions, thinly sliced on diagonal

1. Heat 1 tbsp (15 mL) oil in a Dutch oven or large, deep ovenproof skillet on medium heat. Add onion and garlic and cook gently for 3 to 5 minutes, or until tender and fragrant. Add sweet peppers and celery. Cook for 5 minutes. Remove vegetables from pan.

2. Heat remaining oil in pan. Pat chicken dry and cook on medium-high heat for a few minutes, stirring, until pieces brown a little on all sides.

3. Return vegetables to pan. Stir in tomatoes and rice. Cook, stirring, for 3 minutes.

4. Meanwhile, combine tomato juice, stock, hot pepper sauce, salt, pepper, thyme, oregano and cayenne. Stir well.

PEELING AND SEEDING TOMATOES

If you want to peel tomatoes (usually for aesthetic reasons, because the peel comes off when the tomatoes are cooked and can be unattractive in the finished dish), cut a small X in the bottom end and submerge the tomatoes in boiling water for 10 to 15 seconds. When the tomatoes are cool enough to handle, the skins should slip off easily. (Don't bother peeling cherry tomatoes.)

Seed raw tomatoes when you don't want a mixture to become too wet. Cut the tomato in half horizontally and gently squeeze out the seeds.

PER SERVING

Calories	385
Protein	34 g
Fat	8 g
Saturates	2 g
Cholesterol	71 mg
Carbohydrate	44 g
Fibre	5 g
Sodium	570 mg
Potassium	764 mg

Excellent: Niacin; Vitamin B6; Vitamin C
Good: Vitamin B12; Thiamine

5. Add liquid to pan and bring to a boil. Reduce heat, cover and bake in a preheated 350°F (180°C) oven for 30 to 35 minutes, or until liquid is absorbed and rice is tender.

6. Add shrimp, cover and bake for 5 to 10 minutes longer, or until shrimp are opaque and curled. Sprinkle with green onions.

CHICKEN BREASTS WITH BLACK BEAN SAUCE

Students often bring me wonderful recipes, and this dish from Irene Tam is one of the best, as it is so easy to prepare and the flavours are so dynamic. It is great served hot or cold, so it is perfect for picnics. The sauce can also be used on pork tenderloin, salmon (cook salmon for only 10 to 15 minutes, depending on thickness) or a whole roast chicken. Serve with steamed brown rice or couscous and steamed green vegetables.

Makes 6 servings

2 tbsp (25 mL) black bean sauce (page 73)
2 tbsp (25 mL) water
1 tsp (5 mL) orange juice concentrate
1/2 tsp (2 mL) hot Asian chili paste
1 tsp (5 mL) dark sesame oil, optional
6 single chicken breasts, bone-in, skin removed
2 tbsp (25 mL) chopped fresh cilantro or parsley

1. In a small bowl, combine black bean sauce, water, orange juice concentrate, hot chili paste and sesame oil.

2. Pat chicken breasts dry. Rub black bean mixture all over chicken and arrange chicken bone side down on a baking sheet lined with parchment paper.

3. Cover with foil and bake in a preheated 350°F (180°C) oven for 15 minutes. Uncover and bake for 15 to 20 minutes longer, or until chicken is cooked through. Sprinkle with cilantro before serving.

PER SERVING	
Calories	153
Protein	28 g
Fat	3 g
Saturates	1 g
Cholesterol	72 mg
Carbohydrate	1 g
Fibre	0 g
Sodium	105 mg
Potassium	363 mg

Excellent: Niacin; Vitamin B6
Good: Vitamin B12

ROAST CORNISH HENS WITH HERBS

This dish looks sophisticated yet comforting, so it is perfect for entertaining. To serve, place birds on a large platter lined with fresh sage or bay leaves. Garnish with lemon slices and serve with a rice pilaf or mashed potatoes. Fresh figs also make a lovely garnish.

Makes 8 servings

8 small Cornish hens (about 1 lb/500 g each)
16 cloves garlic, peeled but left whole
16 lemon wedges
2 tbsp (25 mL) olive oil
3 cloves garlic, minced
2 tbsp (25 mL) chopped fresh rosemary, or 1 tsp (5 mL) dried
2 tbsp (25 mL) chopped fresh sage, or 1 tsp (5 mL) dried
2 tbsp (25 mL) chopped fresh tarragon, or 1 tsp (5 mL) dried
2 tbsp (25 mL) chopped fresh thyme, or 1 tsp (5 mL) dried
1 tsp (5 mL) salt
1/2 tsp (2 mL) pepper
2 cups (500 mL) homemade chicken stock (page 109) or water
2 tbsp (25 mL) soy sauce
2 tbsp (25 mL) Worcestershire sauce
2 tbsp (25 mL) all-purpose flour
1 tbsp (15 mL) soft non-hydrogenated margarine or unsalted butter

1. Pat hens dry. Place 2 cloves garlic and 2 lemon wedges in each hen.
2. Combine oil, minced garlic, rosemary, sage, tarragon, thyme, salt and pepper. Gently separate skin from breast and thigh of each hen. Rub meat with herb mixture. Rub extra herb mixture over skin. Arrange birds on parchment-lined baking sheets.
3. Roast birds in a preheated 400°F (200°C) oven for 45 minutes, or until well browned and cooked through. Baste occasionally during roasting.
4. Place birds on a platter. Transfer pan juices to a wide saucepan and skim off fat. Add stock, soy sauce and Worcestershire to saucepan and bring to a boil. Cook for a few minutes.
5. In a small bowl, combine flour and margarine. Stir into sauce and cook for a few minutes until just slightly thickened. Taste and adjust seasonings. Serve hens with sauce.

PER SERVING (WITHOUT SKIN)	
Calories	322
Protein	43 g
Fat	13 g
Saturates	3 g
Cholesterol	182 mg
Carbohydrate	6 g
Fibre	0 g
Sodium	727 mg
Potassium	549 mg

Excellent: Riboflavin; Niacin; Vitamin B6; Vitamin B12; Zinc
Good: Iron

CUMIN

For the most flavourful cumin, buy cumin seeds rather than ground cumin. Toast the seeds in a dry skillet over medium-high heat for about 2 minutes, or until the seeds become slightly reddish and very aromatic. Cool, then grind the seeds in a spice grinder or with a mortar and pestle.

PER SERVING

Calories	185
Protein	24 g
Fat	7 g
Saturates	2 g
Cholesterol	86 mg
Carbohydrate	6 g
Fibre	1 g
Sodium	297 mg
Potassium	340 mg

Excellent: Niacin
Good: Riboflavin; Vitamin B6; Vitamin B12

INDIAN-FLAVOURED GRILLED CHICKEN THIGHS

If I go to Vancouver and do not go to Vij's restaurant, I don't feel as though I have been in Vancouver. This recipe is adapted from a fabulous dish served there.

Tamarind is a sour, acidic paste made from the pods of a hardy tropical tree and is used in Worcestershire and HP sauce. It is available in most Asian markets and some health food stores.

Makes 6 servings

12 boneless, skinless chicken thighs (about 3 oz/90 g each)
3/4 cup (175 mL) low-fat unflavoured yogurt
4 cloves garlic, minced
2 tbsp (25 mL) tamarind paste
1 tbsp (15 mL) garam masala (page 100) or roasted ground cumin
1 tsp (5 mL) cayenne
1/2 tsp (2 mL) salt
1 lemon, cut into slices
Fresh cilantro sprigs

1. Pat chicken dry. In a large bowl, combine yogurt, garlic, tamarind paste, garam masala, cayenne and salt. Add chicken and turn to coat well. Cover and refrigerate for 4 to 8 hours.
2. Grill chicken for 4 minutes per side. (You could also brown chicken in a grill pan, place on a parchment-lined baking sheet and finish cooking in a preheated 375°F/190°C oven for 20 to 30 minutes, or just until cooked.)
3. Serve chicken garnished with lemon and cilantro.

TURKEY BURGERS WITH OLD-FASHIONED COLESLAW

These burgers are popular with most kids, but for really fussy eaters, grill the burgers without the oyster sauce. You can omit the coleslaw entirely or serve it on the side.

You can also make these with ground chicken.

Makes 6 burgers

1 lb (500 g) lean ground turkey breast
1 small onion, finely chopped
1 clove garlic, minced
2 egg whites, or 1 whole egg
1 cup (250 mL) fresh whole wheat or white breadcrumbs
1 tsp (5 mL) salt
1/2 tsp (2 mL) pepper
1/2 tsp (2 mL) ground cumin
2 tbsp (25 mL) ketchup
2 tbsp (25 mL) oyster sauce
1 cup (250 mL) coleslaw
6 whole wheat or regular kaiser rolls or sesame buns

1. In a large bowl, combine turkey, onion, garlic, egg whites, breadcrumbs, salt, pepper, cumin and ketchup. Mix well and shape into 6 patties about 1/2 inch (1 cm) thick.
2. Brush burgers all over with oyster sauce. Barbecue or broil until cooked through, about 5 minutes per side. Top each burger with large spoonful of coleslaw and serve in buns.

OLD-FASHIONED COLESLAW

Combine 1 grated small cabbage, 1 grated carrot and 3 finely chopped green onions.

In a small saucepan, bring 1/3 cup (75 mL) cider vinegar, 2 tbsp (25 mL) granulated sugar and 2 tbsp (25 mL) vegetable oil (optional) to a boil. Toss cabbage mixture with hot dressing and season with salt and pepper to taste.

Makes about 4 cups (1 L).

PER SERVING

Calories	347
Protein	27 g
Fat	5 g
Saturates	1 g
Cholesterol	47 mg
Carbohydrate	48 g
Fibre	2 g
Sodium	1048 mg
Potassium	453 mg

Excellent: Niacin
Good: Thiamine; Riboflavin; Vitamin B6; Folate; Iron

TURKEY AND SWEET POTATO SHEPHERD'S PIE

This is a great way to use leftover turkey. Use potatoes, sweet potatoes or a combination in the topping—you will need about 4 cups (1 L). You can also use diced leftover cooked vegetables in the turkey mixture. Leftover roast chicken, beef or lamb would work well, too.

If you prefer a chunky filling, do not grind the turkey in the food processor.

Makes 6 servings

1 lb (500 g) Yukon Gold or baking potatoes, peeled and cut in chunks
1 lb (500 g) sweet potatoes, peeled and cut in chunks
2 cloves garlic, thinly sliced
1/2 cup (125 mL) milk, hot
Salt and pepper to taste
4 cups (1 L) diced cooked turkey
1 tbsp (15 mL) olive oil
1 onion, chopped
1 carrot, diced
1 cup (250 mL) peas
3/4 cup (175 mL) tomato sauce (page 151) or gravy
3/4 cup (175 mL) ketchup
1 tbsp (15 mL) Worcestershire sauce
1 tbsp (15 mL) soy sauce
1/2 tsp (2 mL) hot red pepper sauce, optional

PER SERVING	
Calories	356
Protein	32 g
Fat	7 g
Saturates	2 g
Cholesterol	69 mg
Carbohydrate	41 g
Fibre	4 g
Sodium	766 mg
Potassium	952 mg

Excellent: Vitamin A; Niacin; Vitamin B6
Good: Thiamine; Riboflavin; Vitamin B12; Vitamin C; Folate; Iron

1. Cook potatoes, sweet potatoes and garlic in a large saucepan of boiling water until tender. Drain well. Mash with hot milk and season with salt and pepper.
2. Meanwhile, place turkey in a food processor and chop finely.
3. Heat oil in a large, deep non-stick skillet on medium heat. Add onion and carrot and cook gently for 5 to 8 minutes, or until tender. Add peas and turkey and heat thoroughly. Add tomato sauce and ketchup and bring to a boil. Stir in Worcestershire, soy sauce and hot pepper sauce.
4. Place turkey mixture in a lightly oiled 8-inch (1.5 L) square baking dish. Spread with mashed potatoes. Place on a large baking sheet and bake in a preheated 350°F (180°C) oven for 30 to 40 minutes, or until very hot and crusty on top.

ROLLED TURKEY BREAST WITH GRAVY

This is a great recipe for families who want roast turkey but don't care for dark meat. I add mushrooms to the gravy for flavour and colour, but you can strain them out before serving if your kids don't like the texture (or even the idea) of mushrooms.

Makes 8 servings

1 3-lb (1.5 kg) rolled boneless turkey breast
1 tbsp (15 mL) chopped fresh thyme, or 1 tsp (5 mL) dried
¼ tsp (1 mL) salt
¼ tsp (1 mL) pepper
3 tbsp (45 mL) olive oil, divided
1 onion, chopped
1 stalk celery, chopped
1 carrot, chopped
3 cups (750 mL) homemade chicken stock (page 109) or
      low-sodium commercial broth
2 tbsp (25 mL) soy sauce
2 tsp (10 mL) Worcestershire sauce
½ lb (250 g) cremini mushrooms, sliced (about 3 cups/750 mL)
3 tbsp (45 mL) all-purpose flour

1. Pat turkey dry and rub with thyme, salt and pepper.

2. In a roasting pan or Dutch oven, heat 1 tbsp (15 mL) oil on medium-high heat. Brown roast on all sides—5 to 10 minutes. Add onion, celery and carrot and cook for a few minutes.

3. Add stock and bring to a boil. Transfer to a preheated 350°F (180°C) oven. Cook, covered, for 1½ hours, or until a meat thermometer reaches 165°F (74°C). Turn roast once halfway through cooking time.

4. Remove turkey to a carving board and cover with foil. Strain juices from pan into a large measuring cup. (Discard pan veggies.) Add soy sauce and Worcestershire. Add water (or additional stock) until you have about 2 cups (500 mL) liquid.

5. To prepare gravy, heat remaining 2 tbsp (25 mL) oil in a saucepan on medium-high heat. Add mushrooms and cook for about 10 minutes, or until any liquid has evaporated. Add flour and cook, stirring, for a few minutes.

6. Add reserved liquid and bring to a boil. Cook for 5 minutes. Taste and adjust seasonings if necessary. Slice turkey and serve with gravy.

PER SERVING	
Calories	273
Protein	40 g
Fat	9 g
Saturates	2 g
Cholesterol	88 mg
Carbohydrate	7 g
Fibre	2 g
Sodium	453 mg
Potassium	635 mg

Excellent: Niacin;
Vitamin B6; Vitamin B12
Good: Vitamin A;
Riboflavin; Iron

ROAST TURKEY BREAST WITH ROSEMARY AND GARLIC

This is a terrific way to prepare a small turkey dinner, and it is much faster. When you cook a whole turkey, the breast meat often becomes dry by the time the dark meat is thoroughly cooked. But when the breast is cooked by itself, it stays tender and juicy, as it does not have to be cooked too long.

Leftover roast turkey is never quite as good reheated; instead, use it in sandwiches, fajitas, soups, casseroles and stir-fries.

Serve this with cherry tomato sauce (page 176), cranberry sauce (page 275) or gravy (page 270).

Makes 8 servings

1 3-lb (1.5 kg) turkey breast, bone in, skin removed
2 cloves garlic, cut in slivers
Tiny sprigs fresh rosemary, or ½ tsp (2 mL) dried
3 tbsp (45 mL) honey
1 tbsp (15 mL) Dijon mustard
1 tbsp (15 mL) olive oil
1 tbsp (15 mL) lemon juice
½ tsp (2 mL) pepper
¼ tsp (1 mL) salt

PER SERVING	
Calories	196
Protein	30 g
Fat	5 g
Saturates	1 g
Cholesterol	70 mg
Carbohydrate	7 g
Fibre	0 g
Sodium	192 mg
Potassium	338 mg
Excellent: Niacin;	
Vitamin B6	
Good: Vitamin B12	

1. Trim any fat from turkey and pat turkey dry. Make small slits in top of breast and insert garlic slivers and rosemary. (If you don't have fresh rosemary, add dried rosemary to honey mixture.)
2. In a small bowl, combine honey, mustard, oil, lemon juice, pepper and salt. Brush all over turkey breast.
3. Place turkey in a baking dish, meaty side up, and cover loosely with foil. Roast in a preheated 350°F (180°C) oven for 20 minutes. Remove foil and continue to roast for 30 to 40 minutes, or until a meat thermometer registers 165°F (74°C). Baste every 10 to 15 minutes.
4. To carve, slice meat off bone on diagonal.

OLD-FASHIONED WHOLE ROAST TURKEY

After trying hundreds of this-is-the-only-way-to-roast-a-turkey recipes, I have found that the real secret to a great roast turkey is to buy a fresh bird (preferably naturally raised or organic) and don't overcook it.

I like to roast the turkey with the skin on and then remove it before eating. The skin keeps the turkey moist as it cooks, and the bird looks great when you take it to the table. And when it comes to stuffing, I prefer simply to bake it on the side (page 274).

If you are cooking a smaller turkey (14 lb/6.5 kg or less), cook it breast side down for the first half hour, then turn it over. Although it is hard to turn the turkey when it is hot in the pan, the breast meat stays very juicy. You can turn it using folded tea towels, extra pot holders, oven mitts or large spoons, but the easiest way is to use heavy-duty rubber kitchen gloves (page 260).

This recipe will make sixteen servings, though I usually make it for twelve so I can enjoy the leftovers in sandwiches or turkey pot pie (page 252).

Use the cooked turkey carcass to make congee (page 275), a soothing Chinese snack or breakfast soup that can be eaten any time of the day.

Makes 16 servings

1 15-lb (7 kg) fresh turkey
1 tbsp (15 mL) olive oil
1/2 tsp (2 mL) salt
1/4 tsp (1 mL) pepper
1 orange, quartered
1 lemon, quartered
1 onion, quartered
3 sprigs fresh rosemary
3 sprigs fresh sage
1 large onion, sliced
1 cup (250 mL) Port or water

Stock and Gravy
Turkey neck and giblets
1 onion, chopped
1 carrot, chopped

PER SERVING	
Calories	414
Protein	63 g
Fat	14 g
Saturates	4 g
Cholesterol	161 mg
Carbohydrate	3 g
Fibre	0 g
Sodium	303 mg
Potassium	692 mg

Excellent: Riboflavin; Niacin; Vitamin B6; Vitamin B12; Iron

1 stalk celery, chopped
1 cup (250 mL) dry white wine or water
3 cups (750 mL) water
$^1/_2$ cup (125 mL) Port or water
2 tbsp (25 mL) olive oil
$^1/_4$ cup (50 mL) all-purpose flour
1 tbsp (15 mL) soy sauce
1 tbsp (15 mL) Worcestershire sauce
$^1/_2$ tsp (2 mL) hot red pepper sauce
Salt and pepper to taste

1. Rinse turkey inside and out and pat dry with paper towels. Reserve neck and giblets. Rub turkey with olive oil and sprinkle with salt and pepper. Fill cavity with orange, lemon, onion, rosemary and sage. Tie legs together to close cavity.

2. Scatter sliced onions in a roasting pan. Place turkey on onions and roast in a preheated 400°F (200°C) oven for 30 minutes. Add Port.

3. Reduce heat to 350°F (180°C) and continue to roast for 2 hours, or until a thermometer inserted into thigh reads 165°F (74°C). Baste every 20 to 30 minutes. If turkey becomes too brown, cover loosely with foil.

4. Meanwhile, to prepare stock, combine neck, giblets, chopped onion, carrot and celery in a large lightly oiled saucepan on medium-high heat and cook until lightly browned. Add wine and bring to a boil. Cook until wine is reduced by about half. Add water, bring to a boil and simmer for about 1 hour. Strain. You should have about 2$^1/_2$ cups (625 mL) stock.

5. When turkey is ready, remove to a serving platter or carving board. Remove orange, lemon, onion and herbs from cavity and discard. Place foil over turkey and allow to rest while making gravy. Strain pan juices and transfer to a large measuring cup.

6. Add Port to roasting pan. Place on heat and scrape bottom of pan to deglaze. Add to pan juices. Spoon any fat from surface of juices. You should have about 1 cup (250 mL) pan juices. Add enough turkey stock to make 3 cups (750 mL) liquid.

7. Heat olive oil in a saucepan on medium-high heat. Add flour and cook for a few minutes until lightly browned. Add turkey stock mixture and bring to a boil. Add soy sauce, Worcestershire and hot pepper sauce. Cook for 5 minutes. Taste and add salt and pepper.

8. Carve turkey and drizzle with gravy. Pass remaining gravy at table.

BREAD STUFFING WITH HERBS

I like to bake stuffing on the side rather than in the bird. This stops the fat from being absorbed into the stuffing and also means I can take the turkey out at 165°F (74°C). If the turkey is stuffed, it should be cooked until the stuffing reaches 165°F, which means the breast meat will probably be overcooked.

If you want more turkey flavour in the stuffing, simply drizzle a few spoonfuls of the cooked defatted turkey juices over the stuffing before serving.

You can also add two heads of roasted garlic (page 67) to this; squeeze the garlic out of the cloves and add to the bread cubes. Use a mix of wild and cultivated mushrooms.

Makes 12 servings

1 tbsp (15 mL) olive oil
2 onions, chopped
4 cloves garlic, finely chopped
4 stalks celery, chopped
4 leeks, trimmed and chopped
1 ½ lb (750 g) mushrooms, trimmed and sliced
      (about 9 cups/2.25 L)
1 lb (500 g) crusty bread, cut in 1-inch (2.5 cm) cubes
      (about 6 cups/1.5 L)
4 cups (1 L) homemade chicken or turkey stock (page 109 or 272)
½ cup (125 mL) chopped fresh parsley
½ cup (125 mL) chopped fresh sage, or 1 tbsp (15 mL) dried
2 tbsp (25 mL) chopped fresh thyme, or 1 tsp (5 mL) dried
Salt and pepper to taste

1. Heat oil in a large, deep non-stick skillet on medium-high heat. Add onions and garlic and cook for 5 to 8 minutes, or until fragrant. Add celery and leeks. Cook for 5 minutes, or until softened.
2. Add mushrooms and cook until any liquid evaporates—about 10 minutes.
3. Add bread cubes, stock, parsley, sage and thyme and combine well. Season with salt and pepper.
4. Spoon stuffing into a lightly oiled 13- x 9-inch (3.5 L) baking dish. (If you want the top crusty, leave uncovered. If you want it moist, cover with foil.) Bake in a preheated 350°F (180°C) oven for 30 to 40 minutes, or until heated through.

PER SERVING	
Calories	161
Protein	6 g
Fat	3 g
Saturates	1 g
Cholesterol	0 mg
Carbohydrate	29 g
Fibre	4 g
Sodium	248 mg
Potassium	407 mg

Excellent: Folate
Good: Thiamine;
Riboflavin; Niacin;
Vitamin C; Iron

LAID-BACK ROAST TURKEY

Try this easy technique for roasting a turkey. The stuffing is cooked outside the bird but still becomes infused with delicious turkey juices, the bird is easy to carve, and you can make the gravy (page 270) ahead instead of at the last minute.

Buy a 14-lb (7 kg) fresh organic or naturally raised turkey and have your butcher open it up and bone out the carcass and thighs, leaving the wings and drumsticks intact. Lay the butterflied turkey flat, skin side down, on a large parchment-lined baking sheet.

Combine a little olive oil with smoked paprika (page 228) and salt and brush over turkey. Roast turkey in a preheated 425°F (220°C) oven for 15 minutes. Reduce oven temperature to 350°F (180°C).

Spread your favourite stuffing over the bottom of a parchment-lined roasting pan. Lay the butterflied turkey, skin side up, on top of the stuffing. Brush with more olive oil mixture. Return to oven and roast for 1¹/₄ to 1¹/₂ hours, or until a meat thermometer registers 165°F (74°C) when inserted into thickest part of thigh.

Makes 8 to 10 servings.

CRANBERRY SAUCE

In a saucepan, combine ³/₄ lb (375 g) fresh or frozen cranberries, ¹/₂ cup (125 mL) dried cranberries (optional), 1 cup (250 mL) granulated sugar and 1 cup (250 mL) cranberry, orange, or apple juice. Stir in grated peel of 1 orange.

Bring to a boil, reduce heat and simmer gently for 10 to 15 minutes, or until cranberries pop open and sauce thickens. (Sauce will continue to thicken as it cools.)

Makes about 2 cups (500 mL).

CONGEE

Every year magazines and newspapers are filled with suggestions about what to do with your leftover Thanksgiving or Christmas turkey. You can, of course, use it in pot pies (page 252) or shepherd's pies (page 269), as well as in soups, salads, sandwiches and quesadillas, but my current favourite turkey leftover dish is congee, a thick, rice-based soup often eaten for breakfast in Asian countries.

Place leftover cooked turkey carcass in a large pot with 16 cups (4 L) water, or just enough to cover carcass. Add 2 1-inch (2.5 cm) pieces peeled fresh ginger root and 1 tbsp (15 mL) salt. Bring to a boil and cook for 1 hour.

Add 1¹/₂ cups (375 mL) rinsed long-grain rice (and any leftover turkey if you wish) and cook for 1 hour longer. Rice should be very soft and soup should thicken.

Remove carcass. Pick off any meat and return meat to soup. Discard carcass and ginger. Add ¹/₄ tsp (1 mL) pepper. Taste and adjust seasonings if necessary. If congee is too thick, add boiling water. (When you eat the soup, watch out for any small bones that may have fallen off the carcass.)

Makes 6 to 8 servings.

Churrasco Flank Steak with Chimichurri
Big Braised Meatballs
Meatloaf with Chickpeas
Moroccan Meatballs
Sweet and Sour Meatballs
Grilled Steak Sandwiches with Melted Onions
Southwestern Barbecued Brisket
Striploin Roast with Wild Mushrooms
Teriyaki Noodles with Beef
Texas Chili
Polenta with Wild Mushroom and Meat Ragout
Calgary Baked Beans
Beef Sukiyaki
Korean Flank Steak
Pot Roast of Beef with Root Vegetables
Sirloin Steak with Mustard Pepper Crust
Sweet and Sour Cabbage Casserole
Pork Tenderloin with Apricot Glaze
Involtini with Asparagus and Fontina
Sugar Cane Pork Chops
Boneless "Sparerib" Roast with Polenta
Braised Lamb Shanks with White Bean Puree

Pot Roast of Lamb with Tomatoes and Orzo
Cantonese-style Grilled Leg of Lamb
Roast Lamb with Rosemary and Potatoes
Balsamic Maple-glazed Lamb Chops with Sweet Potatoes
Shishkebab-flavoured Butterflied Leg of Lamb
Osso Bucco (Braised Veal Shanks)

HEART SMART

MEAT

ASIAN-FLAVOURED BRAISED SHORTRIBS

I first had something like this at the Spice Market, a fantastic restaurant in New York City. Shortribs used to be a cheap cut of beef that nobody wanted; now they are all the rage in restaurants and at home (and they're no longer cheap!). You can buy them cut in chunky pieces or strips and braise them slowly, or you can have them sliced very thinly and grill them.

This Asian-flavoured version tastes great served over mashed sweet potatoes (page 341) or rice. Make it the night before and refrigerate the meat and juices separately. The excess fat will rise and solidify so that it can be removed easily. Reheat the ribs in the defatted juices.

Star anise is a beautiful-looking spice used whole and found in Asian markets. It adds an exotic anise taste to Asian-flavoured dishes. Remove it before serving.

Makes 10 servings

5 lb (2.5 kg) shortribs, cut in 2-inch (5 cm) chunks
1 tsp (5 mL) salt
$^1/_2$ tsp (2 mL) pepper
1 tbsp (15 mL) olive oil
1 large onion, chopped
2 tbsp (25 mL) chopped fresh ginger root
4 cloves garlic, chopped
$^1/_4$ tsp (1 mL) hot red pepper flakes, optional
3 cups (750 mL) homemade chicken or beef stock (page 109)
1 cup (250 mL) dry sherry
1 cup (250 mL) orange juice
3 tbsp (45 mL) soy sauce
2 tbsp (25 mL) honey
5 pieces star anise
3 tbsp (45 mL) chopped fresh cilantro

1. Sprinkle ribs with salt and pepper.
2. Heat oil in a large Dutch oven or roasting pan on medium-high heat and cook ribs for about 15 minutes, or until well browned on all sides (cook in batches if necessary). Remove ribs from pan.
3. Discard all but 1 tbsp (15 mL) oil from pan. Add onion, ginger, garlic and hot pepper flakes. Cook for 5 to 8 minutes, or until browned.

CILANTRO

Cilantro is also known as Chinese parsley or fresh coriander. Some people love its fresh, citrusy flavour; others think it tastes like soap! But if it is given a fair chance and eaten in small quantities at first, most people come to love it. In some Thai, Indian and Asian recipes the stems and roots are also used, especially in soups, curries, stews and marinades.

If you cannot find cilantro, you can use fresh parsley, mint or basil, but there is really no substitute. (Do not even consider using dried cilantro.)

Ground coriander is made from the dried seeds of the cilantro plant. It is often used in curry blends but is not a substitute for fresh cilantro.

PER SERVING	
Calories	256
Protein	24 g
Fat	13 g
Saturates	5 g
Cholesterol	55 mg
Carbohydrate	9 g
Fibre	1 g
Sodium	441 mg
Potassium	382 mg

Excellent: Vitamin B12
Good: Vitamin B6; Iron

4. Add stock, sherry, orange juice, soy sauce, honey and star anise. Bring to a boil. Add shortribs, preferably in a single layer. Place a round of parchment paper directly on surface of meat and then cover with a lid. Cook in a preheated 350°F (180°C) oven for 2 to 3 hours, or until meat is very, very tender.

5. Remove ribs from pan. Strain juices. You should have at least 2 cups (500 mL). Reduce liquid or add water as necessary. Refrigerate ribs and juices separately.

6. Remove and discard fat from surface of juices. Reheat ribs and juices together. Serve sprinkled with cilantro.

CHURRASCO FLANK STEAK WITH CHIMICHURRI

Flank steak is lean, but tender if you cook it rare and slice it thinly. Count on about 4 oz (125 g) meat per serving, as there are no bones, fat or gristle.

Chimichurri is a spicy pesto-type mixture from Latin America. If you like hot food, leave the seeds in the jalapeño.

Serve this with mashed sweet potatoes (page 341).

Makes 6 servings

1/2 cup (125 mL) fresh cilantro leaves and stems
1/3 cup (75 mL) fresh mint leaves
2 cloves garlic
1 jalapeño, seeded and roughly chopped
1/4 cup (50 mL) lime juice
2 tbsp (25 mL) olive oil
1/2 tsp (2 mL) salt
1 1/2 lb (750 g) flank steak or sirloin

PER SERVING

Calories	236
Protein	26 g
Fat	13 g
Saturates	4 g
Cholesterol	46 mg
Carbohydrate	2 g
Fibre	1 g
Sodium	253 mg
Potassium	413 mg

Excellent: Niacin; Vitamin B12
Good: Vitamin B6; Iron

1. In a food processor, chop cilantro and mint. Add garlic and jalapeño and blend in. Add lime juice, oil and salt. Puree. You should have about 3/4 cup (175 mL).

2. Pat steak dry and smear with 1/2 cup (125 mL) marinade. Marinate for 1 hour at room temperature or up to overnight in refrigerator.

3. Grill steak for 4 to 5 minutes per side for medium rare. Serve with remaining sauce.

BIG BRAISED MEATBALLS

These days the style for meatballs seems to be really tiny or really big. In Italian cooking these big meatballs are often deep-fried to brown them thoroughly, but I prefer not to deep-fry, and in this case I don't think the extra calories are necessary.

Serve these with mashed potatoes, spaghetti or crusty bread.

Makes 6 servings

1/2 cup (125 mL) milk
1 cup (250 mL) fresh whole wheat or regular breadcrumbs
1 1/2 lb (750 g) extra-lean ground beef, or
    a combination of ground beef, veal and pork
1 egg
1/4 cup (50 mL) chopped fresh parsley, divided
1 tsp (5 mL) salt
1/2 tsp (2 mL) pepper
1/2 cup (125 mL) grated Parmesan cheese, optional
1 tbsp (15 mL) olive oil
1 onion, chopped
2 cloves garlic, finely chopped
2 28-oz (796 mL) cans plum tomatoes, with juices,
    broken up or pureed

1. In a large bowl, combine milk, breadcrumbs, beef, egg, 2 tbsp (25 mL) parsley, salt, pepper and cheese. Shape mixture into 12 large meatballs.

2. Heat oil in a large, deep non-stick skillet on medium-high heat. Cook meatballs for 5 to 10 minutes, or until brown on all sides. Remove meatballs from skillet.

3. Add onion and garlic to skillet, reduce heat to medium and cook gently for about 5 minutes, or until fragrant and tender. Add tomatoes with juices and bring to a boil.

4. Return meatballs to skillet. Cover, reduce heat and cook for 25 minutes. Uncover and cook for about 15 minutes, or until tomatoes thicken. Taste and adjust seasonings if necessary. Serve meatballs sprinkled with remaining 2 tbsp (25 mL) parsley.

COOKING GROUND BEEF

According to the Beef Information Centre, the only way to be sure ground meat is thoroughly cooked is to use a thermometer.

Meatloaves, burgers and meatballs should be cooked until an instant-read thermometer inserted into the centre measures 160°F (71°C).

PER SERVING

Calories	299
Protein	29 g
Fat	13 g
Saturates	4 g
Cholesterol	92 mg
Carbohydrate	18 g
Fibre	3 g
Sodium	953 mg
Potassium	1020 mg

Excellent: Riboflavin; Niacin; Vitamin B6; Vitamin B12; Vitamin C; Iron
Good: Vitamin A; Thiamine; Folate

MEATLOAF WITH CHICKPEAS

Adding chickpeas to a traditional meatloaf reduces the fat and the cost as well as adding an interesting flavour to a comforting and delicious favourite (though you can also replace the chickpeas with an additional pound of beef). Use one 19-oz (540 mL) can chickpeas (rinsed and well drained) or cook your own dried chickpeas (page 42).

Makes 6 servings

1 large onion, chopped
3 cloves garlic, chopped
1 lb (500 g) extra-lean ground beef
2 cups (500 mL) cooked chickpeas
3/4 cup (175 mL) fresh whole wheat or regular breadcrumbs
1 egg
1/2 cup (125 mL) commercial (e.g., Heinz) or
        homemade chili sauce or ketchup
2 tbsp (25 mL) Dijon mustard
1 1/2 tsp (7 mL) Worcestershire sauce
1 tsp (5 mL) hot red pepper sauce
1 tsp (5 ml) ground cumin
1/2 tsp (2 mL) salt
1/2 tsp (2 mL) pepper
2 tbsp (25 mL) chopped fresh parsley

Topping
2 tbsp (25 mL) commercial chili sauce or ketchup
1 tbsp (15 mL) Dijon mustard

1. In a food processor, combine onion and garlic and process until pureed (or mince by hand). Add chickpeas and chop very finely.
2. In a large bowl, combine onion mixture, chickpeas, beef, breadcrumbs, egg, chili sauce, mustard, Worcestershire, hot pepper sauce, cumin, salt, pepper and parsley. Knead together lightly.
3. Transfer mixture to a 9- x 5-inch (2 L) loaf pan and smooth top. Cover with foil and bake in a preheated 350°F (180°C) oven for 45 minutes.
4. To prepare topping, combine chili sauce and mustard. Spread topping over loaf and continue to bake, uncovered, for 45 minutes, or until meat thermometer reaches 160°F (71°C). Cool for 15 minutes before removing from pan (don't worry if it crumbles a bit when you serve it).

PER SERVING

Calories	317
Protein	22 g
Fat	13 g
Saturates	4 g
Cholesterol	71 mg
Carbohydrate	27 g
Fibre	5 g
Sodium	866 mg
Potassium	520 mg

Excellent: Niacin; Vitamin B12; Folate; Iron
Good: Thiamine; Riboflavin; Vitamin B6

MOROCCAN MEATBALLS

Serve these delicious meatballs over couscous, soft polenta, rice, spaghetti or mashed potatoes. You can use ground chicken or turkey in place of the beef. If you want this plain rather than with a Middle Eastern flavour, just omit the cumin, cinnamon, turmeric and honey in the meatballs and sauce.

Makes 6 servings

Meatballs

3/4 lb (375 g) extra-lean ground beef or lamb
3/4 cup (175 mL) cooked chickpeas, very finely chopped
1 small onion, finely chopped
1 clove garlic, finely chopped
1 egg
1/3 cup (75 mL) dry whole wheat or regular breadcrumbs
1/2 tsp (2 mL) ground cumin
1/2 tsp (2 mL) salt
1 tbsp (15 mL) olive oil

Tomato Sauce

1 onion, chopped
2 cloves garlic, finely chopped
1 tsp (5 mL) ground cumin
1 tsp (5 mL) ground turmeric
Pinch ground cinnamon
Pinch hot red pepper flakes, optional
1 tbsp (15 mL) honey
1 28-oz (796 mL) can plum tomatoes, with juices,
    broken up or pureed

1. In a large bowl, combine beef, chickpeas, onion, garlic, egg, breadcrumbs, cumin and salt. Shape into about 20 meatballs.
2. Heat oil in a large, deep non-stick skillet on medium-high heat. Add meatballs and cook for about 5 minutes, or until brown on all sides.
3. Add onion, garlic, cumin, turmeric, cinnamon and hot pepper flakes to skillet. Reduce heat and cook gently for 5 to 8 minutes, or until onions wilt and are tender.
4. Add honey and tomatoes to pan. Bring to a boil. Reduce heat, cover and simmer gently for 15 minutes. If sauce is not thick enough, remove lid and cook for 5 minutes longer.

PER SERVING	
Calories	240
Protein	18 g
Fat	9 g
Saturates	2 g
Cholesterol	61 mg
Carbohydrate	24 g
Fibre	4 g
Sodium	529 mg
Potassium	649 mg

Excellent: Niacin; Vitamin B12; Folate; Iron
Good: Riboflavin; Vitamin B6; Vitamin C

SWEET AND SOUR MEATBALLS

Serve these delicious meatballs over mashed potatoes or steamed brown rice. Breadcrumbs are used in ground meat mixtures (meatballs, hamburgers and meatloaves) to bind them together and help hold their shape.

You can make tiny meatballs and serve them with toothpicks as appetizers.

Makes 6 servings
Meatballs
1 lb (500 g) extra-lean ground beef
1 egg
3/4 cup (175 mL) fresh whole wheat or regular breadcrumbs
1/4 cup (50 mL) ketchup
1 tsp (5 mL) salt

Sweet and Sour Sauce
1 tbsp (15 mL) vegetable oil
1 onion, chopped
3 cloves garlic, finely chopped
Pinch hot red pepper flakes
1 28-oz (796 mL) can plum tomatoes, with juices, pureed
2 tbsp (25 mL) rice vinegar or lemon juice
2 tbsp (25 mL) brown sugar
2 tbsp (25 mL) chopped fresh parsley

PER SERVING	
Calories	228
Protein	19 g
Fat	9 g
Saturates	3 g
Cholesterol	71 mg
Carbohydrate	18 g
Fibre	2 g
Sodium	812 mg
Potassium	637 mg

Excellent: Niacin; Vitamin B12
Good: Thiamine; Riboflavin; Vitamin B6; Vitamin C; Iron

1. To prepare meatballs, in a large bowl, combine ground beef, egg, breadcrumbs, ketchup and salt. Shape into about 20 balls.
2. Heat oil in a large, deep non-stick skillet on medium heat. Add onion, garlic and hot pepper flakes and cook gently for a few minutes, or until fragrant but not brown.
3. Add tomatoes, vinegar and sugar. Bring to a boil, reduce heat and cook gently for 5 minutes.
4. Gently add meatballs to sauce. Cover and cook on medium-low heat for 15 to 20 minutes, or until meatballs are cooked. Stir occasionally to prevent sticking. Serve meatballs sprinkled with parsley.

GRILLED STEAK SANDWICHES WITH MELTED ONIONS

These sandwiches are perfect for a casual barbecue, but for a fancier dinner, just serve the sliced steak over mashed potatoes or polenta with the onions on top. Either way it is delicious.

When you grill a whole steak rather than individual smaller ones, the results are often juicier (and the thin slices look like more). You can also make this with flank steak (you may need two). Add 2 tbsp (25 mL) balsamic vinegar to the marinade and marinate in the refrigerator overnight.

Use diced leftover steak in salads, stir-fries, wraps, burritos or tacos.

Makes 8 servings

1 tbsp (15 mL) brown sugar
2 cloves garlic, minced
1 tsp (5 mL) coarse salt
1 tsp (5 mL) coarsely ground pepper
2-lb (1 kg) sirloin steak, about 1 ½ inches (4 cm) thick, trimmed
1 tsp (5 mL) olive oil

Melted Onions
2 tbsp (25 mL) olive oil
4 large onions, thinly sliced
1 tbsp (15 mL) brown sugar
¼ cup (50 mL) balsamic vinegar
Salt and pepper to taste

2 whole wheat or regular baguettes
    (each about 16 inches/40 cm long)
1 bunch arugula, trimmed

1. In a small bowl, combine sugar, garlic, coarse salt and pepper. Pat steak dry, brush with 1 tsp (5 mL) oil and rub with sugar mixture. Marinate for 1 hour at room temperature or up to overnight in refrigerator.
2. To prepare onions, heat 2 tbsp (25 mL) oil in a large, deep non-stick skillet on medium-high heat. Add onions. Cook for 10 minutes, without stirring, until onions begin to brown. Reduce heat to medium and cook, stirring occasionally, for 30 minutes. Onions should be very brown. Add sugar and vinegar and cook gently, adding water if necessary, until onions are very tender and "melted." Season with salt and pepper. Keep warm or reheat before serving.

PER SERVING	
Calories	470
Protein	32 g
Fat	12 g
Saturates	3 g
Cholesterol	51 mg
Carbohydrate	63 g
Fibre	8 g
Sodium	764 mg
Potassium	829 mg

Excellent: Niacin;
Vitamin B6;
Vitamin B12; Iron
Good: Thiamine;
Riboflavin

3. Cut each baguette into four pieces and then cut each piece in half horizontally.

4. Grill steak for 4 to 6 minutes per side for medium-rare. Let steak rest on a carving board for at least 5 minutes and then slice thinly on diagonal.

5. Drape slices of steak on bread and smear with onions. Top with arugula.

Grilled Lamb Sandwiches

Use a boneless, butterflied leg of lamb instead of steak. Double the marinade. Cook lamb for about 10 to 15 minutes per side for rare. (Check temperature with a meat thermometer; the internal temperature should be 130°F/54°C.)

Grilled Turkey Sandwiches

Use a boneless, skinless turkey breast instead of steak. Grill for about 15 to 20 minutes per side, or until cooked through (internal temperature should be 165°F/74°C).

COOKING TIME FOR STEAKS AND CHOPS

When you order a medium-rare steak in a restaurant, it never arrives at the table with little slits that the chef cut into it to see whether it was ready. An experienced grill chef can tell when a steak or chop is ready just by pressing the top of the meat, and you can do this, too.

Rest your forearm on a surface in front of you. Relax and feel your biceps muscle. That's what a rare steak feels like. Now lift your forearm off the table but do not flex it. Feel your biceps. That's what a medium steak feels like. Now flex your muscle and feel the biceps. That's well done. (Of course, this method may have to be adjusted slightly, depending on how much resistance training you have been doing!)

SOUTHWESTERN BARBECUED BRISKET

Growing up in a Jewish household, I often had brisket, but never one even remotely this daring! (For a more traditional version, see the variation.) One of the best things about this dish is the leftovers, which you can make into a shepherd's pie, burritos (top with yogurt cheese and lots of fresh cilantro) or quesadillas (add smoked mozzarella). I like to make this the day before serving; I can then chill it so it will slice better, and I can easily defat the juices. (The brisket can also be frozen.)

Serve the brisket slices draped over diamond-shaped slices of polenta (page 180), with a spoonful of guacamole (page 46) and a drizzle of Goat Cheese Cream (page 251).

Makes 16 servings

4-lb (2 kg) beef brisket, trimmed
1 tbsp (15 mL) paprika
1 tsp (5 mL) ground cumin
1 tsp (5 mL) salt
1 tsp (5 mL) pepper
1/2 tsp (2 mL) cayenne
3 large onions, sliced
2 carrots, sliced
1 head garlic, separated (about 12 cloves), peeled
1 1/2 cups (375 mL) beer, homemade beef stock (page 109) or water
1 cup (250 mL) ketchup
1 cup (250 mL) commercial (e.g., Heinz) or homemade chili sauce
1 chipotle or jalapeño, seeded and minced
2 tbsp (25 mL) Dijon mustard
2 tbsp (25 mL) brown sugar
2 tbsp (25 mL) red wine vinegar or sherry vinegar

1. Pat brisket dry. In a small bowl, combine paprika, cumin, salt, pepper and cayenne. Rub on brisket. Allow to marinate for 5 minutes or up to overnight in refrigerator.

2. Place onions, carrots and garlic cloves in bottom of a large roasting pan. Place brisket on top of vegetables.

3. Combine beer, ketchup, chili sauce, chipotle, mustard, sugar and vinegar. Pour over brisket. Cover tightly and cook in a preheated 350°F (180°C) oven for 4 hours, checking every 45 minutes to make

PER SERVING	
Calories	216
Protein	19 g
Fat	9 g
Saturates	3 g
Cholesterol	45 mg
Carbohydrate	16 g
Fibre	2 g
Sodium	648 mg
Potassium	413 mg
Excellent: Vitamin A; Niacin; Vitamin B12	
Good: Vitamin B6; Iron	

sure there is always about 2 cups (500 mL) liquid in pan. Add water if necessary. Uncover and roast for 30 minutes longer.

4. Transfer roast to a carving board. Skim fat from juices. Carve roast and serve with juices. If you are not serving immediately, cool and then chill meat and vegetables. Put juices in a bowl and chill as well. Before reheating, slice brisket against grain into thin slices. Place in a baking dish with vegetables. Remove and discard any fat from juices (it will have come to surface and solidified). Spoon juices on top of meat. Cover and reheat in a 350°F (180°C) oven for about 45 minutes.

Friday Night Brisket

Add 3 more carrots to onions and garlic. Omit cumin and cayenne from rub. Omit chipotle from sauce and use water or ginger ale instead of beer.

Beef Shepherd's Pie

Combine 3 cups (750 mL) cubed leftover brisket or pot roast (page 296) with 3 cups (750 mL) leftover cooked vegetables. Chop finely by hand or in a food processor. Spoon mixture into a deep 10-inch (25 cm) pie dish or 9-inch (2.5 L) square baking dish. Beat 3 cups (750 mL) cooked mashed potatoes, mashed sweet potatoes or other root vegetable until spreadable and spoon over top of meat and vegetables. Dust with paprika. Bake at 350°F (180°C) for 30 to 45 minutes, or until hot.

Makes 8 servings.

STRIPLOIN ROAST WITH WILD MUSHROOMS

A striploin roast is amazingly tender and has great flavour. If your butcher does not have one, use a boneless rib roast of about the same size and weight. You can also use a filet roast, but reduce the cooking time to only 40 minutes in total for medium-rare (start checking with a meat thermometer after about 30 minutes, depending on the thickness of the roast). Or you can use a flank steak and grill it for 3 to 4 minutes per side.

Leftover beef can be used in sandwiches or served cold with potato salad.

Makes 10 to 12 servings

1 tbsp (15 mL) Dijon mustard
2 cloves garlic, minced
1 tbsp (15 mL) pepper
1 tbsp (15 mL) Worcestershire sauce
1 tbsp (15 mL) chopped fresh rosemary, or 1/2 tsp (2 mL) dried
4-lb (2 kg) striploin roast, well trimmed and tied
        (about 2 1/2 inches/6 cm thick)
1 tsp (5 mL) salt
1 tsp (5 mL) olive oil
1 lb (500 g) shallots (about 12), peeled (page 248) and quartered
2 tbsp (25 mL) balsamic vinegar
2 cups (500 mL) dry red wine
1 lb (500 g) wild mushrooms (portobello, shiitake, oyster, or
        a combination), trimmed and cut in 1/2-inch (1 cm) slices
1/3 cup (75 mL) oyster sauce
2 tbsp (25 mL) coarsely chopped fresh parsley

1. In a small bowl, combine mustard, garlic, pepper, Worcestershire and rosemary. Pat roast dry and rub mustard mixture into roast. Marinate for 30 minutes at room temperature or longer in refrigerator. Just before cooking, sprinkle roast with salt.

2. Heat oil in a large, deep non-stick skillet on medium-high heat. Brown roast well on all sides; this should take about 10 minutes. Transfer roast to a baking sheet lined with parchment paper. Discard all but 1 tbsp (15 mL) fat from skillet.

3. Roast meat in a preheated 375°F (190°C) oven for 45 to 60 minutes, or until a meat thermometer inserted in thickest part of meat registers

PER SERVING	
Calories	341
Protein	40 g
Fat	13 g
Saturates	5 g
Cholesterol	80 mg
Carbohydrate	12 g
Fibre	2 g
Sodium	584 mg
Potassium	808 mg

Excellent: Niacin; Vitamin B6; Vitamin B12; Iron; Zinc
Good: Riboflavin

about 135°F (57°C) for medium-rare. Allow roast to rest for 10 to 20 minutes before carving. Remove fat from surface of pan juices.

4. Meanwhile, return skillet to heat. Add shallots, vinegar and any defatted pan juices. Cook, stirring, until vinegar evaporates and shallots begin to brown. Add wine. Cook on medium-high heat, scraping pan, until wine reduces to about 1/2 cup (125 mL) and shallots are tender.

5. Add mushrooms to skillet and cook for about 10 minutes, or until wilted and browned. Add oyster sauce and cook for 5 minutes. Add parsley and taste and adjust seasonings if necessary.

6. Remove string from roast and carve into slices. Top with mushrooms, shallots and juices.

WILD MUSHROOMS

These days you can usually find fresh portobellos (cultivated porcini mushrooms), cremini (small portobellos that are less expensive than the larger version), shiitake and oyster mushrooms. Morels, trumpets, chanterelles and enoki are a bit harder to find, and they can be quite expensive, but they will add a lot of flavour to a special dish.

The stems of some wild mushrooms (e.g., shiitake) are too tough to use in most recipes; freeze them and save for stocks. The stems of other mushrooms, such as portobellos, are flavourful and tender. If a recipe calls only for the caps, use the stems in rice dishes, stuffings, soups or sauces.

Store wild mushrooms in a single layer covered with a damp tea towel. They should keep in the refrigerator for a few days.

Dried wild mushrooms are concentrated in flavour and are used in small quantities. They are more easily available than fresh, and while they can be expensive, just a half ounce adds a ton of flavour. To reconstitute them, place them in a bowl and cover with hot water. Allow to rest for 30 minutes, or until softened. Strain the flavourful liquid through cheesecloth, a paper towel or coffee filter set in a strainer and use it in the recipe, or save for soups or sauces. Rinse the mushrooms and chop.

TERIYAKI NOODLES WITH BEEF

This is a recipe that everyone in the family will love. You can use bone-less, skinless chicken breasts or pork tenderloin instead of the beef.

Makes 6 servings

1 lb (500 g) flank steak, partially frozen
1/3 cup (75 mL) teriyaki sauce, divided
1/2 lb (250 g) whole wheat spaghetti or soba noodles
2 tbsp (25 mL) vegetable oil, divided
1 onion, thinly sliced
1 carrot, thinly sliced
1 sweet red pepper, seeded and thinly sliced
1 stalk celery, thinly sliced
3 fresh shiitake or regular mushrooms, stemmed and sliced
1 1/2 cups (375 mL) broccoli florets
2/3 cup (150 mL) boiling water
4 green onions, sliced on diagonal

1. Slice flank steak as thinly as possible on diagonal against grain. Cut each slice into thirds crosswise. Marinate in 2 tbsp (25 mL) teriyaki sauce for about 10 minutes or up to a few hours in refrigerator.

2. Bring a large pot of water to a boil. Add noodles and cook until tender.

3. Meanwhile, heat 1 tbsp (15 mL) oil in a large, deep non-stick skillet or wok on medium-high heat. Add steak and cook for about 2 minutes, or until meat loses its raw appearance. Remove steak from pan.

4. Clean pan if necessary, and heat remaining oil. Add onion, carrot, red pepper, celery, mushrooms and broccoli. Stir-fry for 3 to 4 minutes, or until vegetables are bright and almost tender.

5. Return steak to pan and add remaining teriyaki sauce and boiling water. Bring to a boil, reduce heat and simmer for 2 minutes.

6. Drain noodles well and add to pan. Cook for a few minutes, tossing everything together, until noodles absorb juices but dish is still very moist. Add green onions.

TERIYAKI SAUCE

In a small saucepan, combine 3 tbsp (45 mL) soy sauce, 3 tbsp (45 mL) water, 3 tbsp (45 mL) rice wine, 3 tbsp (45 mL) granulated sugar, 1 peeled and smashed clove garlic, 1-inch (2.5 cm) piece smashed fresh ginger root and 1-inch (2.5 cm) piece lemon peel. Bring to a boil and cook until mixture is reduced by half. Cool and remove garlic, ginger and lemon peel.

Makes about 1/3 cup (75 mL).

PER SERVING

Calories	371
Protein	26 g
Fat	11 g
Saturates	3 g
Cholesterol	30 mg
Carbohydrate	44 g
Fibre	3 g
Sodium	655 mg
Potassium	510 mg

Excellent: Vitamin A; Niacin; Vitamin C; Vitamin B12
Good: Thiamine; Vitamin B6; Iron; Folate

TEXAS CHILI

This recipe uses small cubes of meat, but you can also use ground meat. Serve it over rice and top with yogurt cheese (page 391) and chopped green onions, or wrap in flour tortillas. Add 1 tbsp (15 mL) chipotle puree (page 183) if you like your chili hot.

Make this for a crowd, or freeze any extra.

Makes 12 servings

1 1/2 lb (750 g) lean stewing beef, diced
1 1/2 lb (750 g) lean stewing pork, diced
1/2 cup (125 mL) all-purpose flour
1 tbsp (15 mL) vegetable oil
4 large onions, finely chopped
6 cloves garlic, finely chopped
3 tbsp (45 mL) chili powder
1 tbsp (15 mL) ground cumin
1 tbsp (15 mL) dried oregano
1 tsp (5 mL) cayenne
1/2 tsp (2 mL) pepper
3 cups (750 mL) homemade beef stock (page 109), or
        1 28-oz (796 mL) can plum tomatoes, with juices, broken up
1 cup (250 mL) beer or water
4 cups (1 L) cooked red kidney beans, or
        2 19-oz (540 mL) cans, rinsed and drained
1 cup (250 mL) grated light Cheddar cheese

PER SERVING

Calories	344
Protein	35 g
Fat	11 g
Saturates	4 g
Cholesterol	66 mg
Carbohydrate	25 g
Fibre	7 g
Sodium	235 mg
Potassium	952 mg

Excellent: Thiamine; Niacin; Vitamin B6; Vitamin B12; Folate; Iron
Good: Riboflavin

1. Pat beef and pork dry and toss with flour.
2. Heat oil in a Dutch oven on medium-high heat. Brown meat in batches, removing each batch from skillet once browned.
3. Discard all but 1 tbsp (15 mL) fat from skillet and return to heat. Add onions and garlic. Reduce heat to medium and cook gently until tender and fragrant, about 10 minutes. Add chili powder, cumin, oregano, cayenne and pepper.
4. Return meat to skillet and combine well. Add stock and beer and bring to a boil. Cook gently, uncovered, for 2 to 3 hours, until meat is very tender and mixture is thick. Stir in beans. Taste and adjust seasonings if necessary.
5. Transfer chili to a 3-qt (3 L) casserole, top with cheese and bake, uncovered, in a preheated 350°F (180°C) oven for 30 minutes, or until thoroughly heated.

POLENTA WITH WILD MUSHROOM AND MEAT RAGOUT

This is a delicious all-purpose meat sauce. It is also wonderful served over pasta. Just a little bit of sausage adds a lot of flavour, but you can omit it if you prefer.

Serve the ragout over the hot polenta in individual bowls. The polenta can also be made ahead, poured into a lightly oiled 13- x 9-inch (3.5 L) baking dish, topped with sauce, cheese and parsley and reheated at 350°F (180°C) oven for 30 minutes.

Makes 4 servings
Wild Mushroom and Meat Ragout
½ oz (15 g) dried wild mushrooms
1 cup (250 mL) warm water
2 tsp (10 mL) olive oil
1 onion, chopped
3 cloves garlic, finely chopped
¼ tsp (1 mL) hot red pepper flakes, optional
1 sweet red pepper, seeded and diced
½ lb (250 g) extra-lean ground beef
1 extra-lean Italian sausage, removed from casing
        (about 2 oz/60 g), optional
1 28-oz (796 mL) can plum tomatoes, with juices,
        pureed or broken up
Salt and pepper to taste

Polenta
6 cups (1.5 L) water
1 tsp (5 mL) salt
½ tsp (2 mL) pepper
1 cup (250 mL) cornmeal (regular or quick-cooking)

Garnish
2 tbsp (25 mL) grated Parmesan cheese
2 tbsp (25 mL) chopped fresh parsley

1. Cover dried mushrooms with warm water and let soak for 30 minutes. Strain liquid through a paper towel–lined sieve and reserve. Rinse mushrooms thoroughly and chop.
2. Heat oil in a large, deep non-stick skillet on medium heat. Add onion, garlic and hot pepper flakes and cook gently for 5 to 8 minutes, or until tender but not brown.

BACON AND SAUSAGES
If you love high-fat foods such as bacon or sausages, use them in small quantities as an ingredient in dishes, rather than as a main food. Use a half slice of bacon per person, crisply cooked and well drained, and crumble it into salads. Or cook a small amount of sausage and add it to soups or pasta sauces. You will get the flavour you crave without a large amount of fat.

PER SERVING

Calories	314
Protein	18 g
Fat	8 g
Saturates	3 g
Cholesterol	32 mg
Carbohydrate	43 g
Fibre	5 g
Sodium	1006 mg
Potassium	764 mg

Excellent: Vitamin A; Vitamin C; Niacin; Vitamin B6; Vitamin B12
Good: Thiamine; Riboflavin; Folate; Iron

BARBECUE SAUCE

Heat 2 tsp (10 mL) olive oil in a saucepan on medium heat. Add 1 chopped onion and 2 finely chopped cloves garlic and cook gently for about 5 minutes. Add 1¹/₂ cups (375 mL) tomato sauce or ketchup, ¹/₄ cup (50 mL) cider vinegar, ¹/₄ cup (50 mL) brown sugar, 1 tbsp (15 mL) Worcestershire sauce, 1 tbsp (15 mL) Dijon mustard and 1 tsp (5 mL) chipotle puree or hot red pepper sauce (optional). Bring to a boil, reduce heat and simmer, stirring often, for 10 minutes. Taste and adjust seasonings if necessary.

Makes about 1¹/₂ cups (375 mL).

PER SERVING

Calories	235
Protein	12 g
Fat	4 g
Saturates	1 g
Cholesterol	11 mg
Carbohydrate	39 g
Fibre	6 g
Sodium	639 mg
Potassium	718 mg

Excellent: Thiamine; Folate

Good: Niacin; Vitamin B6; Folate; Iron

3. Add red pepper and cook for a few minutes. Add beef and sausage meat and cook for 8 to 10 minutes, or until brown. Drain off and discard any excess fat.

4. Add mushrooms, mushroom liquid and tomatoes. Bring to a boil and cook for 30 minutes, or until sauce is quite thick. Add salt and pepper.

5. Meanwhile, to prepare polenta, combine water, salt and pepper in a large pot and bring to a boil. Slowly whisk in cornmeal. Stirring with a long-handled spoon, cook over medium heat for 25 to 30 minutes for regular cornmeal or 5 to 10 minutes for quick-cooking. Polenta should be tender. Taste and adjust seasonings if necessary.

6. Serve polenta topped with sauce and sprinkle with cheese and parsley.

CALGARY BAKED BEANS

A few years ago my friend Carole Martin took me to the Calgary Stampede, where we had so much fun— eating, of course. Carole told me her friend Judy Brovald had the easiest and most delicious recipe for baked beans. Here's my version. Using canned beans gives you a head start, but of course you could also cook your own (page 179).

Makes 12 servings

1 tbsp (15 mL) olive oil
1 boneless pork chop (about 6 oz/175 g), trimmed and diced
1 onion, diced
1 14-oz (398 mL) can plum tomatoes, with juices,
    pureed (about 1¹/₂ cups/375 mL)
1 cup (250 mL) barbecue sauce or ketchup
¹/₄ cup (50 mL) brown sugar
¹/₄ cup (50 mL) molasses
2 tbsp (25 mL) prepared yellow mustard
3 14-oz (398 mL) cans navy beans, rinsed and drained
    (about 5 cups/1.25 L)

1. Heat oil in a Dutch oven on medium-high heat. Add pork and cook for a few minutes, or until brown. Add onion and cook for about 5 minutes, or until softened.

2. Add tomatoes, barbecue sauce, sugar, molasses and mustard. Bring to a boil.

3. Stir in beans. Bake, covered, in a preheated 350°F (180°C) oven for 1 hour, or until thick and saucy.

BEEF SUKIYAKI

This is a soothing, nourishing, sweet-tasting broth full of delicious treasures. Vary the recipe according to your own tastes.

You can make this ahead up to the point of adding the softened noodles and the beef. Reheat before adding the noodles and raw beef, and be sure not to overcook.

Makes 6 servings

3/4 lb (375 g) lean sirloin steak, about 1 inch (2.5 cm) thick, trimmed
1 large onion, thinly sliced
1 lb (500 g) fresh baby spinach, Swiss chard or beet greens,
    torn in pieces
1/4 lb (125 g) very fresh bean sprouts
1/4 lb (125 g) mushrooms, trimmed and sliced
    (about 1 1/2 cups/375 mL)
1 carrot, thinly sliced
1/2 lb (250 g) extra-firm tofu, cut in 1-inch (2.5 cm) pieces
6 green onions, chopped
3 cups (750 mL) homemade beef stock (page 109),
    water or dashi
1 tbsp (15 mL) granulated sugar
3 tbsp (45 mL) soy sauce
3 tbsp (45 mL) dry sherry, optional
3 oz (90 g) rice vermicelli noodles

1. Freeze meat for 20 minutes. Slice very thinly on diagonal.
2. Meanwhile, spread onion slices over bottom of a 4-qt (4 L) saucepan or Dutch oven. Place spinach, bean sprouts, mushrooms, carrot, tofu and green onions on top.
3. Combine stock, sugar, soy sauce and sherry and pour over vegetables. Bring to a boil and simmer gently for 5 to 10 minutes, or until onions are tender.
4. Meanwhile, soak noodles in warm water for 5 minutes. Drain well.
5. Stir softened noodles into vegetables and arrange beef on top. Cook for another 5 minutes. Taste and adjust seasonings if necessary.

DASHI
Dashi is a clear, mild, slightly smoky Japanese soup stock made from kelp and dried fish (most often bonito). Instant dashi is available in powdered or cube form and can be found in Japanese or Asian markets.

PER SERVING

Calories	235
Protein	24 g
Fat	4 g
Saturates	1 g
Cholesterol	28 mg
Carbohydrate	27 g
Fibre	5 g
Sodium	531 mg
Potassium	951 mg

Excellent: Vitamin A; Niacin; Riboflavin; Iron; Vitamin B6; Folate; Vitamin B12
Good: Thiamine; Calcium

SESAME SPINACH

Heat 1 tsp (5 mL) dark sesame oil in a large non-stick skillet on medium heat. Add 1 finely chopped clove garlic and 1 tbsp (15 mL) water. Cook gently for a few minutes until fragrant. Add 2 lb (1 kg) fresh baby spinach and cook for about 5 minutes. (Gradually add spinach to skillet in about three batches, turning until it wilts before adding more. And don't worry, it will reduce in volume!) Season to taste with salt and pepper and sprinkle with 1 tsp (5 mL) toasted sesame seeds (page 384).

Makes 4 to 6 servings.

PER SERVING

Calories	245
Protein	27 g
Fat	10 g
Saturates	4 g
Cholesterol	46 mg
Carbohydrate	10 g
Fibre	trace
Sodium	610 mg
Potassium	387 mg

Excellent: Niacin; Vitamin B12
Good: Vitamin B6

KOREAN FLANK STEAK

This is a delicious way to treat a reasonably priced lean cut of beef. Flank steak can be tough, so it benefits from marinating, but because it is quite thin, it doesn't need to marinate for too long. Serve it with rice or rice vermicelli noodles and spinach.

This marinade also works well with a round steak cut about 3/4 inch (2 cm) thick (marinate it in the refrigerator for 8 to 12 hours) or with a blade or cross-rib steak (marinate for 18 to 24 hours).

Makes 4 to 6 servings
1-lb (500 g) flank steak
1/4 cup (50 mL) soy sauce
1/4 cup (50 mL) granulated sugar
2 tbsp (25 mL) lemon juice
2 tsp (10 mL) dark sesame oil
4 cloves garlic, minced
1/2 tsp (2 mL) pepper

1. Pat steak dry and, very lightly, make horizontal slits in top of meat about 1/8 inch (2 mm) deep.
2. Combine soy sauce, sugar, lemon juice, sesame oil, garlic and pepper. Combine with steak in a flat dish or heavy-duty plastic bag. Marinate in refrigerator, turning two or three times, for 4 to 8 hours or overnight.
3. Just before cooking, remove steak from marinade and pat dry. Place marinade in a small saucepan and bring to a boil. Cook for a few minutes until slightly syrupy.
4. Grill steak for 3 to 4 minutes per side for medium-rare if steak is about 1 inch (2.5 cm) thick. Brush once or twice with reduced marinade during cooking. Allow steak to rest for 5 minutes before carving. Slice thinly on diagonal.

Korean-style Miami Ribs

Instead of flank steak, use 2 lb (1 kg) Miami ribs (thinly sliced short-ribs). Grill for 3 minutes per side.

POT ROAST OF BEEF WITH ROOT VEGETABLES

For many people, pot roast means beef, but this roast will work well with lamb or pork, too. Leftovers can be made into shepherd's pie.

Makes 10 to 12 servings

4-lb (2 kg) boneless cross-rib roast of beef, tied
½ tsp (2 mL) salt
¼ tsp (1 mL) pepper
1 tbsp (15 mL) olive oil
2 onions, chopped
2 cloves garlic, finely chopped
2 tbsp (25 mL) chopped fresh rosemary, or 1 tsp (5 mL) dried
2 tbsp (25 mL) chopped fresh thyme, or 1 tsp (5 mL) dried
2 cups (500 mL) dry red wine or homemade beef stock (page 109)
2 cups (500 mL) homemade beef stock, chicken stock or water
2 tbsp (25 mL) balsamic vinegar or red wine vinegar
2 onions, cut in chunks
2 carrots, cut in chunks
2 parsnips, peeled and cut in chunks
4 Yukon Gold or baking potatoes, peeled and cut in chunks
1 sweet potato, peeled and cut in chunks
1 tbsp (15 mL) all-purpose flour, optional
1 tbsp (15 mL) soft non-hydrogenated margarine or unsalted butter, optional
2 tbsp (25 mL) chopped fresh parsley

1. Pat roast dry and season with salt and pepper.
2. Heat oil in a Dutch oven on medium-high heat. Add roast and brown well on all sides (this should take 10 to 15 minutes). Remove roast from pan.
3. Discard all but 2 tsp (10 mL) oil from pan. Add chopped onions and garlic. Cook until tender, about 4 minutes. Add rosemary, thyme and wine and bring to a boil. Cook, uncovered, for 10 to 15 minutes, or until wine reduces to about 1 cup (250 mL).
4. Add stock and vinegar. Bring to a boil and return beef to pan. Cover tightly and cook in a preheated 350°F (180°C) oven for 1½ hours.

PER SERVING	
Calories	353
Protein	34 g
Fat	11 g
Saturates	4 g
Cholesterol	74 mg
Carbohydrate	28 g
Fibre	4 g
Sodium	302 mg
Potassium	919 mg

Excellent: Vitamin A; Niacin; Vitamin B6; Vitamin B12; Iron
Good: Vitamin C; Riboflavin; Folate

5. Arrange onions, carrots, parsnips, potatoes and sweet potato around roast. Cover and continue to cook for 1 1/2 hours, or until vegetables and beef are tender.

6. Remove beef to a carving board and vegetables to a serving platter. Skim any fat from juices and simmer juices on top of stove. If juices are not thick enough, cook, uncovered, until thick, or mix flour and margarine in a small bowl and add to simmering liquid a teaspoon at a time, stirring, until juices are just slightly thickened.

7. Slice meat, arrange over vegetables and spoon juices on top. Sprinkle with parsley.

SIRLOIN STEAK WITH MUSTARD PEPPER CRUST

Real meat lovers sometimes feel deprived when they try to get used to smaller portions of meat, but if you slice a large sirloin very thinly on the diagonal, a small portion looks like a lot.

You can also use flank steak in this recipe, but marinate it in the refrigerator for 4 to 8 hours or overnight, and cook it for 3 to 4 minutes per side for rare.

Makes 6 to 8 servings

2 tbsp (25 mL) Dijon mustard
1 tbsp (15 mL) Worcestershire sauce
1 tbsp (15 mL) pepper
2 cloves garlic, minced
1/4 tsp (1 mL) hot red pepper sauce
1 1/2-lb (750 g) sirloin steak, about 1 inch (2.5 cm) thick, preferably boneless

1. Combine mustard, Worcestershire, pepper, garlic and hot pepper sauce.

2. Trim steak and pat dry. Spread marinade over steak and marinate in refrigerator for a few hours.

3. Grill steak for 5 to 6 minutes per side for medium-rare. Allow steak to rest for few minutes before carving.

4. Carve steak in thin slices slightly on diagonal (to make a wider slice). Serve 3 or 4 slices per person.

PER SERVING	
Calories	173
Protein	27 g
Fat	6 g
Saturates	2 g
Cholesterol	65 mg
Carbohydrate	1 g
Fibre	trace
Sodium	117 mg
Potassium	365 mg
Excellent: Niacin; Vitamin B12	
Good: Riboflavin; Iron; Vitamin B6	

SWEET AND SOUR CABBAGE CASSEROLE

Cabbage rolls are very popular, but it takes time to roll up all those cabbage leaves. In this recipe you just layer the cabbage with the stuffing and sauce, for the same traditional flavours without the fuss.

The meat and rice mixture can also be made into meatballs. You can poach them in the sauce without even browning them first.

Makes 6 to 8 servings

1 head cabbage
1 lb (500 g) extra-lean ground beef
2 cups (500 mL) cooked brown or white rice
1 clove garlic, minced
1 egg
1/4 cup (50 mL) dry whole wheat or regular breadcrumbs
1/4 cup (50 mL) ketchup
1 tsp (5 mL) salt
1/4 tsp (1 mL) pepper
6 tbsp (75 mL) chopped fresh parsley, divided
1 tsp (5 mL) vegetable oil
1 onion, chopped
1 clove garlic, finely chopped
1/4 cup (50 mL) brown sugar
2 tbsp (25 mL) lemon juice
1 28-oz (796 mL) can plum tomatoes, with juices
1/2 cup (125 mL) cranberry juice or pineapple juice
Salt and pepper to taste

1. Place cabbage in freezer and freeze for 2 days. Completely defrost, remove core and separate leaves. (Instead of freezing, you can separate leaves and cook in a large pot of boiling water for 5 minutes.)
2. In a large bowl, combine ground beef, cooked rice, minced garlic, egg, breadcrumbs, ketchup, salt, pepper and 2 tbsp (25 mL) parsley.
3. To prepare sauce, heat oil in a large non-stick saucepan on medium heat. Add onion and chopped garlic and cook gently for a couple of minutes until fragrant but not brown.
4. Add sugar, lemon juice, tomatoes and cranberry juice and bring to a boil. Add 2 tbsp (25 mL) parsley and cook for 15 minutes,

PER SERVING	
Calories	394
Protein	22 g
Fat	10 g
Saturates	4 g
Cholesterol	75 mg
Carbohydrate	54 g
Fibre	7 g
Sodium	875 mg
Potassium	1083 mg
Excellent: Niacin; Vitamin B6; Vitamin B12; Vitamin C; Folate; Iron	
Good: Thiamine; Riboflavin	

breaking up tomatoes with a spoon. If sauce is too thick, add about ¹/₂ cup (125 mL) water or juice. Season with salt and pepper.

5. Cut tough ribs from cabbage leaves and line bottom of an 11- x 7-inch (2 L) baking dish with a few layers of the nicest leaves. Spread with half of the meat mixture and one-third of the sauce. Repeat with cabbage, meat and sauce. Top with final few layers of leaves and spread with remaining sauce.

6. Place casserole on a baking sheet and cover with foil. Bake, covered, in a preheated 350°F (180°C) oven for 40 minutes. Uncover and bake for 10 minutes longer. Sprinkle with remaining 2 tbsp (25 mL) parsley and allow to rest for 10 minutes before serving. Cut into squares, being careful to cut right through all the cabbage leaves. (Don't worry if casserole is a little watery; just drain off any extra liquid.)

PORK TENDERLOIN WITH APRICOT GLAZE

In the past few years pork has become popular even in upscale restaurants. You can also use this glaze with pork loin roasts, pork chops and chicken.

PER SERVING

Calories	196
Protein	24 g
Fat	4 g
Saturates	1 g
Cholesterol	57 mg
Carbohydrate	15 g
Fibre	trace
Sodium	123 mg
Potassium	476 mg

Excellent: Thiamine; Niacin
Good: Riboflavin; Vitamin B6; Vitamin B12

Makes 6 to 8 servings

¹/₂ cup (125 mL) apricot jam
2 tbsp (25 mL) Dijon mustard
2 tbsp (25 mL) balsamic vinegar or cider vinegar
2 tsp (10 mL) Worcestershire sauce
1 ¹/₂ lb (750 g) pork tenderloin

1. In a small bowl, combine jam, mustard, vinegar and Worcestershire sauce.
2. Pat pork dry and coat with glaze.
3. Place pork on a rack set over a foil-lined baking sheet. Roast in a preheated 375°F (190°C) oven for 40 to 50 minutes, or until cooked through (internal temperature should be about 160°F/71°C).

INVOLTINI WITH ASPARAGUS AND FONTINA

I got this idea from a fun restaurant in Toronto. Rosa, the chef and owner with her sons at Seven Numbers, provides Italian home cooking at very reasonable prices in a crazy environment. Her dishes are simple yet delicious, and really make you feel as though your mother is cooking for you.

You can fill these adorable pork bundles with green beans or thin sticks of red pepper or carrots instead of the asparagus. You can also use Swiss or Cheddar cheese in place of the Fontina. Use flattened chicken breasts or veal scallopini instead of the pork if you wish.

Makes 4 servings

1 lb (500 g) pork tenderloin
1/4 tsp (1 mL) salt
1/4 tsp (1 mL) pepper
8 thin slices Fontina cheese (about 2 oz/60 g total)
24 thin spears asparagus, about 6 inches (15 cm) long
1/4 cup (50 mL) all-purpose flour
1 tbsp (15 mL) olive oil
1/2 cup (125 mL) dry white wine or
     homemade chicken stock (page 109)

1. Slice tenderloin into 8 pieces and pat dry. Pound each piece thinly between pieces of heavy plastic wrap or parchment paper. Pieces should be about 4 inches (10 cm) in diameter. Season with salt and pepper.
2. Top each pork slice with a piece of cheese and three asparagus spears. Roll up and secure with a toothpick. Dredge lightly in flour.
3. Heat oil in a large non-stick skillet on medium-high heat. Brown pork rolls on all sides—about 5 minutes. Remove from skillet.
4. Add wine to skillet and scrape bottom of pan to incorporate any browned bits of pork into sauce. (If wine evaporates too quickly, add some water.) Return rolls to skillet, cover and cook for 3 minutes, or until just cooked through. Taste and adjust seasonings if necessary.
5. Remove toothpicks and serve rolls with sauce spooned over top.

PER SERVING	
Calories	313
Protein	34 g
Fat	13 g
Saturates	5 g
Cholesterol	80 mg
Carbohydrate	11 g
Fibre	2 g
Sodium	321 mg
Potassium	590 mg

Excellent: Thiamine; Riboflavin; Niacin; Vitamin B6; Vitamin B12; Folate
Good: Iron

SUGAR CANE PORK CHOPS

These Southern-style pork chops were inspired by Regina Charboneau, who runs the Twin Oaks bed and breakfast in Natchez, Mississippi. Serve them with mashed or roasted sweet potatoes and mango chutney.

Makes 8 servings

¼ cup (50 mL) brown sugar
1 tsp (5 mL) salt
1 tsp (5 mL) pepper
1 tsp (5 mL) garlic powder
1 tsp (5 mL) onion powder
1 tsp (5 mL) paprika
8 pork loin chops, bone-in, trimmed (about 1 inch/2.5 cm thick)
1 tbsp (15 mL) olive oil

1. In a small bowl, combine sugar, salt, pepper, garlic powder, onion powder and paprika.
2. Pat pork dry and rub sugar mixture into both sides of chops.
3. Heat oil in a large non-stick skillet on medium-high heat. Brown chops for a few minutes per side, in batches if necessary. Transfer to a baking sheet lined with parchment paper. Bake in a preheated 350°F (180°C) oven for 8 minutes, or until just cooked through. Do not overcook.

PER SERVING

Calories	196
Protein	21 g
Fat	9 g
Saturates	3 g
Cholesterol	59 mg
Carbohydrate	7 g
Fibre	0 g
Sodium	338 mg
Potassium	348 mg

Excellent: Thiamine; Niacin; Vitamin B12
Good: Riboflavin; Vitamin B6

BONELESS "SPARERIB" ROAST WITH POLENTA

Pot roasts sound and smell like home. And they are great for entertaining, because you can make them ahead and they taste even better reheated. Defat the sauce when it is cold; the fat will rise to the surface and solidify, making it easy to remove.

This roast tastes like barbecued spareribs, but has much less fat. The sauce is also excellent with chicken or a boneless cross-rib roast of beef. You can add potatoes and carrots along with the other vegetables.

Leftovers can be cut up and served as a stew, or shredded or ground and used as a filling for tacos, fajitas, quesadillas or shepherd's pie. You could also add beans and serve over rice or mashed potatoes as a chili.

Makes 10 to 12 servings

4-lb (2 kg) boneless pork loin roast, tied
1/2 tsp (2 mL) salt
1/4 tsp (1 mL) pepper
2 tsp (10 mL) olive oil
1 cup (250 mL) barbecue sauce (page 293)
2 tbsp (25 mL) Dijon mustard
2 tbsp (25 mL) brown sugar
2 tbsp (25 mL) Worcestershire sauce
2 tbsp (25 mL) red wine vinegar
1 cup (250 mL) water
2 tbsp (25 mL) chipotle puree (page 183), or 2 chopped jalapeños,
    optional
2 onions, cut in chunks
2 carrots, cut in chunks on diagonal
2 stalks celery, cut in chunks on diagonal

Polenta

10 cups (2.5 L) water or milk, or a combination
1 tsp (5 mL) ground cumin
1 tsp (5 mL) salt
1/2 tsp (2 mL) pepper
2 cups (500 mL) cornmeal (regular or quick-cooking)
Sprigs fresh parsley

PER SERVING	
Calories	384
Protein	39 g
Fat	10 g
Saturates	3 g
Cholesterol	96 mg
Carbohydrate	32 g
Fibre	4 g
Sodium	731 mg
Potassium	647 mg

Excellent: Vitamin A; Thiamine; Niacin; Vitamin B6; Vitamin B12
Good: Iron; Riboflavin

1. Pat roast dry and season with salt and pepper.

2. Heat oil in a Dutch oven on medium-high heat. Brown roast well on all sides; this should take 10 to 15 minutes. Discard any fat from pan.

3. Meanwhile, combine barbecue sauce, mustard, brown sugar, Worcestershire, vinegar, water and chipotle. Pour over roast. Cover tightly and cook in a preheated 350°F (180°C) oven for 1 1/2 hours.

4. Arrange onions, carrots and celery around roast, cover and cook for 1 1/2 hours longer, or until meat temperature reaches 160°F (71°C).

5. Remove meat to a carving board. Skim any fat from surface of sauce. If sauce is thin, place on medium-high heat and cook, uncovered, until liquid reduces. You should have about 2 cups (500 mL) sauce. Keep warm if not serving immediately.

6. Meanwhile, to prepare polenta, in a large pot, combine water, cumin, salt and pepper and bring to a boil. Whisk in cornmeal slowly and then, stirring constantly, cook gently for 30 minutes for regular polenta or 5 to 10 minutes for quick-cooking. Taste and adjust seasonings if necessary.

7. Transfer polenta to a large serving platter and arrange sliced pork, vegetables and sauce over top. Garnish with parsley.

KITCHEN USES FOR PLASTIC ZIPPER BAGS

- Use zipper bags as makeshift piping bags for frostings and meringues. Cut a hole in a bottom corner and insert a piping nozzle if you wish. Fill the bag with frosting and twist the top of the bag to force the frosting out the hole. (Use small bags—with small holes—to write on cakes and cookies.)

- Freeze leftover coconut milk, pesto, chipotles, tomato paste, etc., flat in a small zipper bag, so you can snap off what you need a bit at a time. (Store all the small bags in one big one, so they don't get lost in your freezer.)

- When you are rolling sushi with the rice on the outside (as in a California roll), place your sudari mat inside the plastic bag (the large zipper bag is the perfect size) so the rice doesn't stick to the mat.

- Use large zipper bags to pound meat or chicken. Cut the sides of a large bag to make a single long sheet. Place the chicken or meat on one side and fold over the second side. The bags are strong and will not split or tear.

BRAISED LAMB SHANKS WITH WHITE BEAN PUREE

Lamb shanks are often served on the bone, but they can take over the entire plate and look somewhat intimidating! I like to cook the shanks on the bone for the wonderful flavour. Then I take the cooked meat off the bone, reheat it in the sauce and serve it over bean puree, mashed potatoes or polenta, with beets on the side.

The bean puree also makes a great dip or spread.

Makes 8 servings

1 onion, chopped
2 cloves garlic, minced
2 cups (500 mL) dry red wine or homemade chicken stock (page 109)
1 tbsp (15 mL) chopped fresh rosemary, or 1/2 tsp (2 mL) dried
1 tbsp (15 mL) chopped fresh thyme, or 1/2 tsp (2 mL) dried
1/2 tsp (2 mL) pepper
6 lamb shanks (about 8 oz/250 g each), trimmed

Sauce

1 tsp (5 mL) olive oil
6 onions, sliced
6 cloves garlic, finely chopped
1/4 tsp (1 mL) hot red pepper flakes
1 tbsp (15 mL) chopped fresh rosemary, or 1/2 tsp (2 mL) dried
1 tbsp (15 mL) chopped fresh thyme, or 1/2 tsp (2 mL) dried
1/2 tsp (2 mL) pepper
1 28-oz (796 mL) can plum tomatoes, with juices
Salt to taste

White Bean Puree

2 19-oz (540 mL) cans white kidney beans, rinsed and drained, or
    4 cups (1 L) cooked beans (page 179)
3 cloves garlic, finely chopped
1 tsp (5 mL) ground cumin
1/2 tsp (2 mL) pepper
6 cups (1.5 L) water
1 tbsp (15 mL) lemon juice
1/2 tsp (2 mL) hot red pepper sauce
1/2 cup (125 mL) chopped fresh parsley

PER SERVING	
Calories	299
Protein	26 g
Fat	7 g
Saturates	3 g
Cholesterol	56 mg
Carbohydrate	34 g
Fibre	11 g
Sodium	509 mg
Potassium	751 mg

Excellent: Niacin; Folate; Vitamin B12; Iron
Good: Vitamin C; Thiamine; Riboflavin; Vitamin B6

1. In a large bowl, combine chopped onion, minced garlic, wine, rosemary, thyme and pepper. Add lamb and marinate in refrigerator for 2 hours or up to overnight.

2. Drain shanks well and pat dry. Strain juices and reserve.

3. To prepare sauce, heat oil in a Dutch oven on medium-high heat. Add lamb shanks and brown for about 10 minutes, in batches if necessary. Remove and discard all but 1 tbsp (15 mL) fat from pan.

4. Add sliced onions, chopped garlic and hot pepper flakes to pan. Reduce heat to medium and cook gently until tender and fragrant, about 10 minutes.

5. Add rosemary, thyme, pepper, strained marinade juices and tomatoes. Bring to a boil.

6. Return lamb to pan, cover and cook in a preheated 350°F (180°C) oven for 2 to 3 hours, or until lamb is very tender. Skim fat from sauce. If sauce is too liquidy, remove shanks and cook sauce over medium-high heat until thickened. Add salt to taste.

7. Cool lamb shanks slightly and remove meat from bones. Return meat to sauce.

8. Meanwhile, to prepare bean puree, in a large saucepan, combine beans, garlic, cumin, pepper and water. Bring to a boil, reduce heat and cook gently for 20 minutes. Drain, reserving cooking liquid.

9. In a food processor, puree beans with lemon juice and hot pepper sauce. Add enough cooking liquid to achieve desired consistency.

10. Spread bean puree on each plate and top with lamb, onions and juices. Sprinkle with parsley.

POT ROAST OF LAMB WITH TOMATOES AND ORZO

This recipe is always a big hit. It has Greek flavours and tastes wonderfully hearty and robust. You could also make it with a beef pot roast instead of lamb. Serve it sprinkled with crumbled feta cheese if you wish.

Orzo is rice-shaped pasta, but you can use any small pasta in this, or you could use rice (precook it for 10 minutes and then finish cooking in the sauce until tender). You can also omit the pasta, reduce the sauce until it thickens and serve this over mashed potatoes or polenta. Use leftovers in wraps, or chop and serve as a stew.

This is a perfect make-ahead dish. Slice the lamb when cold and reheat in reserved sauce. Reheat orzo or cook before serving.

Makes 10 to 12 servings

4-lb (2 kg) boneless leg or shoulder of lamb, trimmed,
    rolled and tied
1 tsp (5 mL) salt
¼ tsp (1 mL) pepper
1 tbsp (15 mL) olive oil
3 onions, coarsely chopped
20 cloves garlic, peeled but left whole
2 tbsp (25 mL) ground cumin
1 tbsp (15 mL) dried oregano
1 28-oz (796 mL) can plum tomatoes, with juices
1 cup (250 mL) dry white or red wine, homemade chicken stock
    (page 109) or water
1 lb (500 g) orzo or other small pasta (about 3 cups/750 mL)
Bunch of fresh parsley

1. Pat lamb dry and season with salt and pepper.
2. Heat oil in a Dutch oven on medium-high heat. Add lamb and brown well on all sides. This should take about 10 to 15 minutes. Remove roast from pan. Discard all but 1 tbsp (15 mL) fat from pan.
3. Add onions and garlic to pan. Reduce heat to medium and cook for a few minutes. Add cumin and oregano and cook for 2 minutes.
4. Add tomatoes and wine and bring to a boil. Break up tomatoes with a spoon. Return roast to pan, spooning some tomato mixture on top. Cover and cook in a preheated 350°F (180°C) oven for 3 to 4 hours, or until meat is very tender. Check every 30 minutes or so to be sure there are always a few cups of liquid in pan.

PER SERVING	
Calories	447
Protein	45 g
Fat	10 g
Saturates	3 g
Cholesterol	132 mg
Carbohydrate	43 g
Fibre	4 g
Sodium	447 mg
Potassium	655 mg

Excellent: Riboflavin; Niacin; Iron
Good: Vitamin B6; Folate

5. Meanwhile, cook orzo in a large pot of boiling water for 5 minutes. Drain, rinse with cold water and drain again.

6. Remove roast from pan to a carving board. Skim any fat from surface of sauce and discard. Place pan on stove and bring to a boil. Cook over medium-high heat until you have about 5 cups (1.25 L) sauce (if there isn't enough sauce, add some stock or water).

7. Reserve about 1 cup (250 mL) sauce. Add orzo to remaining 4 cups (1 L) liquid in pan and cook for 5 minutes, or until very tender. Taste and adjust seasonings if necessary.

8. Slice roast, place in a large, deep serving dish and moisten with reserved sauce. Spoon orzo around lamb and garnish with parsley.

COOKING TIME FOR ROASTS

The cooking time for roasts depends on the weight, thickness and shape of the cut. Although experienced cooks can usually make an educated guess, a meat thermometer is the only sure way to know whether your meat is cooked to the desired doneness.

The thin-stemmed instant-read thermometers work the best. When you think the meat is ready, insert the thermometer into the centre of the roast, being careful not to let it touch the pan, a bone or piece of fat. The thermometer will register in about 10 seconds. There are also digital thermometer/timers that you can set and leave in the roast; the thermometer will beep when the meat is ready.

I like to cook beef and lamb to 135°F (57°C) for medium-rare. I usually cook pork and unstuffed roast chicken or chicken pieces to 160°F (71°C), but stuffed chicken or turkey should reach 185°F (85°C) to ensure that the raw juices in the stuffing are fully cooked.

CANTONESE-STYLE GRILLED LEG OF LAMB

Lamb is one of the most popular meats served in restaurants, but some people are still reluctant to cook it at home, because they think it will have a strong aroma and taste. But if you buy young lamb, trim it well and cook it medium-rare; the result will be delicious and mild. Trimming the fat also reduces flare-ups on the barbecue. And because the meat is butterflied, it takes only 20 to 30 minutes to cook, depending on the thickness. (If you cannot barbecue this, simply roast it.)

Makes 8 to 10 servings

1 butterflied leg of lamb (about 3 lb/1.5 kg after boning), trimmed
¼ cup (50 mL) hoisin sauce
2 tbsp (25 mL) Dijon mustard
2 tbsp (25 mL) ketchup
2 tbsp (25 mL) honey
1 tbsp (15 mL) soy sauce
1 tsp (5 mL) hot Asian chili paste
1 tsp (5 mL) pepper
2 cloves garlic, minced
1 tbsp (15 mL) minced fresh ginger root

1. Cut lamb open so meat lies as flat as possible. Pat dry.
2. Combine hoisin sauce, mustard, ketchup, honey, soy sauce, chili paste, pepper, garlic and ginger. Smear mixture all over lamb.
3. Grill lamb for 10 to 15 minutes per side for rare, depending on thickness. If you are roasting, preheat oven to 400°F (200°C). Preheat a baking sheet brushed lightly with vegetable oil. Place lamb on hot pan and roast for 30 to 40 minutes. Meat should register about 135°F (57°C) on a meat thermometer.
4. Allow meat to rest for 5 to 10 minutes before carving. Carve in thin slices against grain on diagonal.

SOY SAUCE AND TAMARI

Soy sauce is made from fermented soy beans and wheat. I usually use Kikkoman soy sauce made in Japan or imported Chinese soy sauce. I don't really like low-sodium soy sauce and would rather dilute regular soy sauce with water. If you are allergic to wheat products, use diluted wheat-free tamari instead of soy sauce (check the label to make sure the tamari is wheat free).

PER SERVING

Calories	226
Protein	30 g
Fat	8 g
Saturates	3 g
Cholesterol	105 mg
Carbohydrate	7 g
Fibre	trace
Sodium	329 mg
Potassium	230 mg

Excellent: Niacin; Riboflavin; Vitamin B12
Good: Iron

ROAST LAMB WITH ROSEMARY AND POTATOES

A lot of people prefer to cook butterflied leg of lamb, but cooking the lamb on the bone adds so much flavour.

The potatoes in this dish absorb all the delicious lamb juices.

Makes 10 to 12 servings

2 tbsp (25 mL) Dijon mustard
4 cloves garlic, minced, divided
1 tsp (5 mL) pepper, divided
2 tbsp (25 mL) chopped fresh rosemary, or
        2 tsp (10 mL) dried, divided
4-lb (2 kg) leg of lamb, bone-in, trimmed
3 lb (1.5 kg) Yukon Gold or baking potatoes (6 to 8 large),
        peeled and very thinly sliced
2 large onions, sliced
1/2 tsp (2 mL) salt
1 cup (250 mL) dry white wine,
        homemade chicken stock (page 109) or water

PER SERVING	
Calories	263
Protein	27 g
Fat	6 g
Saturates	3 g
Cholesterol	87 mg
Carbohydrate	23 g
Fibre	2 g
Sodium	191 mg
Potassium	559 mg

Excellent: Niacin;
Riboflavin; Vitamin B12
Good: Thiamine; Iron;
Vitamin B6

1. In a small bowl, combine mustard, 2 cloves garlic, 1/2 tsp (2 mL) pepper and 1 tbsp (15 mL) rosemary.
2. Pat lamb dry. Spread mustard mixture over lamb and allow to marinate while preparing potatoes.
3. Arrange potatoes, onions and remaining garlic in bottom of a roasting pan. Sprinkle with remaining rosemary, pepper and salt. Pour wine over top.
4. Place lamb on top of potatoes. Roast in a preheated 400°F (200°C) oven for 80 to 90 minutes for medium-rare. Meat thermometer should read 135°F (57°C). Turn roast once during cooking.
5. Allow roast to rest for 10 minutes before carving (return potatoes to oven to brown if you wish). Serve lamb with potatoes and onions.

BALSAMIC MAPLE-GLAZED LAMB CHOPS WITH SWEET POTATOES

This is a great way to use a less-expensive balsamic vinegar, as it becomes sweeter when it is reduced (save your better-quality vinegar for salads).

You can also use teriyaki sauce (page 290) instead of the balsamic glaze.

Makes 8 servings

1 tbsp (15 mL) olive oil
3 lb (1.5 kg) sweet potatoes (4 large), peeled and thickly sliced
8 shallots, peeled (page 248) and halved
1 tbsp (15 mL) chopped fresh rosemary, or ½ tsp (2 mL) dried
1 tsp (5 mL) salt, divided
¼ tsp (1 mL) pepper
2 cups (500 mL) balsamic vinegar
3 tbsp (45 mL) maple syrup
1 tsp (5 mL) Dijon mustard
1-inch (2.5 cm) piece orange peel
16 thin rib lamb chops (about 2½ to 3 oz/75 to 90 g each),
    trimmed

1. Brush a large sheet of heavy-duty foil with oil. Arrange sweet potato slices, overlapping slightly, over centre of foil. Sprinkle sweet potatoes with shallots, rosemary, ½ tsp (2 mL) salt and pepper. Fold over foil and seal and place package in or on barbecue. Cook for about 35 minutes, turning package once or twice. (Package can also be baked in a 400°F/200°C oven for about 35 minutes, or until tender.)

2. Meanwhile, in a saucepan, combine vinegar, maple syrup, mustard, orange peel and remaining ½ tsp (2 mL) salt. Bring to a boil, reduce heat and simmer, uncovered, for 10 to 15 minutes, or until mixture is syrupy. You should have about 1 cup (250 mL) glaze. Discard orange peel. Reserve ¼ cup (50 mL) glaze for garnish.

3. Pour ½ cup (125 mL) glaze over chops and rub in. Grill lamb for 2 minutes. Brush with ¼ cup (50 mL) glaze, turn and cook for 2 minutes longer for medium-rare.

4. Drizzle plates with reserved glaze. Serve chops on a bed of sweet potatoes.

PER SERVING	
Calories	257
Protein	14 g
Fat	7 g
Saturates	2 g
Cholesterol	45 mg
Carbohydrate	35 g
Fibre	4 g
Sodium	220 mg
Potassium	514 mg

Excellent: Vitamin A; Niacin; Vitamin B12
Good: Vitamin C; Riboflavin; Vitamin B6

SHISHKEBAB-FLAVOURED BUTTERFLIED LEG OF LAMB

This marinade is also great on shishkebabs. Just cut the lamb into 1 1/2-inch (4 cm) cubes and thread on metal skewers, alternating with onion wedges. Grill, turning to cook all sides (8 to 12 minutes total). Serve with rice and carrot salad (page 122).

Makes 8 servings

3-lb (1.5 kg) butterflied leg of lamb
1 onion, cut in quarters
4 cloves garlic, peeled
1 tbsp (15 mL) ground cumin
1 tbsp (15 mL) paprika
1/2 tsp (2 mL) ground ginger
2 tbsp (25 mL) honey
2 tbsp (25 mL) lemon juice
1/4 cup (50 mL) chopped fresh cilantro or parsley
1/2 cup (125 mL) low-fat unflavoured yogurt

PER SERVING	
Calories	211
Protein	30 g
Fat	8 g
Saturates	3 g
Cholesterol	106 mg
Carbohydrate	4 g
Fibre	trace
Sodium	55 mg
Potassium	246 mg
Excellent: Riboflavin; Niacin; Vitamin B12	
Good: Iron	

1. Trim lamb of all fat and pat dry.
2. In a food processor, puree onion, garlic, cumin, paprika and ginger. Stir in honey, lemon juice, cilantro and yogurt.
3. Pour marinade over lamb and marinate for at least 30 minutes or up to overnight in refrigerator.
4. Just before cooking, scrape marinade from lamb. Grill lamb for about 10 minutes per side. (You could also brown lamb in a skillet and finish cooking in a preheated 400°F/200°C oven for 25 to 30 minutes.) Internal temperature should reach 135°F (57°C) for medium-rare. Allow lamb to rest for 5 to 10 minutes before carving on diagonal.

OSSO BUCCO (BRAISED VEAL SHANKS)

Osso bucco ("bone with a hole") is one of the most delicious braised dishes; it is a perfect dish to make ahead and reheat. I like to buy veal shanks cut about 1 1/2 inches (4 cm) thick (thicker shanks take longer to cook). If you want to serve the meat on the bone, this recipe will serve six, but you can easily serve eight if you take the meat off the bone.

Osso bucco is traditionally served with a herb topping called gremolata. Although it often accompanied by a side dish of risotto, I like to serve it with simply cooked short-grain rice and peas, which don't require all that last-minute stirring.

Makes 8 servings

1/4 cup (50 mL) all-purpose flour
1/4 tsp (1 mL) salt
1/2 tsp (2 mL) pepper
6 pieces veal shank (about 8 oz/250 g each), trimmed
2 tsp (10 mL) vegetable oil
2 onions, chopped
4 cloves garlic, finely chopped
2 stalks celery, chopped
2 carrots, chopped
2 cups (500 mL) dry white wine or homemade chicken
        stock (page 109)
1 28-oz (796 mL) can plum tomatoes, with juices
2 tbsp (25 mL) lemon juice
1 tbsp (15 mL) chopped fresh rosemary, or 1/2 tsp (2 mL) dried
1/2 tsp (2 mL) pepper
2 cups (500 mL) short-grain Italian rice
1 cup (250 mL) peas
Salt to taste

Gremolata

1/4 cup (50 mL) chopped fresh parsley
1 tbsp (15 mL) grated lemon peel
2 cloves garlic, finely chopped

PER SERVING	
Calories	437
Protein	32 g
Fat	9 g
Saturates	3 g
Cholesterol	110 mg
Carbohydrate	55 g
Fibre	4 g
Sodium	365 mg
Potassium	908 mg

Excellent: Vitamin A; Niacin; Vitamin B6; Vitamin B12
Good: Vitamin C; Thiamine; Riboflavin; Folate; Iron

1. Combine flour, salt and pepper. Pat veal dry and dust with seasoned flour.

2. Heat oil in a Dutch oven on medium-high heat. Add veal and brown on all sides, about 10 to 15 minutes in total. Remove meat from pan.

3. Add onions, garlic, celery and carrots to pan. Reduce heat to medium and cook gently for about 10 minutes, or until fragrant and tender.

4. Add wine and increase heat. Bring to a boil and cook until half the wine evaporates. Add tomatoes, breaking them up with a spoon. Add lemon juice, rosemary and pepper.

5. Return veal to pan. Cover and cook in a preheated 350°F (180°C) oven for 2 to 4 hours, or until veal is very tender. If sauce is thin, remove veal to a platter and keep warm. Bring sauce to a boil and cook until thickened.

6. About 20 minutes before serving, bring a large pot of water to a boil and add rice. Return to a boil and cook for 10 to 12 minutes, or until tender. Add peas and allow to rest for 2 minutes. Drain rice and peas in a sieve. Season with salt.

7. To prepare topping, in a small bowl, combine parsley, lemon peel and garlic. Remove veal from bones and serve on rice with sauce. Sprinkle with herb topping.

Carrots Glazed with Marmalade
Glazed Cumin Carrots
Balsamic-glazed Asparagus and Carrots
Stir-fried Broccoli with Ginger
Broccoli or Rapini with Raisins and Pine Nuts
Asparagus with Ginger and Sesame
Baked Butternut
Grilled Portobello Mushrooms and Shallots
Wild Mushrooms with Herbs
Vegetable Stir-fry
Sauteed Peppers with Garlic
Glazed Fennel with Balsamic
Glazed Rosemary Beets
Sauteed Greens
Caramelized Onions
Grilled Ratatouille
Sauteed Green Beans with Bean Sprouts and Green Onions
Stir-fried Baby Bok Choy
Maxwell Street Market Grilled Corn
Spicy Corn Ragout
Creamy Polenta with Corn and Roasted Garlic
Glazed Winter Vegetables with Maple and Ginger
Roasted Root Vegetables

Golden Harvest Mash
Cauliflower Puree
Braised Red Cabbage and Apples
Sweet Potato Maple Mash
Lynn's Lemon Potatoes
Buttermilk Mashed Potatoes
Stuffed Baked Potato Casserole
Israeli Roasted Fries
Faux Hugh Fried Rice
Edamame Fried Rice
Chinese Sticky Rice Stuffing
Mixed Grain Pilaf
Wild Mushroom Risotto
Beet Risotto
Barley and Wild Mushroom Risotto
Risotto with Butternut
Rice with Pasta and Chickpeas
Middle Eastern Couscous
Israeli Couscous with Squash and Peppers

HEART SMART

VEGETABLES
AND
SIDE DISHES

CARROTS GLAZED WITH MARMALADE

Here's a great idea from one of Canada's top French chefs, Jean-Pierre Challet. It is a version of Vichy carrots, originally cooked in sparkling mineral water from the city of Vichy. Instead of glazing carrots with the traditional sugar or honey, Jean-Pierre uses his own marmalade made with exotic spices. But it tastes great even made with a good store-bought marmalade.

Makes 4 to 6 servings

1 1/2 lb (750 g) baby or regular carrots
1 tbsp (15 mL) vegetable oil
2 tbsp (25 mL) orange marmalade
1 cup (250 mL) sparkling mineral water, homemade chicken stock (page 109) or water
1/2 tsp (2 mL) salt
1 tbsp (15 mL) chopped fresh parsley

PER SERVING	
Calories	120
Protein	1 g
Fat	4 g
Saturates	trace
Cholesterol	0 mg
Carbohydrate	21 g
Fibre	3 g
Sodium	359 mg
Potassium	484 mg
Excellent: Vitamin A	
Good: Vitamin C;	
Folate	

1. Cut carrots on diagonal into slices about 1/2 inch (1 cm) thick.
2. Heat oil in a large, deep non-stick skillet on medium-high heat. Add carrots and marmalade and cook, stirring, until carrots are well coated.
3. Add sparkling water and salt and bring to a boil. Cook carrots, uncovered, for 15 to 20 minutes, or until liquid has evaporated and carrots are glazed. Sprinkle with parsley.

GLAZED CUMIN CARROTS

Cumin, which gives this sweet dish its mysterious taste, is used in many cuisines, including East Indian, Southwestern and Middle Eastern dishes. If you don't have it, substitute 1/2 tsp (2 mL) curry powder or chili powder. Use maple syrup or brown sugar instead of honey if you wish.

Makes 4 to 6 servings

2 tsp (10 mL) vegetable oil
1 clove garlic, finely chopped
1 tbsp (15 mL) finely chopped fresh ginger root
1 1/2 tsp (7 mL) ground cumin
2 lb (1 kg) carrots, thinly sliced on diagonal
1 tbsp (15 mL) honey
Pinch salt
1 1/2 cups (375 mL) homemade vegetable stock (page 109) or water

PER SERVING	
Calories	130
Protein	2 g
Fat	1 g
Saturates	trace
Cholesterol	0 mg
Carbohydrate	31 g
Fibre	5 g
Sodium	138 mg
Potassium	535 mg
Excellent: Vitamin A;	
Vitamin B6	

1. Heat oil in a large, deep non-stick skillet on medium heat. Add garlic and ginger and cook gently for 1 minute. Add cumin and cook for 30 seconds.

2. Add carrots, honey, salt and stock. Cook, uncovered, for about 20 to 25 minutes, or until all liquid evaporates and carrots are tender and glazed. (If liquid evaporates before carrots are tender, simply add a bit of water.) Taste and adjust seasonings if necessary.

BALSAMIC-GLAZED ASPARAGUS AND CARROTS

This is a beautiful and delicious combination.

Makes 4 servings

1 tbsp (15 mL) vegetable oil
1 lb (500 g) baby or regular carrots, cut on diagonal
1 lb (500 g) thick asparagus, trimmed and cut in thirds
1/4 cup (50 mL) water
2 tbsp (25 mL) balsamic vinegar
1 tbsp (15 mL) honey
1/2 tsp (2 mL) salt
1 cup (250 mL) cherry tomatoes

PER SERVING	
Calories	119
Protein	3 g
Fat	4 g
Saturates	trace
Cholesterol	0 mg
Carbohydrate	20 g
Fibre	4 g
Sodium	347 mg
Potassium	535 mg
Excellent: Vitamin A; Folate	
Good: Vitamin C	

1. Heat oil in a large, deep non-stick skillet or wok on medium-high heat. Add carrots and cook, stirring, for about 3 minutes.

2. Add asparagus and cook for a minute longer. Add water and cook for a few minutes, or until liquid evaporates.

3. Add vinegar, honey and salt. Cook for 2 minutes, or until glazed.

4. Add cherry tomatoes and cook for 2 to 3 minutes, or just until tomatoes are heated through.

STIR-FRIED BROCCOLI WITH GINGER

If there's one vegetable that's good for you and that everyone loves, it's broccoli. You can also prepare this recipe with rapini.

Makes 4 to 6 servings

1 bunch broccoli (about 1 1/2 lb/750 g)
1 tsp (5 mL) vegetable oil
1 tbsp (15 mL) finely chopped fresh ginger root
3 green onions, chopped
1 clove garlic, finely chopped
3 tbsp (45 mL) water
1 tbsp (15 mL) soy sauce
1 tbsp (15 mL) hoisin sauce

1. Trim broccoli and cut into 1-inch (2.5 cm) chunks. Keep stems and florets separate.
2. Heat oil in a large, deep non-stick wok or skillet on medium-high heat. Add ginger, green onions and garlic and stir-fry for about 20 seconds, or until fragrant.
3. Add broccoli stems and stir-fry for about 2 minutes.
4. Add florets, water, soy sauce and hoisin sauce and bring to a boil. Cook, stirring, for 3 to 4 minutes, or until broccoli is bright green and glazed with sauce.

PER SERVING	
Calories	60
Protein	4 g
Fat	2 g
Saturates	trace
Cholesterol	0 mg
Carbohydrate	9 g
Fibre	3 g
Sodium	324 mg
Potassium	385 mg
Excellent: Vitamin C; Folate	
Good: Vitamin A	

BROCCOLI OR RAPINI WITH RAISINS AND PINE NUTS

This southern Italian style of preparing vegetables is sure to be a hit. Broccoli is always popular, but rapini, a cross between broccoli and turnip greens, is becoming more common as people discover how delicious and healthful it is. Trim the ends but use all the leafy parts as well as the stalks and florets.

Makes 4 servings

1 large bunch broccoli or rapini (about 1 1/2 lb/750 g), trimmed and
cut in 2-inch (5 cm) chunks
1 tsp (5 mL) olive oil
1 small onion, chopped
1 clove garlic, finely chopped
1/4 cup (50 mL) raisins
1 tbsp (15 mL) pine nuts, toasted (page 219)

1. Bring a large pot of water to a boil. Add broccoli. Return to a boil and cook for 3 to 5 minutes, or until just tender. Rinse with cold water to stop cooking and set colour and texture. Drain well.
2. Meanwhile, in a large, deep non-stick skillet or wok, heat oil on medium heat. Add onion and garlic and cook gently for 5 to 8 minutes, or until tender (add a bit of water if necessary to prevent browning). Add raisins and pine nuts and cook for a few minutes longer.
3. Add broccoli and toss gently until heated through and coated with onion mixture. Serve hot or at room temperature.

PER SERVING

Calories	101
Protein	5 g
Fat	3 g
Saturates	trace
Cholesterol	0 mg
Carbohydrate	18 g
Fibre	4 g
Sodium	39 mg
Potassium	535 mg

Excellent: Vitamin C; Folate
Good: Vitamin A; Vitamin B6

ASPARAGUS WITH GINGER AND SESAME

This recipe is also delicious made with sugar snap peas or broccoli.

Makes 6 servings

1 tsp (5 mL) dark sesame oil
1 tbsp (15 mL) finely chopped fresh ginger root
3 green onions, chopped
1 1/2 lb (750 g) asparagus, trimmed and cut in 2-inch (5 cm) lengths
1 tbsp (15 mL) soy sauce
1 tbsp (15 mL) balsamic vinegar
1/2 tsp (2 mL) honey

1. Heat oil in a wok or large, deep non-stick skillet on medium heat. Add ginger and green onions and cook gently for 1 minute, or until fragrant.
2. Add asparagus and stir-fry for about 2 to 3 minutes, or just until it loses its rawness.
3. Combine soy sauce, vinegar and honey. Add to skillet and cook for 1 minute, or just until asparagus is tender. Taste and adjust seasonings if necessary.

PER SERVING	
Calories	27
Protein	2 g
Fat	1 g
Saturates	trace
Cholesterol	0 mg
Carbohydrate	4 g
Fibre	1 g
Sodium	146 mg
Potassium	125 mg
Excellent: Folate	

ASPARAGUS

Try to buy asparagus with tightly closed tips. I like fat, juicy asparagus rather than the pencil-thin ones. Trim (rather than break) about 1 inch (2.5 cm) from the tough bottom ends and peel an inch or two up the stalks if you wish. Although the peeling takes time, the peeled stalks are very tender.

I cook asparagus in a skillet, covered with water, rather than steaming it upright. The tender tips and peeled stalks will cook at the same rate. Cook the asparagus for 3 to 5 minutes, until it is bright green and a spear just begins to bend over when it is held upright. After cooking, serve the asparagus immediately if you are serving it hot. If you are serving it cold, rinse in cold water to set the texture and colour and then pat dry.

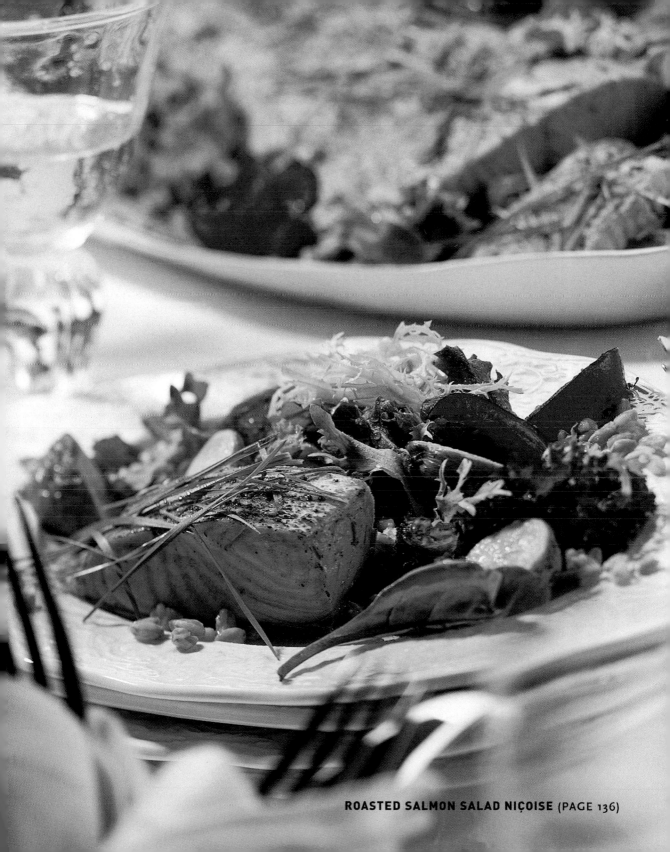

ROASTED SALMON SALAD NIÇOISE (PAGE 136)

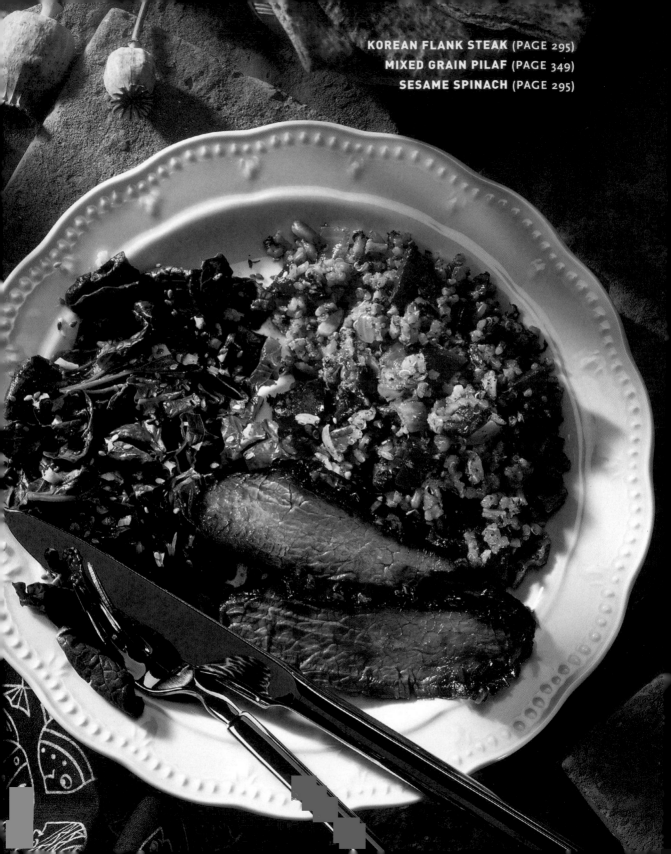

KOREAN FLANK STEAK (PAGE 295)
MIXED GRAIN PILAF (PAGE 349)
SESAME SPINACH (PAGE 295)

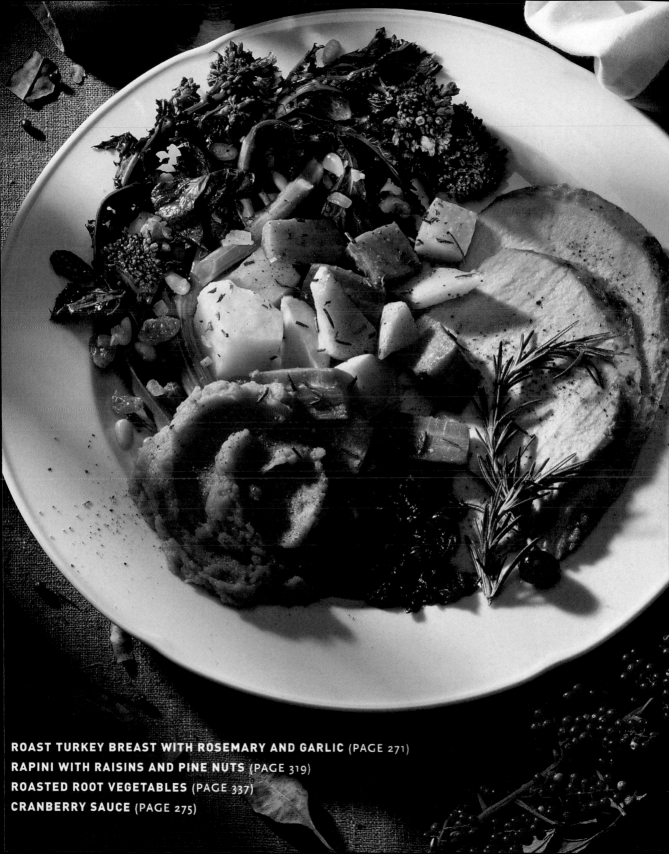

ROAST TURKEY BREAST WITH ROSEMARY AND GARLIC (PAGE 271)
RAPINI WITH RAISINS AND PINE NUTS (PAGE 319)
ROASTED ROOT VEGETABLES (PAGE 337)
CRANBERRY SAUCE (PAGE 275)

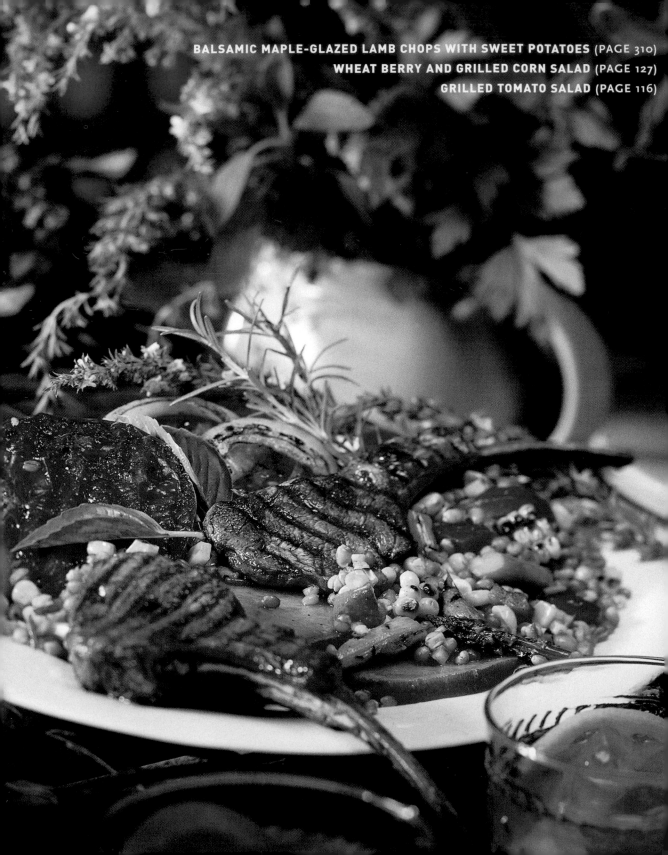

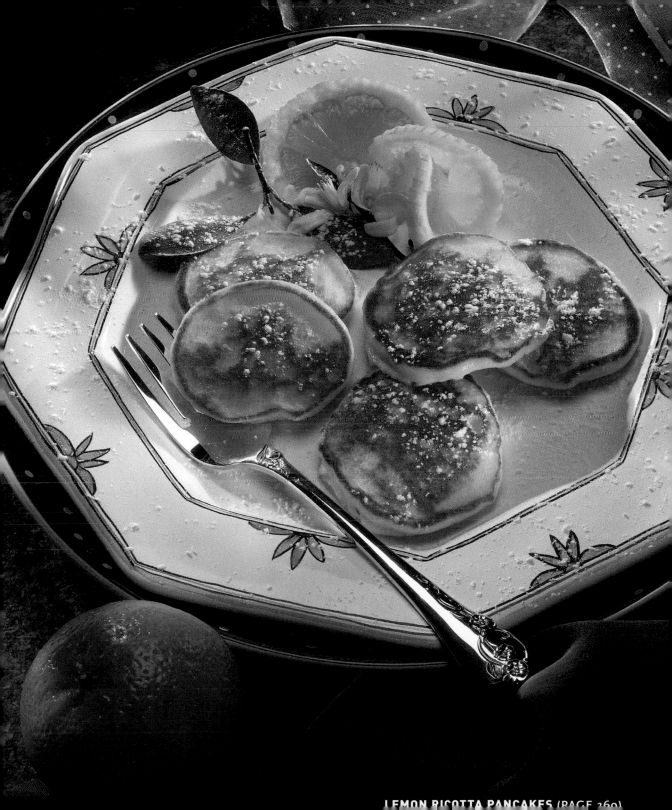

LEMON RICOTTA PANCAKES (PAGE 360)

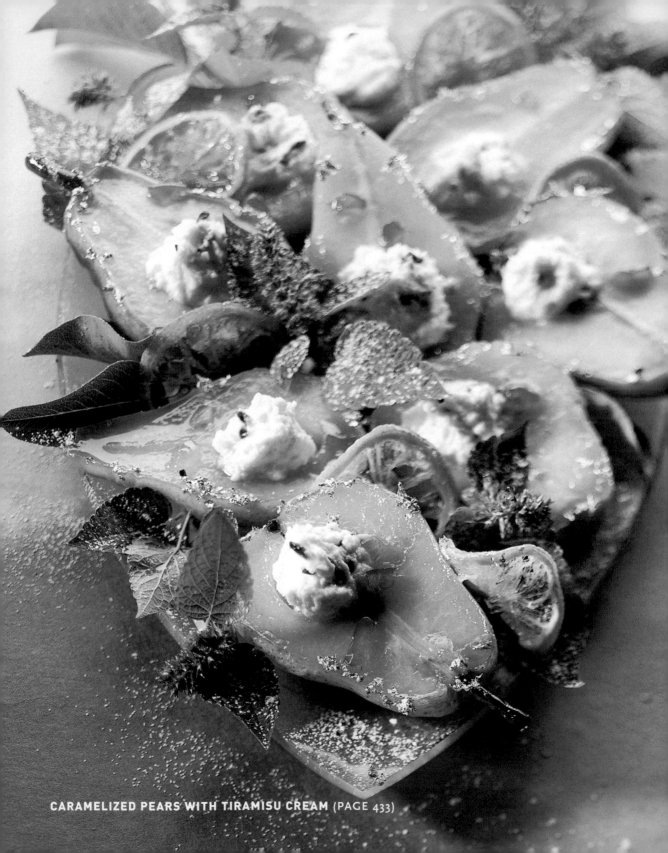

CARAMELIZED PEARS WITH TIRAMISU CREAM (PAGE 433)

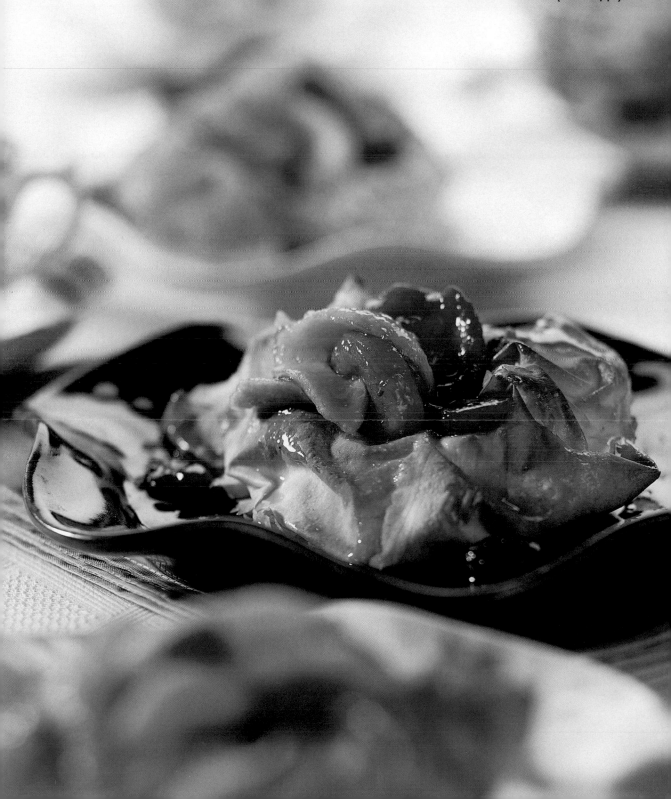

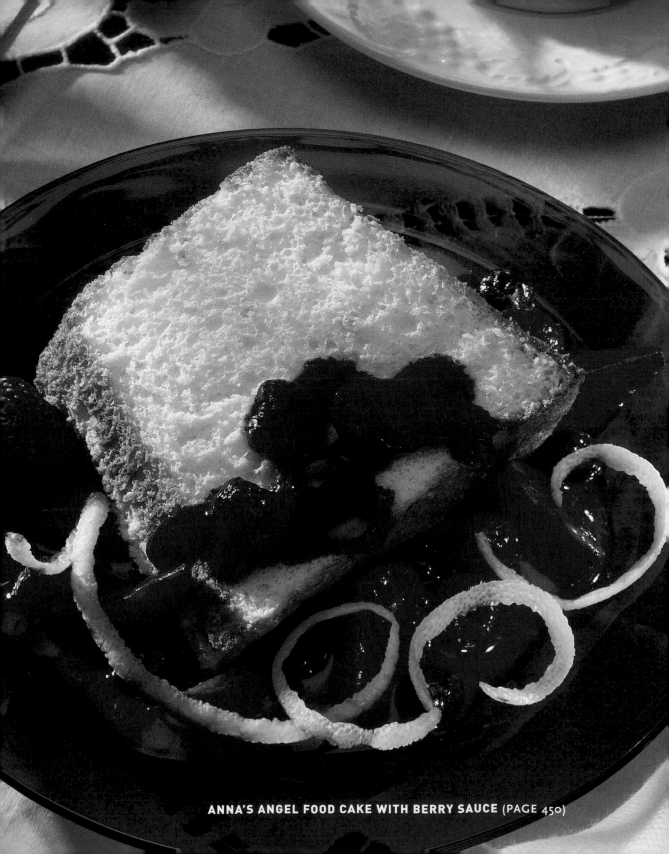

ANNA'S ANGEL FOOD CAKE WITH BERRY SAUCE (PAGE 450)

BAKED BUTTERNUT

Any kind of winter squash can be used in this recipe, but butternut or buttercup are particularly rich in texture and taste.

Makes 6 servings

3 lb (1.5 kg) butternut squash (about 2 lb/1 kg peeled and seeded)
2 tbsp (25 mL) brown sugar or maple sugar
1 tsp (5 mL) ground cinnamon
¼ tsp (1 mL) ground nutmeg
¼ tsp (1 mL) salt
¼ tsp (1 mL) pepper

PER SERVING	
Calories	103
Protein	2 g
Fat	trace
Saturates	0 g
Cholesterol	0 mg
Carbohydrate	27 g
Fibre	trace
Sodium	105 mg
Potassium	619 mg
Excellent: Vitamin A; Vitamin C	
Good: Vitamin B6; Folate	

1. Cut squash in half. Scoop out seeds and stringy pulp.
2. Place squash, cut side down, on a baking sheet. Bake in a preheated 350°F (180°C) oven for 45 to 50 minutes, or until very tender.
3. Meanwhile, in a large bowl, combine brown sugar, cinnamon, nutmeg, salt and pepper.
4. Scoop squash into bowl and mash coarsely with brown sugar mixture. Taste and adjust seasonings if necessary. Serve immediately, or spoon into a casserole dish and keep warm until ready to serve.

SQUASH AND PUMPKIN

When a recipe calls for summer squash, it usually refers to yellow or green zucchini or other soft-seeded squash like patty pan or crookneck. Winter squashes include butternut, buttercup, Hubbard, acorn and spaghetti. Butternut and buttercup are my favourite winter squashes because they are sweeter and less watery than most, but they are also a bit more expensive.

Summer squash has thin, edible skins and does not need peeling, but winter squash sometimes does. You can peel the squash before cooking, or bake it in the oven or microwave. Cut the squash in half, scoop out the seeds and bake cut side down on a parchment-lined baking sheet. After baking, scoop out the flesh and mash or puree.

Pumpkin has become very popular recently because of its healthful properties (a good source of fibre, beta carotene, vitamin E, calcium and iron), but be sure to buy the small pie or sugar pumpkins—usually only available around Thanksgiving. (To add to the confusion, what we call squash is called pumpkin in some countries.) You can usually use squash in any recipe that calls for pumpkin.

GRILLED PORTOBELLO MUSHROOMS AND SHALLOTS

At the teppanyaki bar in the Four Seasons Hotel in Tokyo, I watched the chef prepare all sorts of delicious vegetable dishes, including these simple mushrooms. He cooked the whole mushrooms on a big grill, but I just use the barbecue or grill pan. You can also use regular (white button) mushrooms or cremini (brown button) in this recipe.

Makes 6 to 8 servings
1 lb (500 g) fresh wild mushrooms (shiitake, portobello or a
        combination)
1 tbsp (15 mL) vegetable oil, divided
2 shallots, thinly sliced
2 tbsp (25 mL) soy sauce
Salt and pepper to taste

1. Trim mushrooms and clean well. Remove stems of shiitakes. If you are using portobellos, gently scrape out gills if you wish.
2. Brush mushrooms with 1 1/2 tsp (7 mL) oil. Grill for about 5 minutes, or until lightly browned. Slice mushrooms.
3. Heat remaining 1 1/2 tsp (7 mL) oil in a large, deep non-stick skillet. Add shallots and cook gently for a few minutes until tender.
4. Increase heat to medium-high and add mushrooms and soy sauce. Combine well with shallots. Cook for a few minutes, or until pan is dry. Season with salt and pepper.

SHALLOTS

Shallots have a very special flavour, not unlike a combination of onion with a little garlic. For some reason, some cooks confuse them with scallions, the American term for green onions.

Shallots look like small bulbs, and they pack a lot of flavour for their size. If you can't find them and a recipe calls for raw shallots, substitute green onions; if a recipe calls for a cooked shallot, you can substitute a small onion plus a small clove of garlic.

PER SERVING

Calories	36
Protein	1 g
Fat	3 g
Saturates	trace
Cholesterol	0 mg
Carbohydrate	3 g
Fibre	1 g
Sodium	347 mg
Potassium	161 mg

WILD MUSHROOMS WITH HERBS

Serve these as a side dish, as a topping for steaks, chops or bruschetta, in mashed potatoes or rice, or on top of greens for a warm salad. Different wild mushrooms can be found at different times of the year, but if they are too expensive or you can't find them, simply substitute plain brown mushrooms (cremini).

Makes 4 to 6 servings

2 tsp (10 mL) olive oil
2 shallots, finely chopped
4 cloves garlic, finely chopped
1 lb (500 g) fresh wild mushrooms,
    trimmed and sliced (about 6 cups/1.5 L)
1 tsp (5 mL) chopped fresh rosemary, or pinch dried
1 tsp (5 mL) chopped fresh thyme, or pinch dried
2 tbsp (25 mL) chopped fresh parsley
2 tbsp (25 mL) chopped fresh chives or green onions
Salt and pepper to taste

PER SERVING	
Calories	50
Protein	2 g
Fat	3 g
Saturates	trace
Cholesterol	0 mg
Carbohydrate	6 g
Fibre	2 g
Sodium	4 mg
Potassium	321 mg

Good: Riboflavin; Niacin

1. Heat oil in a large, deep non-stick skillet on medium heat. Add shallots and garlic and cook gently for a few minutes, or until very fragrant.
2. Add mushrooms. When mushrooms begin to release their juices, increase heat to medium-high. Cook, stirring often, for about 10 minutes, or until mushrooms are cooked and any juices have evaporated. Add rosemary and thyme after mushrooms have cooked for a few minutes.
3. Sprinkle mushrooms with parsley, chives, salt and pepper.

VEGETABLE STIR-FRY

This is an easy dish that you can make with any vegetables you have on hand. Dely Balagtas, who works with me at the cooking school, often makes this for staff lunches (she likes to use oyster sauce as the flavouring). Serve it as a side dish or with rice as a vegetarian main course.

Makes 6 to 8 servings

2 tsp (10 mL) vegetable oil
1 tbsp (15 mL) finely chopped fresh ginger root
3 green onions, sliced
2 cloves garlic, finely chopped
1 onion, sliced
2 carrots, sliced on diagonal
1 zucchini, sliced on diagonal
1 sweet red, green or yellow pepper, seeded and sliced
1 cup (250 mL) green beans, trimmed and sliced on diagonal
8 shiitake mushrooms, stemmed and sliced
1 small head broccoli, trimmed, with stems sliced
        and florets broken into pieces
1/4 cup (50 mL) homemade vegetable stock (page 109) or water
1 cup (250 mL) snow peas, trimmed
2 tbsp (25 mL) hoisin sauce, teriyaki sauce (page 290),
        soy sauce or oyster sauce
1/2 tsp (2 mL) dark sesame oil

1. Heat vegetable oil in a wok or large, deep non-stick skillet on medium-high heat. Add ginger, green onions and garlic. Stir-fry for 30 seconds but do not brown.
2. Add onion, carrots, zucchini and pepper. Stir-fry for 2 minutes.
3. Add green beans, mushrooms, broccoli and stock. Cook for 2 minutes. Cover and cook for 1 more minute if necessary to help cook broccoli.
4. Add snow peas and hoisin sauce and bring to a boil. Cook for 1 minute. Stir in sesame oil.

PER SERVING	
Calories	101
Protein	4 g
Fat	3 g
Saturates	0 g
Cholesterol	0 mg
Carbohydrate	18 g
Fibre	5 g
Sodium	125 mg
Potassium	497 mg

Excellent: Vitamin A; Vitamin C; Folate
Good: Vitamin B6

SAUTEED PEPPERS WITH GARLIC

This gorgeous mix of peppers is great on its own, in frittatas, as a sauce for pastas or pasta salads or served on top of grilled chicken or chops. You can also chop it and stir it into risotto or use it as a topping for bruschetta or pizza. Use multi-coloured peppers or all one kind.

You don't have to peel the peppers, but they're much sweeter if you do. Use a vegetable peeler and buy peppers that are squarish, to make peeling easier. The peppers could also be grilled or roasted (page 146) and then peeled, but if you grill or roast them first, shorten the cooking time.

Makes 8 servings

2 tsp (10 mL) olive oil
3 cloves garlic, finely chopped
1 hot banana pepper or jalapeño, seeded and chopped, optional
3 sweet red peppers, peeled, seeded and cut in 1-inch (2.5 cm)
      chunks
3 sweet yellow peppers, peeled, seeded and cut in 1-inch (2.5 cm)
      chunks
3 sweet green peppers, peeled, seeded and cut in 1-inch (2.5 cm)
      chunks
2 tbsp (25 mL) balsamic vinegar
Salt and pepper to taste
1/3 cup (75 mL) shredded fresh basil

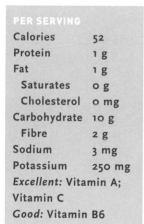

PER SERVING

Calories	52
Protein	1 g
Fat	1 g
Saturates	0 g
Cholesterol	0 mg
Carbohydrate	10 g
Fibre	2 g
Sodium	3 mg
Potassium	250 mg

Excellent: Vitamin A; Vitamin C
Good: Vitamin B6

1. Heat oil in a large, deep non-stick skillet on medium heat. Add garlic and banana pepper and cook, stirring, for 1 minute.
2. Add sweet peppers and combine well. Cook for 5 minutes, or until peppers begin to wilt. Cover and cook for 10 to 15 minutes, or until peppers are very tender. Add a few spoonfuls of water if pan becomes too dry. Uncover and cook until any liquid in pan has evaporated.
3. Add balsamic vinegar. Bring to a boil and cook for a few minutes. Add salt and pepper. Stir in basil.

GLAZED FENNEL WITH BALSAMIC

Cooked fennel is very tender and has a gentle anise flavour.

Instead of balsamic you could use vincotto, an Italian vinegar made by gently boiling the must of grapes in the wine-making process. It comes plain or flavoured (e.g., raspberry, fig or lemon), and you use it as you would a good-quality balsamic.

Makes 4 to 6 servings

2 bulbs fennel (about 2 lb/1 kg total)
1 tbsp (15 mL) olive oil
3 tbsp (45 mL) honey, brown sugar or maple syrup
1/3 cup (75 mL) balsamic vinegar
1/2 tsp (2 mL) salt
1/2 cup (125 mL) water

1. Trim fennel. Cut into wedges through core so wedges stay together.
2. Heat oil in a large, deep non-stick skillet on medium-high heat. Add fennel and cook for a few minutes, without stirring, until it is lightly browned. Turn and brown second side.
3. Add honey and vinegar and coat fennel well. Sprinkle with salt and add water.
4. Bring to a boil, reduce heat to medium and cook, stirring occasionally, until liquid evaporates and fennel is glazed, about 25 minutes. (If liquid evaporates before fennel is tender, add a bit more water.)

FENNEL

Fennel has a texture like celery and a sweet, delicate, anise flavour. The taste is usually more pronounced when the fennel is raw and very mild when it is cooked.

Use the bulb part only, as the stalks tend to be stringy and tough. The dill-like fronds can be used for a garnish or seasoning.

Raw fennel has a wonderful crunch and can be served in salads, as part of a vegetable tray with dips or even on a fruit platter for dessert.

PER SERVING

Calories	146
Protein	2 g
Fat	4 g
Saturates	1 g
Cholesterol	0 mg
Carbohydrate	29 g
Fibre	5 g
Sodium	367 mg
Potassium	637 mg

GLAZED ROSEMARY BEETS

Beets have been underrated and ignored in the past, but they are enjoying a renaissance. It's about time. They have stunning colour (you can now find them in different colours and shapes), great texture and a sweet taste. If you cook them in the oven, their colour and flavour will not leach out into the cooking water.

Makes 6 servings

2 lb (1 kg) beets (about 6 medium), washed and trimmed
2 tsp (10 mL) olive oil
1/4 cup (50 mL) balsamic vinegar
2 tbsp (25 mL) brown sugar
1 tsp (5 mL) chopped fresh rosemary, or pinch dried
1/2 cup (125 mL) water
Salt and pepper to taste
1/4 cup (50 mL) chopped fresh chives or green onions

PER SERVING	
Calories	68
Protein	1 g
Fat	2 g
Saturates	trace
Cholesterol	0 mg
Carbohydrate	13 g
Fibre	3 g
Sodium	58 mg
Potassium	389 mg
Excellent: Folate	

1. Wrap beets in foil in a single layer. Bake in a preheated 400°F (200°C) oven for about 1 hour, or until very tender. (Pierce beets with tip of a sharp knife to see if they are ready.)
2. Cool beets slightly. Rub or scrape off skins while beets are still warm (it is easier). Cut into wedges.
3. Heat oil in a large, deep non-stick skillet on medium-high heat. Add beets and toss to coat with oil. Add vinegar and sugar. Bring to a boil.
4. Add rosemary and water. Cook for 5 to 8 minutes, or until liquid evaporates and beets are well glazed. Season with salt and pepper. Sprinkle with chopped chives.

SAUTEED GREENS

Many leafy green vegetables can be cooked in this healthful and delicious way. Use beet greens, bok choy, kale, curly endive, Swiss chard or any combination. (If you are using spinach, don't add any liquid and cook for only a minute or two.)

The greens can be served as a side dish, or under grilled fish or chicken. Don't be alarmed at the large amount of raw greens; they cook down very quickly!

Makes 6 servings

2 tsp (10 mL) olive oil
2 shallots, peeled and finely chopped
2 cloves garlic, finely chopped
2 lb (1 kg) leafy greens (12 to 16 cups/3 to 4 L)
½ cup (125 mL) homemade vegetable stock (page 109) or water
Salt and pepper to taste

PER SERVING	
Calories	54
Protein	3 g
Fat	2 g
Saturates	trace
Cholesterol	0 mg
Carbohydrate	6 g
Fibre	3 g
Sodium	107 mg
Potassium	625 mg
Excellent: Vitamin A; Vitamin C; Folate	
Good: Iron	

1. Heat oil in large, deep non-stick skillet or wok on medium heat. Add shallots and garlic and cook gently for a few minutes until soft and fragrant (add a bit of water if vegetables start to stick).

2. Add greens and toss with garlic mixture.

3. Add stock and bring to a boil. When greens start to wilt, stir, cover and cook for a few minutes longer. Season with salt and pepper.

CARAMELIZED ONIONS

Caramelized onions can be used in so many ways—on top of steaks, chops or bruschetta, in quesadillas with a little smoked cheese and diced grilled chicken, in frittatas and omelettes or beaten into mashed potatoes. You can also serve them on their own as a side dish. You can double this recipe, but cook the onions in two large skillets, or they will not brown properly. Have patience, and cook them slowly. They freeze well in zipper-style plastic bags (page 303).

Makes about 1 cup (250 mL)

2 tsp (10 mL) olive oil
4 onions, thinly sliced (about 1 lb/500 g)
2 cloves garlic, finely chopped
1 tbsp (15 mL) granulated sugar
1 tbsp (15 mL) balsamic vinegar
Salt to taste
1 tbsp (15 mL) chopped fresh parsley

PER 1/4 CUP (50 ML)	
Calories	76
Protein	1 g
Fat	2 g
Saturates	trace
Cholesterol	0 mg
Carbohydrate	13 g
Fibre	2 g
Sodium	3 mg
Potassium	170 mg

1. Heat oil in a large, deep non-stick skillet on medium-high heat. Add onions and garlic, reduce heat to medium and cook for a few minutes without stirring to allow onions to brown a little on bottom. Stir and cook for 5 minutes longer, until onions are evenly golden and wilted.
2. Sprinkle onions with sugar and vinegar. Continue to cook for 10 minutes, until onions are browned, tender and very fragrant.
3. Season with salt and stir in parsley. Serve warm or at room temperature.

GRILLED RATATOUILLE

This modern version of ratatouille, which was traditionally cooked like a stew, is light and lively tasting. It can be tossed with a vinaigrette and served as a salad or can be used in sandwiches. The vegetables will keep in the refrigerator for about a week.

You can also roast the vegetables to make a roasted ratatouille (page 180).

Makes 4 to 6 servings
2 tbsp (25 mL) mL) olive oil
2 cloves garlic, minced
1 tbsp (15 mL) chopped fresh thyme, or 1/2 tsp (2 mL) dried
3/4 tsp (4 mL) salt
1/4 tsp (1 mL) pepper
1 large onion, peeled
2 zucchini, trimmed
2 Asian eggplants, trimmed
2 tomatoes
1 sweet red pepper
1 tbsp (15 mL) balsamic vinegar
2 tbsp (25 mL) chopped fresh parsley

1. In a small bowl, combine oil, garlic, thyme, salt and pepper.
2. Cut onion, zucchini and eggplants lengthwise into slices 1/4 inch (5 mm) thick. Cut tomatoes into slices 1/2 inch (1 cm) thick. Brush onion, zucchini, eggplants and tomatoes with olive oil mixture. Reserve any extra marinade for dressing.
3. Grill vegetable slices on both sides until lightly browned. Onions will take 3 to 4 minutes per side, eggplants and zucchini 2 to 3 minutes, and tomatoes only about 1 minute per side.
4. Grill red pepper on all sides until blackened (do not brush pepper with oil). Cool. Rub off skin. Cut pepper in half, discard core, ribs and seeds and slice into strips.
5. Toss vegetables together gently or layer them on a serving platter.
6. Combine any leftover marinade with balsamic vinegar and drizzle over vegetables. Sprinkle with parsley.

PER SERVING	
Calories	136
Protein	3 g
Fat	7 g
Saturates	1 g
Cholesterol	0 mg
Carbohydrate	18 g
Fibre	5 g
Sodium	452 mg
Potassium	652 mg
Excellent: Vitamin C	
Good: Vitamin A; Thiamine; Vitamin B6; Folate	

SAUTEED GREEN BEANS WITH BEAN SPROUTS AND GREEN ONIONS

Serve this under lamb chops, salmon or thinly sliced steak. Leftovers can be added to a salad or to clear broth and served as a soup.

If you can't find really fresh bean sprouts, omit them. (In Asia at the markets you can buy cleaned bean sprouts that have had the ends removed. You can do this, too; it's time-consuming, but the sprouts end up looking like translucent jewels.)

Enoki mushrooms come in little shrink-wrapped packages. You cut off the stem ends and cut open the package at the same time.

Makes 6 to 8 servings

PER SERVING	
Calories	50
Protein	3 g
Fat	2 g
Saturates	0 g
Cholesterol	0 mg
Carbohydrate	8 g
Fibre	2 g
Sodium	265 mg
Potassium	279 mg
Good: Vitamin B6; Folate	

2 tsp (10 mL) vegetable oil
3/4 lb (375 g) green beans, thinly sliced on diagonal
1 1/2 tbsp (20 mL) soy sauce
1/2 lb (250 g) very fresh bean sprouts
1 package enoki mushrooms (about 3 1/2 oz/100 g)
4 green onions, thinly sliced on diagonal

1. Heat oil in a large, deep non-stick skillet or wok on medium-high heat. Add green beans and stir-fry for 2 minutes.
2. Add soy sauce and bring to a boil. Add bean sprouts and cook for 30 seconds.
3. Stir in mushrooms and green onions. Cook for 30 seconds.

STIR-FRIED BABY BOK CHOY

Bok choy has become very popular. Even kids love it. Use it in main course stir-fries or prepare it like this and serve as a side dish.

If you use regular bok choy, cut each one into quarters.

Makes 6 servings

1 tsp (5 mL) olive oil
1 clove garlic, finely chopped
1 lb (500 g) baby bok choy, halved if necessary
1 tbsp (15 mL) soy sauce
¼ cup (50 mL) water

1. Heat oil in a large, deep non-stick skillet or wok on medium-high heat. Add garlic and cook, stirring, for about 10 seconds. Do not brown.
2. Add bok choy and stir together for 1 minute.
3. Add soy sauce and water and bring to a boil. Cook, stirring often, for about 5 minutes, or until bok choy wilts slightly and becomes tender.

PER SERVING	
Calories	18
Protein	1 g
Fat	1 g
Saturates	0 g
Cholesterol	0 mg
Carbohydrate	2 g
Fibre	1 g
Sodium	196 mg
Potassium	274 mg
Good: Vitamin A; Vitamin C	

WOKS

Woks are useful for low-fat cooking, as you can cook a lot of food in very little oil.

Buy a large wok so you have plenty of room to stir things around. Choose one with handles on both sides (easier to lift) and a lid (so you can also use it for steaming).

The wok should be very hot before you add the food. To help prevent sticking, season your new wok by washing it well. Fill it half full with a neutral-tasting vegetable oil, then heat the wok on the stove and let it cool down. Do this a few times, brushing the unoiled areas occasionally. Pour out the oil and wipe out the wok. After using, wash it only with water. Reseason as necessary.

CORN

Corn cut off the cobs adds a delicious taste and crunch to salads. Cobs of corn can also be grilled. Remove the husks and silk (a damp paper towel works well) and grill the cobs directly on the barbecue until they brown.

Frozen corn has already been blanched, so it only needs to be defrosted. If you are using it in a cooked dish, you don't even need to defrost it.

Although you can use canned corn, I think frozen is superior, and it doesn't contain as much salt.

MAXWELL STREET MARKET GRILLED CORN

I tasted this corn in Chicago at the Maxwell Street Market. The Market is as close as you'll get to Mexico without going there, and it's definitely worth a visit.

Don't be tempted to omit the lime juice; it makes the dish.

Makes 8 servings

8 ears corn
⅓ cup (75 mL) light mayonnaise
¼ cup (50 mL) grated Parmesan cheese
2 tbsp (25 mL) chili powder
8 lime wedges

1. Remove husks and silk from corn. Place on a hot barbecue, turning every few minutes, until lightly browned on all sides. (Corn can also be boiled.)
2. Slather mayonnaise on corn with a pastry brush. Combine cheese and chili powder and sprinkle over corn.
3. Serve with a wedge of lime and squeeze lime juice over corn before eating.

PER SERVING	
Calories	166
Protein	4 g
Fat	8 g
Saturates	2 g
Cholesterol	9 mg
Carbohydrate	23 g
Fibre	3 g
Sodium	237 mg
Potassium	248 mg
Good: Thiamine; Folate	

SPICY CORN RAGOUT

This is a great side dish to serve under meatloaf (page 281), grilled chicken or salmon. It tastes delicious even when made with frozen corn, and is a wonderful way to add some sunshine to your plate in the middle of winter.

If you do not like spicy food, leave out the chipotle.

Makes 8 to 10 servings

2 tsp (10 mL) olive oil
1 red onion, diced
2 cloves garlic, finely chopped
2 sweet red peppers, seeded and diced
1 tbsp (15 mL) chipotle puree (page 183), or 1 jalapeño, chopped, optional
8 cups (2 L) corn kernels
1 cup (250 mL) homemade vegetable stock (page 109) or water
3/4 lb (375 g) fresh baby spinach
1/4 tsp (1 mL) pepper
Salt to taste
1/3 cup (75 mL) chopped fresh cilantro or parsley

1. Heat oil in large, deep non-stick skillet or Dutch oven on medium heat. Add onion and garlic and cook gently for a few minutes until fragrant but not brown.
2. Add red peppers and chipotle. Cook for 5 to 8 minutes, or until peppers are tender.
3. Stir in corn and mix together well. Add stock and bring to a boil. Reduce heat and cook gently for 5 minutes. Stir in spinach and cook for 2 to 3 minutes longer, or just until wilted. Add pepper, salt and cilantro. Taste and adjust seasonings if necessary.

PER SERVING	
Calories	182
Protein	7 g
Fat	2 g
Saturates	trace
Cholesterol	0 mg
Carbohydrate	42 g
Fibre	6 g
Sodium	178 mg
Potassium	577 mg

Excellent: Vitamin A; Vitamin C; Folate
Good: Thiamine; Riboflavin; Niacin; Vitamin B6; Iron

POLENTA

When cornmeal is cooked in water, milk or stock, the creamy result is called polenta, a kind of cornmeal porridge. Cook the polenta, stirring often, over low heat (or unattended in a double boiler). Regular cornmeal will take about 30 minutes to become tender. Quick-cooking polenta will cook in about 5 minutes.

PER SERVING	
Calories	128
Protein	4 g
Fat	1 g
Saturates	trace
Cholesterol	2 mg
Carbohydrate	27 g
Fibre	2 g
Sodium	320 mg
Potassium	135 mg

CREAMY POLENTA WITH CORN AND ROASTED GARLIC

I made this in a Southwest cooking class, and it was a knockout. You could serve it as a side dish or as a main course with a salad. It can be made an hour before serving; keep it warm over a double boiler. If you don't have time to roast the garlic, just add 1 minced clove garlic.

Makes 8 to 10 servings

7 cups (1.75 L) water
3/4 tsp (4 mL) salt
1 tsp (5 mL) pepper
1 1/2 cups (375 mL) cornmeal (regular or quick-cooking)
1 head roasted garlic puree (page 67)
1 cup (250 mL) corn kernels
2 tbsp (25 mL) chopped fresh cilantro or parsley, optional
3/4 cup (175 mL) milk, hot

1. In a large saucepan, bring water to a boil. Add salt and pepper. Whisk in cornmeal slowly, stirring constantly. When mixture bubbles, reduce heat and cook on low heat for 5 minutes for quick-cooking cornmeal or 30 minutes for regular. Stir occasionally. If mixture becomes too thick, add some boiling water.

2. Add roasted garlic and corn and cook for 5 minutes.

3. Stir in cilantro and enough milk to reach consistency of very creamy mashed potatoes. Taste and adjust seasonings if necessary.

GLAZED WINTER VEGETABLES WITH MAPLE AND GINGER

The maple and ginger make Brussels sprouts taste so good that even people who don't care for sprouts like this dish.

Makes 6 servings

2 tsp (10 mL) vegetable oil
1 tbsp (15 mL) chopped fresh ginger root
1 lb (500 g) carrots, sliced on diagonal
1 lb (500 g) Brussels sprouts, trimmed and halved
2 tbsp (25 mL) maple syrup
1 cup (250 mL) homemade vegetable stock (page 109), or water
½ tsp (2 mL) salt
¼ tsp (1 mL) pepper

1. Heat oil in a large, deep non-stick skillet on medium heat. Add ginger and cook gently for a few minutes until very fragrant.

2. Add carrots and Brussels sprouts. Drizzle with maple syrup and turn to coat well.

3. Add stock, salt and pepper. Bring to a boil and cook, uncovered, for 15 to 20 minutes, or until liquid evaporates and vegetables are glazed.

PER SERVING	
Calories	92
Protein	2 g
Fat	2 g
Saturates	trace
Cholesterol	0 mg
Carbohydrate	19 g
Fibre	5 g
Sodium	254 mg
Potassium	431 mg
Excellent: Vitamin A; Vitamin C	
Good: Vitamin B6; Folate	

ROASTED ROOT VEGETABLES

Sometimes I make this recipe using just potatoes and/or sweet potatoes. You can also cook cauliflower or asparagus this way; the flavour becomes very concentrated. Roast trimmed asparagus for 15 minutes and cauliflower florets for 25 to 30 minutes.

Makes 4 to 6 servings

1 lb (500 g) Yukon Gold or baking potatoes, peeled or scrubbed
1 lb (500 g) sweet potatoes, peeled
1 large carrot
1 parsnip, peeled
1/4 lb (125 g) rutabaga, peeled
1 1/2 tbsp (20 mL) olive oil
2 cloves garlic, minced
2 tbsp (25 mL) chopped fresh rosemary, or 1 tsp (5 mL) dried
1/2 tsp (2 mL) salt
1/2 tsp (2 mL) pepper
1/4 tsp (1 mL) hot red pepper flakes, optional

PER SERVING	
Calories	253
Protein	4 g
Fat	6 g
Saturates	1 g
Cholesterol	0 mg
Carbohydrate	49 g
Fibre	7 g
Sodium	327 mg
Potassium	831 mg

Excellent: Vitamin A; Vitamin C; Vitamin E; Vitamin B6
Good: Thiamine; Folate

1. Cut potatoes, sweet potatoes, carrot, parsnip and rutabaga into 1 1/2-inch (4 cm) pieces. Place in cold water if they begin to discolour while you are preparing them. Drain vegetables well and pat dry.
2. In a large bowl, combine oil, garlic, rosemary, salt, pepper and hot pepper flakes. Add vegetables and toss well.
3. Spread vegetables in a single layer on a baking sheet lined with parchment paper (use two sheets if necessary). Bake in a preheated 425°F (220°C) oven for 45 to 55 minutes, or until vegetables are browned and tender. Stir a few times during cooking.

GOLDEN HARVEST MASH

Mashed potatoes are practically a Thanksgiving dinner staple, but try this twist—mashing potatoes with other root vegetables.

Makes 8 to 10 servings

1 lb (500 g) Yukon Gold or baking potatoes, peeled and cut in chunks
1/2 lb (250 g) parsnips, peeled and cut in chunks
1/2 lb (250 g) carrots, squash or turnips, peeled and cut in chunks
2 lb (1 kg) sweet potatoes, peeled and cut in chunks
2 tbsp (25 mL) olive oil
1 tsp (5 mL) salt
1 small bunch chives

1. Combine potatoes, parsnips and carrots in a large pot and cover with plenty of cold water. Bring to a boil and cook for 10 minutes. Add sweet potatoes to pot and cook all vegetables for 10 to 15 minutes longer, or until tender. Drain vegetables well.

2. Add oil and salt and mash coarsely. (If mixture is too thick, add a little hot milk.) Taste and adjust seasonings if necessary.

3. Spoon mashed vegetables into a serving dish. Cut chives into 2-inch (5 cm) pieces over vegetables.

PER SERVING	
Calories	183
Protein	3 g
Fat	4 g
Saturates	1 g
Cholesterol	0 mg
Carbohydrate	36 g
Fibre	4 g
Sodium	322 mg
Potassium	440 mg
Excellent: **Vitamin A**	
Good: **Vitamin B6;**	
Vitamin C; Folate	

CAULIFLOWER PUREE

Low-carb diets made this mashed-potato substitute very popular, but it is delicious in its own right. It looks like the real thing (which is why it has been called faux mashed potatoes) but with a fraction of the carbs. This version is based on a recipe from Jane Langdon, who runs Wine Country Cooking School in Niagara-on-the-Lake.

Steaming the cauliflower in a small amount of water helps to prevent it from becoming waterlogged.

Makes 6 servings

1 medium head cauliflower (about 1 1/2 lb/750 g)
1 tbsp (15 mL) soft non-hydrogenated margarine or unsalted butter
1 tsp (5 mL) salt
1/4 tsp (1 mL) pepper
3 tbsp (45 mL) grated Parmesan cheese, optional
1 tbsp (15 mL) chopped fresh parsley

1. Trim cauliflower and cut into florets. Place in a large saucepan with about 1 inch (2.5 cm) water. Cover and bring to a boil. Reduce heat and cook for 15 to 20 minutes, or until cauliflower is very tender.
2. Drain cauliflower well and transfer to a food processor. Process briefly. (Do this in two batches if necessary.) Add margarine, salt, pepper and Parmesan. Process until smooth. Serve garnished with parsley.

PER SERVING	
Calories	29
Protein	1 g
Fat	2 g
Saturates	trace
Cholesterol	0 mg
Carbohydrate	2 g
Fibre	1 g
Sodium	423 mg
Potassium	76 mg
Good: Vitamin C	

BRAISED RED CABBAGE AND APPLES

Red cabbage is a wonderful vegetable that is often overlooked. It can be served raw in a slaw or salad or used as a garnish. Cooked, it is mild and sweet tasting. Use an apple like Golden Delicious, which won't completely fall apart when cooked.

Makes 8 servings

2 tsp (10 mL) olive oil
2 onions, thinly sliced
2 apples, peeled and thinly sliced
1 red cabbage, shredded (about 2 lb/1 kg or 8 cups/2 L)
2 tbsp (25 mL) cider vinegar or red wine vinegar
2 tbsp (25 mL) maple syrup
1 cup (250 mL) apple juice or cider
Salt and pepper to taste
2 tbsp (25 mL) chopped fresh parsley

1. Heat oil in a large, deep non-stick skillet or wok on medium-high heat. Add onions and apples. Cook for 5 minutes, or until tender.
2. Add cabbage, vinegar, maple syrup and apple juice. Bring to a boil. Cook, covered, over medium heat until tender, about 25 minutes. Season with salt and pepper and stir in parsley.

CABBAGE

Cabbage is low in calories as well as being a good source of vitamin C.

Savoy cabbage looks similar to the common white/green cabbage, but it has a deeper colour and crinkly leaves. Red cabbage can be combined with green cabbage to add colour to coleslaws.

Napa cabbage (sometimes called Chinese cabbage) has an elongated shape and delicate flavour. (When you are buying Napa cabbage, make sure the leaves do not have any black spotted mould on them.)

Bok choy, another Chinese green, is also a cabbage. It is usually served cooked and is great in stir-fries.

PER SERVING

Calories	89
Protein	2 g
Fat	2 g
Saturates	0 g
Cholesterol	0 mg
Carbohydrate	19 g
Fibre	4 g
Sodium	11 mg
Potassium	279 mg
Excellent: Vitamin C	

SWEET POTATO MAPLE MASH

One of the good things about the low-carb fad was that it got people eating things like grains and sweet potatoes. Sweet potatoes are perfect for a holiday dinner as they are bright, colourful and sweet.

I like to serve this as a base for Fish in Spicy Cherry Tomato Sauce (page 228). Mound the mashed sweet potatoes on individual plates. Top with spinach and fish. Spoon tomatoes on top of fish.

Makes 6 to 8 servings

2 lb (1 kg) sweet potatoes, peeled and cut in chunks
2 tbsp (25 mL) maple syrup
2 tbsp (25 mL) olive oil
2 tbsp (25 mL) orange juice
1 tsp (5 mL) salt
2 tbsp (25 mL) finely chopped candied ginger, optional

1. Cook sweet potatoes in a large pot of boiling water until tender. Drain well and mash coarsely.
2. Add maple syrup, oil, orange juice and salt and mash until smooth. Stir in candied ginger. Taste and adjust seasonings if necessary.
3. Serve immediately or swirl in a buttered baking dish (or pipe into rosettes) and bake in a 350°F (180°C) oven for 20 to 30 minutes, or until lightly browned and very hot.

PER SERVING	
Calories	174
Protein	2 g
Fat	5 g
Saturates	1 g
Cholesterol	0 mg
Carbohydrate	31 g
Fibre	2 g
Sodium	405 mg
Potassium	224 mg

Excellent: Vitamin A
Good: Vitamin B6; Vitamin C

LYNN'S LEMON POTATOES

One of my best friends, Lynn Saunders, was so excited to give me a recipe for a change. Use ½ cup (125 mL) lemon juice if you like things really lemony. You can also use thyme instead of rosemary, or use half potatoes and half sweet potatoes, celeriac or turnip.

Serve this with roast chicken, lamb or smoked turkey.

Makes 8 servings

3 lb (1.5 kg) Yukon Gold or baking potatoes
1 tbsp (15 mL) chopped fresh rosemary, or ½ tsp (2 mL) dried
½ tsp (2 mL) salt
¼ tsp (1 mL) pepper
1 ½ cups (375 mL) homemade vegetable stock (page 109) or water
⅓ cup (75 mL) lemon juice

1. Peel or scrub potatoes and cut into 2-inch (5 cm) chunks. Place in a 13- x 9-inch (3.5 L) baking dish and sprinkle with rosemary, salt and pepper.
2. Combine stock and lemon juice and pour over potatoes. Bake in a preheated 400°F (200°C) oven for 1 ½ to 2 hours, stirring occasionally, until potatoes are tender, tops are crispy and brown and almost all liquid has evaporated.

POTATOES

There are many different kinds of potatoes. Russets, Idaho, red-skinned potatoes and Yukon Golds are great for mashing or baking (whole or as French fries). New potatoes are good for boiling, steaming and some potato salads.

PER SERVING

Calories	117
Protein	3 g
Fat	0 g
Saturates	trace
Cholesterol	0 mg
Carbohydrate	26 g
Fibre	2 g
Sodium	158 mg
Potassium	147 mg

Good: Vitamin B6

BUTTERMILK MASHED POTATOES

Buttermilk is low in fat but still has a marvellously creamy texture. Heat it gently to prevent it from separating. Although you can substitute unflavoured yogurt, buttermilk does have a distinctive tang and aroma. For dairy-free mashed potatoes, use chicken stock or lactose-free milk.

Instead of cooking the whole garlic cloves with the potatoes, you could squeeze two whole heads of roasted garlic (page 67) into the buttermilk while you are heating it.

Makes 4 to 5 servings

2 lb (1 kg) Yukon Gold or baking potatoes, peeled and halved
6 cloves garlic, peeled but left whole
$1/2$ cup (125 mL) buttermilk
2 tbsp (25 mL) olive oil, optional
Salt and pepper to taste
1 tbsp (15 mL) chopped fresh chives or green onions

1. Place potatoes and garlic in large pot and cover with cold water. Bring to a boil. Reduce heat and cook for 20 to 30 minutes, or until potatoes are tender. Drain well.
2. Meanwhile, in a small saucepan, warm buttermilk gently but do not boil (or it will separate).
3. Mash potatoes and garlic with warm buttermilk and oil. Season with salt and pepper. Stir in chives.

PER SERVING	
Calories	162
Protein	4 g
Fat	trace
Saturates	trace
Cholesterol	1 mg
Carbohydrate	36 g
Fibre	2 g
Sodium	41 mg
Potassium	609 mg
Excellent: Vitamin B6	

STUFFED BAKED POTATO CASSEROLE

This is even easier than stuffed baked potatoes. Make the casserole ahead and reheat just before serving. Use Yukon Golds, russets or baking potatoes. You could also add two slices of crisp bacon, crumbled and sprinkled on with the cheese.

Makes 8 servings

3 large Yukon Gold or baking potatoes (about 10 oz/300 g each)
1 cup (250 mL) yogurt cheese (page 391) or low-fat sour cream
1/2 tsp (2 mL) ground cumin
3 green onions, chopped
1/2 tsp (2 mL) salt
1/4 tsp (1 mL) pepper
1 cup (250 mL) grated old Cheddar cheese

1. Scrub potatoes and place on a baking sheet. Bake in a preheated 400°F (200°C) oven for 1 1/2 hours, or until very tender.
2. Cut potatoes in half lengthwise. Arrange snugly, in a single layer, cut side up, in a lightly oiled 9-inch (2.5 L) square baking dish. Gently loosen potatoes from their skins with a fork and fluff slightly (leaving them in the skins).
3. Combine yogurt cheese and cumin and spread over potatoes. Sprinkle with green onions, salt and pepper. Mash gently into potatoes with a potato masher. Mixture should start looking like a casserole (don't worry about potato skins). Sprinkle with cheese.
4. Bake in a preheated 400°F (200°C) for 20 to 30 minutes, or until thoroughly heated and crusty.

Stuffed Baked Potatoes

Scrub 3 large baking potatoes and place on a baking sheet. Bake in a preheated 400°F (200°C) oven for 1 to 1 1/2 hours, or until very tender. Cut potatoes in half lengthwise and gently scoop out flesh, leaving a shell 1/4 to 1/2 inch (5 mm to 1 cm) thick.

Mash potato flesh with 1/2 cup (125 mL) yogurt cheese (page 391) or sour cream, 1/2 cup (125 mL) grated old Cheddar or crumbled blue cheese, 3 chopped green onions, 1/2 tsp (2 mL) ground cumin, 1/2 tsp (2 mL) salt and 1/4 tsp (1 mL) pepper. Taste and adjust seasonings if necessary. Spoon mashed potatoes back into shells. Reheat at 400°F (200°C) for 20 minutes, or until thoroughly heated.

Makes 6 servings.

BAKED POTATO SKINS

Cut cooked potato skins into thin strips and toss with salt, pepper, seasonings (curry powder, chili powder or other herbs or spices) and a small amount of olive oil if desired. Spread on a baking sheet and bake in a preheated 400°F (200°C) oven for 15 to 20 minutes, or until crispy. Stir every 5 minutes. Crumble and sprinkle on soups and salads, or leave in larger pieces and serve as a snack.

PER SERVING

Calories	169
Protein	9 g
Fat	4 g
Saturates	2 g
Cholesterol	13 mg
Carbohydrate	25 g
Fibre	2 g
Sodium	317 mg
Potassium	511 mg

Good: Vitamin B6; Calcium

ISRAELI ROASTED FRIES

In Israel, French fries are often tossed with a herb mixture after frying, but this technique also works well with oven-roasted fries. You can use baby potatoes in this recipe, too.

Makes 4 servings

2 lb (1 kg) Yukon Gold or baking potatoes,
    peeled and cut as for French fries
2 tbsp (25 mL) olive oil, divided
½ tsp (2 mL) salt, divided
1 clove garlic, minced
2 tbsp (25 mL) chopped fresh parsley

1. Toss potatoes with 1 tbsp (15 mL) oil and ¼ tsp (1 mL) salt. Spread in a single layer on a baking sheet lined with parchment paper. Roast in a preheated 425°F (220°C) oven for 35 to 40 minutes, or until browned, crisp and tender inside.
2. In a large bowl, combine remaining 1 tbsp (15 mL) oil, garlic, parsley and remaining ¼ tsp (1 mL) salt. Toss potatoes in this mixture as soon as they come out of the oven.

PER SERVING	
Calories	207
Protein	4 g
Fat	4 g
Saturates	1 g
Cholesterol	0 mg
Carbohydrate	41 g
Fibre	3 g
Sodium	304 mg
Potassium	688 mg
Excellent: Vitamin B6	
Good: Thiamine; Niacin; Vitamin C	

FAUX HUGH FRIED RICE

Hugh Carpenter, one of our most popular guest teachers, likes to call his own versions of things "faux" (e.g., Faux Tuscan Chicken). His own recipe for fried rice has many different sauces, and when I was making it one day, after a glass of wine, I left out some and then mixed the others together by mistake. It still came out great, so I decided to call my version "faux Hugh."

Makes 8 servings

1 ½ cups (375 mL) basmati rice
2 ½ cups (625 mL) water
4 tsp (20 mL) olive oil, divided
2 eggs
1 small onion, chopped
2 cloves garlic, finely chopped
2 carrots, chopped
½ lb (250 g) thin asparagus spears, very thinly sliced
¼ cup (50 mL) orange juice
2 tbsp (25 mL) rice wine
2 tbsp (25 mL) oyster sauce
1 tbsp (15 mL) sweet Thai chili sauce
2 tsp (10 mL) dark sesame oil
3 green onions, thinly sliced on diagonal

1. Rinse rice in a strainer until water runs clear.
2. Place rice and water in a saucepan and bring to a boil. Cook at medium-high for about 5 minutes, or until almost all surface water has been absorbed. Cover, lower heat and cook for 10 minutes longer. Remove from heat but leave covered for 10 more minutes. Fluff and cool in a large bowl.
3. Heat 2 tsp (10 mL) oil in a large, deep non-stick skillet on medium-high heat. Beat eggs, add to skillet and cook, stirring, for a few minutes, or until scrambled. Remove eggs from skillet.
4. Heat remaining 2 tsp (10 mL) oil in skillet and add onion and garlic. Cook, stirring, for about 3 minutes, or until tender. Add carrots and asparagus and cook for a few minutes longer, or until colours brighten.
5. Add cooked rice and eggs and stir together until hot.
6. Combine orange juice, rice wine, oyster sauce, sweet chili sauce and sesame oil and stir into rice. Sprinkle with green onions before serving.

PER SERVING	
Calories	234
Protein	5 g
Fat	5 g
Saturates	1 g
Cholesterol	47 mg
Carbohydrate	40 g
Fibre	2 g
Sodium	55 mg
Potassium	159 mg
Excellent: Vitamin A	
Good: Folate	

EDAMAME

You can buy edamame (fresh soybeans) frozen in the pod. Cook for 5 minutes in boiling water and drain well. Season with salt. Eat with your fingers as an appetizer by popping the beans out of the shells.

You can also buy edamame shelled; serve them as a vegetable or in a vegetable mélange like succotash.

PER SERVING

Calories	366
Protein	15 g
Fat	11 g
Saturates	2 g
Cholesterol	93 mg
Carbohydrate	52 g
Fibre	3 g
Sodium	60 mg
Potassium	447 mg

Excellent: Folate
Good: Thiamine; Niacin; Vitamin C; Iron

EDAMAME FRIED RICE

Everyone loves fresh soybeans (edamame), and cooks are using them instead of peas or lima beans in many recipes. They are usually sold frozen, either in the pods or shelled, and are easily available now in supermarkets. They are also very healthful.

This is a great way to use cold leftover rice, so make extra the next time you steam rice and save it for this.

Makes 4 servings

1 tbsp (15 mL) vegetable oil
2 cloves garlic, finely chopped
4 cups (1 L) cold cooked long-grain rice
1 cup (250 mL) shelled edamame (fresh or frozen soybeans)
2 tbsp (25 mL) homemade chicken stock (page 109) or water
2 tsp (10 mL) oyster sauce
2 eggs, lightly beaten
2 tsp (10 mL) shredded nori, optional

1. Heat oil in a large, deep non-stick skillet or wok over medium-high heat. Add garlic and cook, stirring, just until fragrant, about 10 seconds. Add rice, separating grains with back of a spoon. Stir in edamame and cook for 2 to 3 minutes, or until rice is heated through.
2. Stir in stock and oyster sauce.
3. Make a hole in centre of rice. Add eggs and gently stir until they form soft curds, about 1 minute. Stir to mix eggs into rice.
4. Sprinkle with shredded nori.

CHINESE STICKY RICE STUFFING

I like to serve this stuffing as a side dish or dressing. You can add edamame (page 347), peas, diced carrots, fresh shiitake mushrooms, dried shrimp, Chinese barbecued sausage or water chestnuts, but Jenny Cheng Burke who works with me says this simple version is the best. I think so, too.

This is also great as a light meal or wrapped in lettuce leaves.

Makes 6 to 8 servings
2 cups (500 mL) sticky rice
6 to 8 dried shiitake mushrooms
2 tbsp (25 mL) vegetable oil
1 onion, chopped
1 cup (250 mL) diced cooked chicken
1 1/2 cups (375 mL) homemade chicken stock (page 109) or water
2 tbsp (25 mL) rice wine
2 tbsp (25 mL) soy sauce
1 tsp (5 mL) dark sesame oil
1/4 tsp (1 mL) pepper

1. Rinse rice twice and then soak in cold water for 30 to 60 minutes.
2. Meanwhile, soak mushrooms in warm water for 30 to 60 minutes, or until softened. (The thicker the mushrooms, the longer they need to soak.) Drain mushrooms well, rinsing off any grit and squeezing out any excess liquid. Discard stems, cut mushrooms in half and slice thinly.
3. Heat vegetable oil in a large saucepan on medium-high heat. Add onion, mushrooms and chicken and cook for 5 minutes.
4. Drain rice and add to saucepan. Combine well and cook for 1 minute.
5. Add stock, rice wine, soy sauce and sesame oil. Bring to a boil. Add pepper. Cover, reduce heat and simmer for 20 minutes. Let rest for 15 minutes before serving. Taste and adjust seasonings if necessary.

PER SERVING	
Calories	319
Protein	9 g
Fat	7 g
Saturates	1 g
Cholesterol	9 mg
Carbohydrate	55 g
Fibre	1 g
Sodium	199 mg
Potassium	190 mg
Good: Niacin	

QUINOA

Quinoa is an ancient, protein-rich grain that can be found at health food stores or bulk food stores. It needs to be thoroughly washed before cooking, as it has a slightly bitter covering (saponin) that should be rinsed away. You can also toast the washed quinoa to add a nutty flavour without adding fat. Before cooking, toast it in a dry skillet, stirring, until it colours slightly.

To cook quinoa, rinse 1½ cups (375 mL) quinoa in cold water until the water runs clear. Bring 3 cups (750 mL) water and 1 tsp (5 mL) soy sauce to a boil. Add the quinoa, cover and simmer for 15 minutes. Fluff gently before serving.

Makes 4 to 6 servings.

PER SERVING

Calories	344
Protein	8 g
Fat	7 g
Saturates	1 g
Cholesterol	0 mg
Carbohydrate	66 g
Fibre	9 g
Sodium	57 mg
Potassium	577 mg

Excellent: Vitamin A; Vitamin C; Iron
Good: Thiamine; Niacin; Vitamin B6; Folate

MIXED GRAIN PILAF

A mix of different grains makes this pilaf particularly interesting, but use just one or two if you cannot find all of them. I got the idea for this from my good friend Mary Risley, who owns the Tante Marie School of Cooking in San Francisco.

Makes 4 to 6 servings

2 tsp (10 mL) vegetable oil
1 onion, chopped
2 cloves garlic, finely chopped
1 tbsp (15 mL) chili powder
1 tsp (5 mL) ground cumin
¼ tsp (1 mL) cayenne
½ cup (125 mL) long-grain brown rice, preferably basmati
½ cup (125 mL) pearl barley
¼ cup (50 mL) quinoa, rinsed
¼ cup (50 mL) wehani rice
3 cups (750 mL) homemade vegetable stock (page 109) or
     chicken stock
2 sweet red peppers, preferably roasted (page 146),
     seeded, peeled and diced
1 tbsp (15 mL) pine nuts, toasted (page 219)
¼ cup (50 mL) chopped fresh cilantro or parsley

1. Heat oil in a large saucepan on medium heat. Add onion and garlic and cook for a few minutes until tender. Stir in chili powder, cumin and cayenne. Cook for about 30 seconds, stirring constantly, until very fragrant.
2. Add brown rice, barley, quinoa and wehani. Stir in well.
3. Add stock and bring to a boil. Reduce heat, cover and cook gently for 40 to 45 minutes, or until liquid is absorbed and rice is very tender.
4. Stir in red peppers, pine nuts and cilantro. Taste and adjust seasonings if necessary.

WILD MUSHROOM RISOTTO

Although risotto must be cooked just before serving, it is well worth the trouble. Cook it for guests you don't mind having in the kitchen while you finish the dish—they can even help you stir. Planning is also important when you are serving risotto. Make sure there isn't anything else on the menu that you have to prepare at the last minute.

When the risotto is ready, it should be a creamy mass, but each grain of rice should still be separate. Serve it right away on hot plates, directly from the pot or a heated serving bowl.

Makes 6 servings

$^{1}/_{2}$ oz (15 g) dried wild mushrooms
1 $^{1}/_{2}$ cups (375 mL) warm water
1 tbsp (15 mL) olive oil
1 onion, chopped
2 cloves garlic, finely chopped
$^{1}/_{2}$ lb (250 g) fresh portobello or other wild mushrooms or
    regular mushrooms, trimmed and sliced
2 cups (500 mL) short-grain rice
6 cups (1.5 L) homemade vegetable stock (page 109) or
    chicken stock
Salt and pepper to taste
1 tbsp (15 mL) white truffle oil, optional
2 tbsp (25 mL) chopped fresh parsley
$^{1}/_{4}$ cup (50 mL) grated Parmesan cheese

1. Cover dried mushrooms with warm water. Allow to rest for about 30 minutes, or until mushrooms have softened. Pour through a strainer lined with cheesecloth or paper towel to remove sand and grit, reserving liquid. Rinse mushrooms well and chop.

2. In a large non-stick saucepan, heat oil on medium heat. Add onion and garlic and cook for 5 minutes, or until tender.

3. Add fresh mushrooms and cook for 5 to 8 minutes, or until any liquid has evaporated.

4. Add chopped wild mushrooms and cook for a few minutes. Stir in rice and cook for a few minutes.

5. Meanwhile, combine stock and reserved mushroom liquid in a saucepan and bring to a simmer.

6. Add 1 cup (250 mL) hot stock to rice. Cook over medium to medium-high heat, stirring constantly, until liquid evaporates or has

WHITE TRUFFLE OIL
White truffle oil is olive oil infused with white truffles. White (and black) truffles are incredibly aromatic fungi found buried at the roots of trees such as oaks and poplars in Italy and France. You can buy the oil in specialty stores. Keep it in the refrigerator and use it up quickly, as the wonderful truffle flavour dissipates once the bottle has been opened.

PER SERVING

Calories	338
Protein	12 g
Fat	5 g
Saturates	2 g
Cholesterol	4 mg
Carbohydrate	59 g
Fibre	2 g
Sodium	111 mg
Potassium	391 mg

Excellent: Niacin
Good: Vitamin B12

been absorbed. Continue adding liquid about ¹/₂ cup (125 mL) at a time, stirring constantly, until rice is tender. This should take about 15 to 18 minutes. Do not worry if you do not need all the liquid, or if you need a little more. Rice should be just barely tender.

7. Season with salt, pepper and truffle oil. Stir in parsley, sprinkle with cheese and serve immediately.

RICE

Use long-grain rice in pilafs or when you want each grain to remain separate. If you want the rice to stick together (sushi) or if you want the dish to be creamy (risottos and rice puddings), use short-grain rice.

Brown rice is more nutritious than white rice, as its outer husk contains bran, fibre and vitamins. But brown rice usually takes longer to cook, and it is more expensive. It doesn't keep as long as white rice, so buy it in small quantities and/or keep it refrigerated.

Basmati Rice

Basmati is a naturally aromatic long-grain rice from India. Before cooking, wash the rice in plenty of cold water until the rinse water runs clear. You can buy brown or white basmati rice, and although both are very good, I find the white more fragrant. Other fragrant rices such as jasmine and Thai-scented are also delicious.

Risotto Rice

Risotto (which is the name of the dish as well as the rice-cooking technique) is made with a special short-grain Italian rice such as Vialone Nano (my favourite), Carnaroli or Arborio. The texture of the finished dish should be creamy, but you should still be able to distinguish each grain in the creamy mass.

Sticky Rice

Sticky rice (also called sweet or glutinous rice) is very white and opaque. (It is quite sticky, but don't worry. You get used to it.) Buy it at Asian markets and serve it as a side dish or in stuffings (page 348).

Sushi Rice

Sushi rice is a short-grain Japanese rice that sticks together when steamed, making it perfect for moulding in dishes like sushi.

Wehani Rice

Wehani is a delicious brown rice that resembles wild rice in taste, appearance and texture. It has a firm outside shell and is very chewy and flavourful. It can be used in any recipe that calls for brown rice or wild rice. Look for it in health food stores, bulk food stores and specialty stores.

When you cook wehani, use twice as much water as you would for regular rice, and steam it for 40 to 50 minutes, or until tender. Or you can cook it in lots of boiling water like pasta. Cook for about 25 to 35 minutes, or until tender and the grains puff, then drain through a sieve.

Wild Rice

Wild rice is actually a grass, not a grain. But when it cooks, it has a texture and flavour very similar to brown rice. Wild rice takes about 50 minutes to cook, so make extra and freeze for another time. It tastes great in salads, rice pudding and pancakes.

BEET RISOTTO

The vibrant colour of this risotto makes it perfect for a romantic dinner, especially if you cook it with your partner! If you have any leftovers, make risotto cakes (page 354).

Makes 4 to 6 servings

1 lb (500 g) red beets, trimmed but not peeled
1 tbsp (15 mL) olive oil
1 large onion, chopped
2 cloves garlic, finely chopped
2 cups (500 mL) short-grain rice
5 cups (1.25 L) homemade vegetable stock (page 109) or
      chicken stock
Salt and pepper to taste
2 tbsp (25 mL) chopped fresh parsley
1/2 cup (125 mL) crumbled soft unripened goat cheese

1. Wrap beets in foil in a single layer. Place in a preheated 400°F (200°C) oven and roast for about 1 hour, or until beets are tender when pierced with a knife. Unwrap, cool for 5 minutes and rub off peels. Dice beets.

2. Heat oil in a large non-stick saucepan on medium heat. Add onion and garlic and cook gently for 5 minutes. Add rice and coat with onion and oil.

3. Meanwhile, heat stock in a saucepan just until simmering.

4. Add 1 cup (250 mL) stock to rice. Stirring constantly, cook on medium or medium-high heat until all liquid has been absorbed or has evaporated. Then, still stirring, add 1/2 cup (125 mL) stock at a time, waiting until pan is almost dry before adding next batch. It should take about 15 to 20 minutes to add all liquid. Add more liquid if necessary or stop adding liquid if rice is tender before all liquid is used. Rice should be just barely tender.

5. Stir in beets when rice is almost tender. Add salt and pepper. Sprinkle with parsley and goat cheese.

PER SERVING	
Calories	539
Protein	18 g
Fat	10 g
Saturates	4 g
Cholesterol	10 mg
Carbohydrate	93 g
Fibre	4 g
Sodium	173 mg
Potassium	658 mg

Excellent: Niacin; Folate
Good: Riboflavin; Vitamin B6; Vitamin B12; Iron

BARLEY AND WILD MUSHROOM RISOTTO

The texture of cooked barley is very much like risotto, so it lends itself easily to the traditional risotto cooking method. Although it takes 30 to 40 minutes for the barley to become tender, you do not have to stir it constantly as with traditional risotto.

This dish is very high in dietary fibre. It makes a great appetizer, side dish or meatless main course.

Makes 4 servings

1 oz (30 g) dried wild mushrooms
2 cups (500 mL) warm water
1 tbsp (15 mL) olive oil
1 onion, finely chopped
2 cloves garlic, finely chopped
1 cup (250 mL) pearl barley
1 cup (250 mL) dry white wine or vegetable stock
6 cups (1.5 L) homemade vegetable stock (page 109) or chicken
    stock, hot
Salt and pepper to taste
1/2 cup (125 mL) grated Parmesan cheese, optional
2 tbsp (25 mL) chopped fresh parsley

PER SERVING	
Calories	199
Protein	5 g
Fat	3 g
Saturates	1 g
Cholesterol	1 mg
Carbohydrate	37 g
Fibre	6 g
Sodium	41 mg
Potassium	430 mg
Excellent: Niacin	
Good: Iron	

1. Soak mushrooms in warm water for 30 minutes. Strain liquid through paper towels to remove sand and grit, and reserve liquid. Rinse mushrooms well and chop.

2. Heat oil in a large non-stick saucepan on medium heat. Add onion and garlic and cook gently for about 5 minutes, or until tender and fragrant. Add barley and coat well with onion mixture. Add mushrooms and combine.

3. Stirring constantly, add wine. Cook until wine has evaporated or been absorbed by barley. Add mushroom liquid and cook, stirring occasionally, for 5 to 8 minutes, or until liquid has been absorbed.

4. Start adding hot chicken stock 1 cup (250 mL) at a time, stirring often, over medium heat. Do not add next batch of liquid until barley is almost dry again. When barley is tender, after about 30 to 40 minutes, stop adding stock, whether it has all been used or not.

5. Add salt and pepper. Stir in cheese and parsley and serve immediately.

RISOTTO WITH BUTTERNUT

Kids may say they don't like squash, but they love butternut. It's all in the name. In this dish the butternut adds a lovely colour and rich and complex flavour and texture. Serve it as a first course, main course or side dish with roasted or grilled meat or fish.

Makes 6 to 8 servings

1 tbsp (15 mL) olive oil
2 leeks or small onions, trimmed and diced
1 clove garlic, finely chopped
1 1/2 cups (375 mL) short-grain rice
2 cups (500 mL) diced, peeled butternut squash
4 cups (1 L) homemade vegetable stock (page 109) or chicken
      stock
1/2 tsp (2 mL) pepper
Salt to taste
2 tbsp (25 mL) chopped fresh chives or green onions

1. Heat oil in a large saucepan on medium heat. Add leeks and garlic and cook gently for 5 minutes until fragrant and tender but not brown.
2. Stir in rice and coat well. Add squash and combine well.
3. Meanwhile, heat stock in a separate saucepan just until simmering.
4. Add 1 cup (250 mL) stock to rice. Stirring constantly, cook on medium or medium-high heat until stock has evaporated. Continue to add stock 1/2 cup (125 mL) at a time. Stirring constantly, cook until each addition is absorbed before adding next. After 15 minutes, begin tasting risotto to see if it is ready (you may need a bit more or less stock). Season with pepper and salt. Stir in chives. Taste and adjust seasonings if necessary. Serve immediately.

Risotto with Rapini

Cook 1 lb chopped rapini or broccoli in a large pot of boiling water for 5 minutes. Add in place of squash.

RISOTTO CAKES

Combine 2 to 3 cups (500 mL to 750 mL) cooked risotto with 1 beaten egg. Shape into patties about 3 inches (7.5 cm) in diameter and 3/4 inch (2 cm) thick. Heat a little olive oil in a non-stick skillet and pan-fry risotto cakes for about 5 minutes per side, or until browned and crusty on the outside and hot in the middle. You can also pack the risotto into a small parchment-lined or oiled loaf pan or ramekins. Cover with parchment paper and bake in a preheated 350°F (180°C) oven for 30 minutes.
      Makes 3 to 4 patties.

PER SERVING

Calories	248
Protein	4 g
Fat	3 g
Saturates	1 g
Cholesterol	0 mg
Carbohydrate	52 g
Fibre	2 g
Sodium	27 mg
Potassium	357 mg

Excellent: Vitamin A

RICE WITH PASTA AND CHICKPEAS

Although using pasta in a rice pilaf seems unusual to North Americans, it is quite common in Middle Eastern recipes. I love the texture of the two together. This makes a great vegetarian main course.

If you are using white rice in this, use 1 1/2 cups (375 mL) liquid and cook for only 15 to 20 minutes.

Makes 4 to 6 servings

1 tbsp (15 mL) olive oil
1 onion, thinly sliced
1 cup (250 mL) long-grain brown or white rice
1/2 cup (125 mL) broken whole wheat spaghetti
2 1/2 cups (625 mL) homemade vegetable stock (page 109) or
    chicken stock
1 19-oz (540 mL) can chickpeas, rinsed and drained, or
    2 cups (500 mL) cooked chickpeas (page 42)
1/4 tsp (1 mL) pepper
Salt to taste
2 tbsp (25 mL) chopped fresh cilantro or parsley

1. Heat oil in a large non-stick saucepan on medium-high heat. Add onion and cook for about 10 to 12 minutes, or until well browned. Remove onion from saucepan.
2. Add rice and pasta to saucepan and cook, stirring, for 2 minutes, or until slightly brown.
3. Add stock and bring to a boil. Reduce heat, cover and simmer gently for 15 minutes.
4. Add chickpeas and cook, covered, for 5 to 10 minutes longer, or until all liquid has been absorbed. Stir in onion, pepper and salt. Sprinkle with cilantro.

PER SERVING	
Calories	404
Protein	13 g
Fat	6 g
Saturates	1 g
Cholesterol	0 mg
Carbohydrate	74 g
Fibre	8 g
Sodium	287 mg
Potassium	344 mg

Excellent: Vitamin B6; Folate
Good: Thiamine; Niacin; Iron

MIDDLE EASTERN COUSCOUS

One of my students, Mary Lou Taylor, gave me this recipe years ago, and I have been making it ever since. Mary Lou, who is a great cook, served the couscous with lamb shanks, but it goes equally well with chicken.

For an attractive presentation, lightly oil six individual ramekins and fill with the couscous mixture. You can invert immediately onto serving plates or make ahead and cover with foil. Before serving, place ramekins in a larger baking dish filled with hot water (the water should reach about halfway up the sides of the ramekins) and reheat in a preheated 350°F (180°C) oven for 15 to 20 minutes before unmoulding.

Makes 6 to 8 servings

1 cup (250 mL) couscous
1 cup (250 mL) boiling water
1 tsp (5 mL) olive oil
2 green onions, chopped
3/4 tsp (4 mL) ground cumin
1/4 tsp (1 mL) turmeric
Pinch ground cinnamon
1 cup (250 mL) drained and chopped canned plum tomatoes
3 tbsp (45 mL) raisins
2 tbsp (25 mL) chopped fresh parsley
2 tbsp (25 mL) chopped pistachio nuts, optional

1. Place couscous in an 8-inch (2 L) square baking dish. Add boiling water. Cover tightly with foil and allow to rest for 10 minutes, or until ready to use. Fluff gently with a fork.
2. Meanwhile, heat oil in large, deep non-stick skillet on medium heat. Add green onions and cook gently for 2 minutes. Add cumin, turmeric and cinnamon and cook for 30 seconds.
3. Add tomatoes and cook for a few minutes, or until very thick. Add raisins, parsley, couscous and pistachios. Combine well. Taste and adjust seasonings if necessary.

COUSCOUS

Although some people think of couscous as a grain, it is really pasta made from a grain (semolina) and is a traditional food of the Middle East. Originally, couscous took hours to cook, as it had to be steamed and dried many times, but today most couscous is instant or quick-cooking, and simply needs to be reconstituted with water.

PER SERVING	
Calories	143
Protein	7 g
Fat	2 g
Saturates	trace
Cholesterol	0 mg
Carbohydrate	30 g
Fibre	5 g
Sodium	73 mg
Potassium	214 mg

ISRAELI COUSCOUS

Israeli couscous is a pearl-shaped pasta made to resemble couscous. It has a texture similar to barley and must be cooked in boiling water rather than simply being reconstituted like regular couscous. Add it to soups or serve it with stews and stir-fries instead of rice.

ISRAELI COUSCOUS WITH SQUASH AND PEPPERS

Israeli couscous is now a favourite ingredient of celebrity chefs everywhere. If it is not available, use regular rice-shaped pasta (orzo), plain rice or any tiny soup pasta.

Makes 6 to 8 servings

1 tbsp (15 mL) olive oil
1 onion, chopped
2 cloves garlic, finely chopped
1 tsp (5 mL) ground cumin
1 1/2 cups (375 mL) Israeli couscous or orzo (about 1/2 lb/250 g)
2 sweet red peppers, seeded and diced
2 cups (500 mL) diced butternut squash
3 cups (750 mL) homemade chicken stock (page 109) or low-
    sodium commercial broth, hot
Salt and pepper to taste
1/3 cup (75 mL) chopped fresh cilantro or parsley

1. Heat oil in large non-stick saucepan on medium heat. Add onion and garlic and cook gently for 5 to 8 minutes, or until golden.
2. Add cumin and couscous and cook for a few minutes, or until lightly browned. Add red peppers and squash and mix together well.
3. Add hot chicken stock and bring to a boil. Reduce heat, cover and simmer gently for 10 to 14 minutes, or until couscous is tender. Taste and season with salt and pepper. Sprinkle with cilantro.

PER SERVING

Calories	237
Protein	9 g
Fat	4 g
Saturates	1 g
Cholesterol	1 mg
Carbohydrate	42 g
Fibre	4 g
Sodium	21 mg
Potassium	384 mg

Excellent: Vitamin C
Good: Vitamin A; Niacin

Grapefruit Calypso
Rocky Mountain Muesli
Pineapple Upside-down French Toast
Baked French Toast
Finnish Pancakes with Strawberry Sauce
Cinnamon Banana Mash Pancakes
Blueberry Double Flax Pancakes
Ina's Whole Wheat Oatmeal Pancakes
Caramelized Apple Puff Pancake
Lemon Ricotta Pancakes
Gingerbread Pancakes with Pear Compote
Southwest Frittata
Portobello Egg Cups with Salsa
Smoked Salmon Soufflé Roll
Shrimp Taco Tapas with Chipotle Mayonnaise
Broccoli and Cheddar Quiche with Mashed Potato Crust
Goat Cheese and Fresh Herb Soufflé
Baked Sweet Potato Hash
Scrambled Tofu with Onions and Mushrooms
Breakfast Pizza
Breakfast Sandwich
Peanut Butter Granola Bars
Mint Tea
Lemon Rosemary Herbal Remedy
Spiced Chai

Strawberry Lemonade
Hot Spiced Apple Cider
Fara's European Fruit Salad "Drink"
Tropical Frozen Smoothie
Yogurt Fruit Shake
Yogurt Cheese

HEART SMART

BREAKFASTS AND BRUNCHES

GRAPEFRUIT CALYPSO

This can be served as an appetizer for brunch or lunch, but it also makes a simple but delicious dessert. I like to use pink grapefruit, but the recipe works equally well with white. If you are nervous about flambéing the rum, you can omit it, or just drizzle the warm rum over the grapefruit and serve without flambéing.

Makes 6 servings

3 pink grapefruit
½ cup (125 mL) brown sugar
½ tsp (2 mL) ground cinnamon
Pinch ground nutmeg
Pinch ground allspice
2 tbsp (25 mL) dark rum, optional

1. Cut grapefruit in half and loosen sections with a grapefruit knife or serrated knife. Do not remove sections from rinds. Place grapefruit cut side up on a baking sheet.
2. Combine sugar, cinnamon, nutmeg and allspice. Press mixture into surface of grapefruit halves.
3. Just before serving, broil grapefruit for 3 to 5 minutes, or until sugar bubbles and grapefruit is hot.
4. Heat rum gently in a small saucepan. When it just bubbles, flambé. Pour over grapefruit.

PER SERVING	
Calories	106
Protein	1 g
Fat	trace
Saturates	0 g
Cholesterol	0 mg
Carbohydrate	27 g
Fibre	2 g
Sodium	6 mg
Potassium	222 mg
Excellent: Vitamin C	

ROCKY MOUNTAIN MUESLI

Muesli is one of my favourite breakfasts. The original Bircher muesli was invented by a Swiss doctor for patients in his health clinic, and it is still very popular (in Australia, for example, it is so common that it is sold in supermarkets in containers just like yogurt).

Muesli may not look that great, but it is really delicious. This version is adapted from one that I enjoyed at the Royal Canadian Lodge in Banff, Alberta.

When you serve the muesli, stir in a spoonful of chopped or sliced nuts and fresh or dried fruit such as sliced bananas, fresh berries, dried apricots or cranberries.

Makes about 4 cups (1 L) or 8 servings

2 cups (500 mL) large-flake rolled oats
1/2 cup (125 mL) barley flakes
1/2 cup (125 mL) milk
1 apple, peeled and grated
3/4 cup (175 mL) orange juice
1/4 cup (50 mL) honey
3/4 cup (175 mL) unflavoured low-fat yogurt

1. Combine oats, barley, milk, apple, orange juice and honey. Refrigerate overnight or for up to 1 week.
2. Stir in yogurt before serving (or stir a little yogurt into individual portions as you serve them).

PER SERVING	
Calories	139
Protein	3 g
Fat	1 g
Saturates	trace
Cholesterol	1 mg
Carbohydrate	30 g
Fibre	2 g
Sodium	10 mg
Potassium	164 mg

HOMEMADE GRANOLA

Today, the terms *muesli* and *granola* are often used interchangeably to refer to any oat-based dry cereal mix (traditionally, muesli is wet). To make a dry granola, in a large bowl, combine 4 cups (1 L) large-flake rolled oats, 1 cup (250 mL) sliced almonds, 1/2 cup (125 mL) unsweetened coconut, 1/2 cup (125 mL) sunflower seeds, 1/2 cup (125 mL) wheat bran and 1/2 tsp (2 mL) ground cinnamon.

In a saucepan, combine 1/2 cup (125 mL) brown sugar and 1/3 cup (75 mL) honey or maple syrup. Bring to a boil. Toss with oat mixture.

Spread granola on a large parchment-lined baking sheet. Bake in a preheated 325°F (160°C) oven for 35 to 40 minutes, or until lightly toasted. Break into chunks, turn over and bake for 10 to 15 minutes longer. Break up again and cool. Stir in 1 cup (250 mL) chopped dried fruit. Store in an airtight container.

Makes about 6 cups (1.5 L).

PINEAPPLE UPSIDE-DOWN FRENCH TOAST

It is hard for me to find a dish that everyone in my family loves, but this one pleases us all. A cross between French toast and upside-down cake, it is sure to be a big hit. Other kinds of fruit can also be used.

To make this easy to prepare in the morning, soak the bread in the egg mixture overnight in the refrigerator. Have the pan with the sugar and pineapple ready to go into the oven as soon as you lay the bread on top.

Makes 8 servings

8 thick (about ³/₄-inch/2 cm) slices whole wheat or
    regular egg bread, crusts removed or not
3 eggs
4 egg whites
1¹/₂ cups (375 mL) milk
¹/₄ cup (50 mL) granulated sugar
1 tsp (5 mL) vanilla
¹/₄ tsp (1 mL) ground cinnamon
1 tbsp (15 mL) soft non-hydrogenated margarine or unsalted butter
¹/₃ cup (175 mL) brown sugar
8 round slices canned pineapple (14-oz/398 mL can)

1. Place bread slices in a large shallow pan.
2. Beat together eggs, egg whites, milk, granulated sugar, vanilla and cinnamon. Strain mixture over bread. Turn bread and allow to soak for at least 10 minutes, or up to overnight in refrigerator.
3. Brush margarine over bottom of a 13- x 9-inch (3.5 L) baking dish. Sprinkle evenly with brown sugar, pressing sugar into bottom of pan. Arrange slices of pineapple on sugar in a single layer. Place a piece of egg-soaked bread over each pineapple slice.
4. Bake in a preheated 350°F (180°C) oven for 30 to 40 minutes, or until bread is puffed and browned. Remove from oven and cool for 5 minutes.
5. To serve, invert baking pan onto a large platter and cut into squares.

PER SERVING	
Calories	276
Protein	9 g
Fat	6 g
Saturates	2 g
Cholesterol	97 mg
Carbohydrate	48 g
Fibre	2 g
Sodium	245 mg
Potassium	265 mg
Good: Thiamine;	
Vitamin B12	

BAKED FRENCH TOAST

I like to bake French toast instead of frying it. You can make this ahead and soak the bread in the refrigerator overnight, but the recipe works well even after soaking the bread for about 15 minutes (which is what I tend to do, as last-minute cooking is my usual style).

Serve this with maple syrup, fruit or sweetened yogurt cheese (page 391).

Makes 6 servings

4 eggs
8 egg whites
1 ½ cups (375 mL) milk
2 tbsp (25 mL) granulated sugar
2 tsp (10 mL) vanilla
½ tsp (2 mL) ground cinnamon
12 slices whole wheat raisin bread, challah or
    whole wheat bread (about ½ inch/1 cm thick)
1 tbsp (15 mL) soft non-hydrogenated margarine or unsalted butter

PER SERVING (2 SLICES)	
Calories	276
Protein	16 g
Fat	8 g
Saturates	2 g
Cholesterol	149 mg
Carbohydrate	37 g
Fibre	5 g
Sodium	370 mg
Potassium	411 mg
Excellent: Riboflavin	
Good: Niacin;	
Vitamin B12	

1. Whisk together eggs, egg whites, milk, sugar, vanilla and cinnamon. (Strain mixture if you wish.)
2. Dip bread in egg mixture and turn to coat well. Soak in egg mixture for at least 15 minutes or as long as overnight in refrigerator.
3. Line baking sheet(s) with parchment paper and brush with margarine. Arrange bread in a single layer on paper. Dot with any remaining margarine.
4. Bake in a preheated 375°F (190°C) oven for 25 to 30 minutes, or until browned and puffed (you can turn bread after 15 minutes, if desired).

FINNISH PANCAKES WITH STRAWBERRY SAUCE

I first had these amazingly tender crêpe-like pancakes at the Scandinavian Home Restaurant in Thunder Bay. I thought the strawberry sauce was a secret recipe until I found out it was simply frozen strawberries in syrup—what a great trick. This version is from Betty Carpick, who invited me to Thunder Bay to participate in a fundraising event for the Northern Heart Research Foundation.

These have become my family's favourite pancake (my kids thought they were "finished" pancakes, so that's what we call them around the house).

Makes 10 pancakes

3 eggs
1/2 cup (125 mL) all-purpose flour
1/4 cup (50 mL) whole wheat flour
1 1/2 cups (375 mL) milk
1 tbsp (15 mL) granulated sugar
5 tsp (25 mL) vegetable oil, divided
1/2 tsp (2 mL) salt
1 10-oz (300 g) package strawberries in syrup, defrosted, or berry sauce (page 450)

1. In a food processor, combine eggs, flours, milk, sugar, 4 tsp (20 mL) oil and salt. Process until smooth. Let batter rest for 30 minutes.

2. Brush remaining 1 tsp (5 mL) oil in a 9-inch (23 cm) non-stick skillet on medium heat. Add 1/3 cup (75 mL) batter and tilt pan to swirl batter over bottom of pan. Cook for 2 to 3 minutes, or until set. Bottom should be lightly browned. Flip pancake and cook second side for 1 to 2 minutes, or until browned. Remove pancake from pan and roll up loosely with nicer side (first side cooked) on outside. Keep warm in a 200°F (100°C) oven until all batter is used. Brush pan with more oil if necessary.

3. Serve pancakes with strawberries.

PER PANCAKE	
Calories	127
Protein	4 g
Fat	5 g
Saturates	1 g
Cholesterol	57 mg
Carbohydrate	17 g
Fibre	1 g
Sodium	155 mg
Potassium	120 mg
Good: Vitamin C	

CINNAMON BANANA MASH PANCAKES

I've been lucky enough to go to New Orleans a few times, and on my last visit I went out for breakfast with Thomas Mann, one of the city's most creative jewellery artists. We had delicious pancakes like these. Serve them with maple syrup or cinnamon sugar. You can make mini pancakes (2 to 3 inches/5 to 7.5 cm in diameter) and stack them. You can also add 1/2 cup (125 mL) chopped macadamia nuts or pecans to the batter with the bananas.

Makes 6 large pancakes

3/4 cup (175 mL) all-purpose flour
3/4 cup (175 mL) whole wheat flour
1/4 cup (50 mL) brown sugar
2 tsp (10 mL) baking powder
1 tsp (5 mL) ground cinnamon
1/2 tsp (2 mL) baking soda
1/2 tsp (2 mL) salt
2 eggs
2 cups (500 mL) buttermilk
1 tsp (5 mL) vanilla
1 tbsp (15 mL) vegetable oil, divided
3 ripe bananas, coarsely mashed

1. In a large bowl, combine flours, sugar, baking powder, cinnamon, baking soda and salt.
2. In a separate bowl, beat eggs, buttermilk, vanilla and 2 tsp (10 mL) oil. Mix in bananas.
3. Add banana mixture to dry ingredients and combine to make a thick batter. Do not overmix; batter can be lumpy.
4. Heat remaining 1 tsp (5 mL) oil in a non-stick skillet on medium heat. Spread about 3/4 cup (175 mL) batter in skillet. Pancake should be about 6 inches (15 cm) in diameter. Cook for 2 to 3 minutes per side, or until bubbles appear on surface. Repeat until all pancakes are made.

PER PANCAKE

Calories	277
Protein	9 g
Fat	5 g
Saturates	1 g
Cholesterol	65 mg
Carbohydrate	50 g
Fibre	3 g
Sodium	393 mg
Potassium	486 mg

Good: Thiamine; Riboflavin; Niacin; Vitamin B6; Folate; Calcium

BLUEBERRY DOUBLE FLAX PANCAKES

These light, fluffy pancakes are not only delicious, but they contain flax, which is so good for you. (Healthy never used to be a selling point, but now healthy can taste good, too.)

Flax is perishable, so store it in the freezer. To get the most out of it, grind it in a small spice or coffee grinder. I like the texture of the seeds whole or lightly crushed, so I usually include those, too, if possible.

If you are using frozen berries, use them while they are still frozen, and add them to the partially cooked pancakes just before you flip them, so the batter doesn't turn blue.

Serve these with maple syrup or blueberry sauce.

Makes 16 pancakes

3/4 cup (175 mL) whole wheat flour
1/2 cup (125 mL) all-purpose flour
1/2 cup (125 mL) ground flax
1/4 cup (50 mL) granulated sugar
2 tsp (10 mL) baking powder
1/2 tsp (2 mL) baking soda
1/4 tsp (1 mL) ground cinnamon
1/4 tsp (1 mL) salt
1 tbsp (15 mL) whole or lightly crushed flax seed, optional
2 eggs
1 1/4 cups (300 mL) buttermilk
1 tbsp (15 mL) vegetable oil, divided
2 cups (500 mL) blueberries

1. In a large bowl, combine flours, ground flax, sugar, baking powder, baking soda, cinnamon, salt and flax seed.
2. In a separate bowl, whisk together eggs, buttermilk and 2 tsp (10 mL) oil. Stir into flour mixture.
3. Heat remaining 1 tsp (5 mL) oil in a large non-stick skillet on medium heat. Drop batter by 1/4 cup (50 mL) measure onto pan. Press blueberries gently into top of each pancake. Cook for 2 to 3 minutes, or until surface loses its sheen. Flip and cook second side for 1 to 2 minutes, or until pancakes are cooked. Repeat until all batter is used.

BLUEBERRY MAPLE SAUCE

Serve this sauce hot or cold over pancakes, waffles, ice cream or angel food cake.

In a saucepan, combine 4 cups (1 L) blueberries, 1 cup (250 mL) cranberry juice, 2 tbsp (25 mL) maple syrup, 1 tsp (5 mL) grated lemon peel and 1/4 tsp (1 mL) ground cinnamon. Bring to a boil, reduce heat and cook gently for about 5 minutes, or until blueberries soften.

In a small bowl, whisk together 2 tbsp (25 mL) cornstarch and 2 tbsp (25 mL) cold water.

Stir cornstarch mixture into blueberries and cook for 1 to 2 minutes, or until thickened.

Makes about 4 cups (1 L).

PER PANCAKE	
Calories	101
Protein	3 g
Fat	3 g
Saturates	1 g
Cholesterol	24 mg
Carbohydrate	15 g
Fibre	2 g
Sodium	139 mg
Potassium	109 mg

INA'S WHOLE WHEAT OATMEAL PANCAKES

Ina Pinkney says the test of a good pancake is that it should taste great on its own without any syrup or topping. And she should know. At Ina's, on West Randolph Street in Chicago, people line up for hours to sample her pancakes. When I was there I had Heavenly Hots and my favourite, these amazing whole wheat oatmeal pancakes made with buttermilk and brown sugar. And although they taste great on their own, I do like a little pure maple syrup on top.

Ina uses butter in her pancakes, but you can also use oil.

Makes 12 pancakes

¾ cup (175 mL) large-flake rolled oats
2 ¼ cups (550 mL) buttermilk
1 egg
3 tbsp (25 mL) brown sugar
2 tbsp (45 mL) vegetable oil, divided
½ cup (125 mL) all-purpose flour
½ cup (125 mL) whole wheat flour
1 tsp (5 mL) baking soda
½ tsp (2 mL) salt

PER PANCAKE	
Calories	116
Protein	4 g
Fat	4 g
Saturates	1 g
Cholesterol	17 mg
Carbohydrate	16 g
Fibre	1 g
Sodium	258 mg
Potassium	131 mg

1. Combine rolled oats and buttermilk, cover and refrigerate overnight.
2. In a large bowl, beat together egg, sugar and 1 tbsp (15 mL) oil.
3. In a separate bowl, combine flours, baking soda and salt. Stir dry ingredients into egg mixture along with soaked oats. Batter should be quite thick.
4. In a large non-stick skillet, heat remaining 1 tbsp (15 mL) oil on medium heat. Add batter in ¼ cup (125 mL) measures. Pancakes should by about 4 inches (10 cm) in diameter. Cook for 3 to 4 minutes, or until little bubbles appear and surface loses its sheen. Flip and cook second side for 2 to 3 minutes, or until cooked through. Repeat until all batter is used.

CARAMELIZED APPLE PUFF PANCAKE

This pancake is so good, I sometimes serve it for dessert. And it is very quick to make. Serve it hot or cold, or try pears instead of apples (you'll need about four) for a great variation. If you do not have a non-stick skillet with an ovenproof handle, transfer the caramelized apples to an 11- x 7-inch (2 L) baking dish and pour the egg mixture on top before baking.

Use apples that hold their shape: Golden Delicious, Fuji and Braeburn are a few of my favourites.

Makes 6 servings

3 tbsp (45 mL) soft non-hydrogenated margarine or unsalted butter
3 apples, peeled and thinly sliced
1/3 cup (75 mL) brown sugar
1/2 tsp (2 mL) ground cinnamon
3 eggs
2 tbsp (25 mL) granulated sugar
1/2 cup (125 mL) milk
1/2 cup (125 mL) all-purpose flour
1 tbsp (15 mL) sifted icing sugar

1. Melt margarine in a large non-stick ovenproof skillet. Remove half from skillet and reserve.

2. Add apples, brown sugar and cinnamon to skillet and cook for 5 minutes.

3. Meanwhile, blend reserved margarine, eggs, granulated sugar, milk and flour.

4. Pour batter over apples and bake in a preheated 425°F (220°C) oven for 20 to 25 minutes, or until browned and puffed.

5. Remove skillet from oven and shake to loosen apples. Invert carefully onto a large plate. Sprinkle with icing sugar. Serve in wedges.

PER SERVING	
Calories	237
Protein	5 g
Fat	9 g
Saturates	2 g
Cholesterol	94 mg
Carbohydrate	36 g
Fibre	2 g
Sodium	122 mg
Potassium	193 mg
Good: Vitamin B12	

LEMON RICOTTA PANCAKES

The lemon flavour in these light and delicate pancakes is wonderful to wake up to. Dust the pancakes with a little extra sifted icing sugar before serving, if you wish.

Makes 6 servings (about 20 3-inch/7.5 cm pancakes)

1 cup (250 mL) light ricotta cheese
3 egg yolks
1/2 cup (125 mL) all-purpose flour
1/4 cup (50 mL) granulated sugar
2 tsp (10 mL) grated lemon peel
Pinch ground nutmeg
1 tbsp (15 mL) soft non-hydrogenated margarine or
        unsalted butter, melted
4 egg whites
1/3 cup (75 mL) lemon juice
1/4 cup (50 mL) sifted icing sugar

PER SERVING	
Calories	194
Protein	10 g
Fat	7 g
Saturates	2 g
Cholesterol	120 mg
Carbohydrate	24 g
Fibre	trace
Sodium	118 mg
Potassium	120 mg
Good: Riboflavin; Vitamin B12	

1. In a large bowl, whisk together ricotta, egg yolks, flour, sugar, lemon peel, nutmeg and melted margarine.
2. In a separate bowl, beat egg whites until light and fluffy. Stir one-third of whites into ricotta batter. Gently fold in remaining whites.
3. Heat a large, lightly oiled non-stick skillet on medium heat. Add batter to pan in large spoonfuls, flattening batter slightly with back of spoon. Cook for about 2 minutes per side, or until just cooked through.
4. In a saucepan, heat lemon juice and stir in icing sugar. Brush lightly over tops of cooked pancakes.

GINGERBREAD PANCAKES WITH PEAR COMPOTE

Pancakes with gingerbread flavours make a very happening break-fast or brunch, but they burn more easily than plain pancakes, so watch them closely and reduce the heat if necessary. Serve with maple syrup flavoured with a little lemon juice or this delicious pear compote. The compote can also be served on other pancakes, ice cream or angel food cake.

For brunch hors d'oeuvres, make baby pancakes using 1 tsp (5 mL) batter for each pancake, and cook for about a minute per side. Cook the compote until thick and sandwich between two mini pancakes. Dust with icing sugar.

Makes 6 servings

Pear Compote

2 pears, peeled and diced
$^1/_2$ cup (125 mL) orange juice
2 tbsp (25 mL) brown sugar
1 tbsp (15 mL) chopped candied ginger

Gingerbread Pancakes

$^3/_4$ cup (175 mL) all-purpose flour
$^3/_4$ cup (175 mL) whole wheat flour
2 tbsp (25 mL) granulated sugar
1 tsp (5 mL) baking soda
$^1/_2$ tsp (2 mL) ground ginger
$^1/_2$ tsp (2 mL) ground cinnamon
Pinch ground nutmeg
Pinch ground allspice
Pinch ground cloves
Pinch salt
2 cups (500 mL) buttermilk
2 eggs
2 tbsp (25 mL) molasses
5 tsp (25 mL) vegetable oil, divided
1 tbsp (15 mL) grated orange peel

PER SERVING	
Calories	304
Protein	9 g
Fat	8 g
Saturates	1 g
Cholesterol	65 mg
Carbohydrate	52 g
Fibre	4 g
Sodium	324 mg
Potassium	497 mg

Good: Thiamine; Riboflavin; Niacin; Folate; Iron

1. To prepare compote, combine pears, orange juice, brown sugar and candied ginger in a non-stick skillet on medium-high heat. Cook, covered, for 5 to 10 minutes, or until tender. Continue to cook, uncovered, for 5 minutes, or until thickened.

2. To prepare pancakes, in a large bowl, combine flours with sugar, baking soda, ginger, cinnamon, nutmeg, allspice, cloves and salt.

3. In a separate bowl, whisk together buttermilk, eggs, molasses, 4 tsp (20 mL) oil and orange peel. Whisk into dry ingredients.

4. Heat remaining 1 tsp (5 mL) oil in a large non-stick skillet on medium heat. Drop batter by spoonful onto hot pan. Cook for 2 to 3 minutes, or until tops of pancakes appear dry with small bubbles. Turn and cook second side for 1 minute. Be careful not to burn pancakes.

GINGER

Ginger is used as a flavouring ingredient in many different kinds of recipes, and it comes in different forms.

Fresh Ginger Root

Look for a firm root with taut skin. Store it at room temperature where the air can circulate around it. To keep it longer, place peeled pieces in a jar of sherry, rice wine, brandy or vodka. They should keep indefinitely. Use the ginger-flavoured spirit instead of rice wine or sherry in stir-fries.

I usually peel or scrape ginger (with the edge of a spoon) before using it (unless it is going to be removed from the dish before serving or is being used in a marinade).

To chop fresh ginger, slice it very thinly and stack the slices on top of each other. Slice again and then slice crosswise. For minced ginger, chop until very fine. Or you can chop or mince the ginger in a food processor, using the on/off technique.

Candied Ginger

Candied ginger is ginger root that has been cooked in a sugar syrup and dusted with sugar. It is delicious in muffins and quickbreads, or just for eating.

Ground Ginger

Ground or powdered ginger is often used in baking, and although it doesn't taste at all like fresh ginger, in some recipes you could substitute 1 tsp (5 mL) ground for 1 tbsp (5 mL) fresh.

Pickled Ginger

Sometimes called pink ginger or sushi ginger, thinly sliced pickled ginger is available at Japanese and Asian food stores or fish markets. The organic varieties are usually golden instead of pink in colour.

SOUTHWEST FRITTATA

A frittata is a cross between an open-faced omelette and a crustless quiche. I like to start a frittata on top of the stove and finish it in the oven, but if you do not have an ovenproof skillet, just pour the egg/vegetable mixture into an oiled 8-inch (2 L) square baking dish and bake at 350°F (180°C) for 30 to 40 minutes.

Serve this hot, at room temperature or even cold. Use leftovers in sandwiches, or dice and use as a garnish for soups or salads.

Makes 6 servings

4 tsp (20 mL) olive oil, divided
1 onion, diced
1 potato, peeled and diced
1 jalapeño, seeded and finely chopped, or 1 tbsp (15 mL) chipotle
    puree (page 183), optional
1 cup (250 mL) corn kernels
1/3 cup (75 mL) chopped fresh cilantro, basil, chives or dill, divided
4 eggs
4 egg whites
1/4 cup (50 mL) water
1 tsp (5 mL) salt
2 tomatoes, seeded and chopped
1 cup (250 mL) chopped red cabbage or radicchio
1/2 cup (125 mL) crumbled soft unripened goat cheese or feta

1. Heat 2 tsp (10 mL) oil in a 10-inch (25 cm) non-stick ovenproof skillet on medium-high heat. Add onion, potato and jalapeño if using. Cook for 10 to 15 minutes, or until potato is just cooked. Add corn and 1/4 cup (50 mL) cilantro and cook for 1 minute.

2. Meanwhile, in a large bowl, whisk together eggs, egg whites, water and salt. Stir in corn mixture.

3. Wipe out skillet and heat remaining 2 tsp (10 mL) oil in skillet on medium-high heat. Add egg mixture and cook for 3 to 5 minutes, or until bottom is set. Transfer to a preheated 350°F (180°C) oven for 15 to 20 minutes, or until bottom is lightly browned and eggs are set.

4. Serve frittata directly from pan or loosen edges and gently slide onto a large serving platter. Sprinkle tomatoes, cabbage, cheese and remaining 2 tbsp (25 mL) cilantro over eggs in circles or strips. Serve in wedges.

PER SERVING	
Calories	181
Protein	11 g
Fat	9 g
Saturates	3 g
Cholesterol	148 mg
Carbohydrate	15 g
Fibre	2 g
Sodium	512 mg
Potassium	336 mg

Good: Vitamin A;
Riboflavin; Folate;
Vitamin B12

PORTOBELLO EGG CUPS WITH SALSA

I love the idea of using big mushroom caps as edible containers. Adding a spoonful of vinegar to the egg-poaching water will help coagulate the whites. You could also fill the mushrooms with scrambled eggs.

Makes 6 servings

6 portobello mushrooms, about 4 inches (10 cm) in diameter
4 tsp (20 mL) olive oil, divided
1 tbsp (15 mL) chopped fresh rosemary, or ½ tsp (2 mL) dried
1 tbsp (15 mL) chopped fresh thyme, or ½ tsp (2 mL) dried
½ tsp (2 mL) salt
½ tsp (2 mL) pepper
3 plum tomatoes, seeded and diced
1 clove garlic, minced
½ small onion, finely chopped
1 jalapeño, seeded and finely chopped
¼ cup (50 mL) chopped fresh basil or cilantro
6 eggs
3 whole wheat or regular English muffins, halved

1. Remove stems from portobellos and save to use in stir-fries or soups. Very gently, with a small spoon, scrape out mushroom gills.
2. In a small bowl, combine 2 tsp (10 mL) oil, rosemary, thyme, salt and pepper. Brush over mushroom caps.
3. Arrange mushrooms on a parchment-lined baking sheet in a single layer. Bake in a preheated 400°F (200°C) oven for 10 to 15 minutes, or until cooked through.
4. Meanwhile, to prepare salsa, combine tomatoes, garlic, onion, jalapeño and basil.
5. Heat remaining 2 tsp (10 mL) oil in a large non-stick skillet. Add salsa. Cook for 1 to 2 minutes, or until hot.
6. Bring a large, deep skillet of water to a boil. Add eggs and poach for 3 to 5 minutes, or until whites are firm and yolks are just slightly runny. Remove eggs from pan with a slotted spoon and drain well. Place on a tray lined with paper towels and trim edges.
7. Meanwhile, toast English muffins. Place a mushroom cap on each muffin half. Place an egg in each cap and spoon salsa over top.

PER SERVING

Calories	198
Protein	12 g
Fat	10 g
Saturates	2 g
Cholesterol	215 mg
Carbohydrate	19 g
Fibre	4 g
Sodium	345 mg
Potassium	408 mg

Excellent: Riboflavin; Niacin
Good: Vitamin B12; Folate; Iron

SMOKED SALMON SOUFFLÉ ROLL

This looks stunning, and it will definitely turn you into a culinary star (garnish the platter with lemon slices and sprigs of fresh dill). You can use prosciutto or thinly sliced ham instead of the salmon, or even fill the roll with chicken, tuna or salmon salad.

This can all be made ahead and refrigerated overnight. Serve it cold or at room temperature. The roll can also be cut into small pieces and served as hors d'oeuvres.

Makes 10 to 12 servings

2 cups (500 mL) cold milk
1/2 cup (125 mL) all-purpose flour
1/2 tsp (2 mL) salt
1/2 tsp (2 mL) pepper
Pinch ground nutmeg
1/4 tsp (1 mL) hot red pepper sauce
2 tbsp (25 mL) chopped fresh dill or chives
4 egg yolks
7 egg whites (about 1 cup/250 mL)
1/2 tsp (2 mL) cream of tartar
1/4 cup (50 mL) grated Parmesan cheese
1 1/2 cups (375 mL) thick yogurt cheese (page 391) or
        low-fat sour cream
1 tbsp (15 mL) honey-style mustard
1/2 lb (250 g) smoked salmon, thinly sliced
3 tbsp (45 mL) chopped fresh chives or green onions

1. Lightly oil a 17- x 11-inch (45 x 29 cm) baking sheet. Line with parchment paper. Lightly oil paper.

2. In a large saucepan, whisk milk and flour until smooth. Bring to a boil slowly, stirring often. Remove from heat and stir in salt, pepper, nutmeg, hot pepper sauce and dill.

3. In a small bowl, beat egg yolks. Stir a little hot milk mixture into yolks and then beat eggs back into saucepan.

4. In a large stainless-steel or glass bowl, beat egg whites and cream of tartar until opaque and firm. Stir one-quarter of whites into sauce to lighten. Then fold sauce back into whites. Fold in Parmesan.

5. Spread mixture over prepared baking sheet and bake in a preheated 400°F (200°C) oven for 15 to 18 minutes, or until firm but not dry. Cool for 10 minutes.

PER SERVING	
Calories	155
Protein	15 g
Fat	6 g
Saturates	2 g
Cholesterol	101 mg
Carbohydrate	11 g
Fibre	0 g
Sodium	456 mg
Potassium	282 mg

Excellent: Vitamin B12
Good: Niacin; Riboflavin; Calcium

6. Meanwhile, combine yogurt cheese and mustard. Taste and add more mustard if you wish.

7. Invert soufflé onto a clean tea towel. Carefully lift off paper. Cool for 10 minutes longer. Spread yogurt cheese mixture over soufflé. Arrange smoked salmon on yogurt cheese in a single layer. Do not worry if it doesn't completely cover cheese. Sprinkle salmon with chives.

8. Using tea towel to help you, gently roll up soufflé lengthwise. Carefully transfer to a long serving tray. Cut into slices (it is traditional to cut the roll on the diagonal, but I like to cut it into rounds).

SAFETY IN THE KITCHEN

Kitchen safety is really just common sense, but when you are busy, sometimes common sense doesn't come as quickly as it should. Here are some reminders:

- Have a healthy respect for knives. I like to keep them in a knife block. Always wash, dry and put them away immediately instead of leaving them in a sink of soapy water. Do not try to catch a knife if it is falling; stand back and let it fall. (In professional kitchens, chefs always wear close-toed shoes or clogs to guard against falling knives or hot spills.)
- If you break a glass or bottle, wrap it in newspaper or put it in a container instead of putting the broken glass straight into the garbage. Mop up broken glass with a sponge or cloth that you plan to throw out immediately, or use paper towels.
- Keep a small fire extinguisher in the kitchen and know how to use it.
- Keep your floor and work area clear. Clean up spills immediately before someone slips on them. Clear boxes and bags from the floor.
- Do not let pot handles stick out from the stove where they might be knocked over. If the handles become hot, sprinkle them with flour as a warning, the way they do in professional kitchens.
- Do not wear dangling bracelets, scarves or necklaces when you are cooking.
- Avoid using wet dish towels or wet oven mitts to pick up hot pans. Do not put glass dishes on the heat or hot coffee pots on cold surfaces.
- When you are cooking, focus on cooking. Try not to get distracted.

SHRIMP TACO TAPAS WITH CHIPOTLE MAYONNAISE

This recipe was inspired by an appetizer we had in Mexico when we went AWOL from our all-inclusive Playa del Carmen resort. The little tacos can be served as appetizers or for brunch (serve two per person).

Makes 8 tacos

1 lb (500 g) cooked shrimp, diced
1/4 cup (50 mL) light mayonnaise
1 tbsp (15 mL) chipotle puree (page 183), or 1 jalapeño,
     seeded and chopped
1/4 cup (50 mL) chopped fresh cilantro
8 8-inch (20 cm) whole wheat or regular flour tortillas
1/2 avocado, peeled and pitted
Juice of 1 lime
8 small leaves Romaine lettuce

1. In a large bowl, combine shrimp, mayonnaise, chipotle and cilantro.
2. Heat a dry skillet on medium heat. Heat tortillas for about 10 to 20 seconds per side. (You can also wrap tortillas in foil and warm in a 350°F/180°C oven for 10 minutes.)
3. Cut avocado into 8 slices and brush with lime juice.
4. Arrange warm tortillas on work surface. Top bottom third of each tortilla with shrimp mixture, avocado slices and lettuce. Roll up tightly.

TORTILLAS

Flour tortillas and corn tortillas are not always interchangeable, but both are delicious. Keep them on hand in the freezer.

Flour tortillas are widely available now and can be used raw or cooked. Use them for pizza crusts, fajitas, rollups, quesadillas and wraps. Or use them in grilled cheese sand-wiches made in a sand-wich machine, grill pan or non-stick skillet.

I often use corn tortillas baked as chips (page 49) or warmed as a bread, but they can also be used in tacos and enchiladas.

PER SERVING (2 TACOS)

Calories	135
Protein	10 g
Fat	8 g
Saturates	1 g
Cholesterol	85 mg
Carbohydrate	5 g
Fibre	1 g
Sodium	205 mg
Potassium	201 mg

Excellent: Vitamin B12
Good: Niacin

BROCCOLI AND CHEDDAR QUICHE WITH MASHED POTATO CRUST

The mashed potato crust is great for those who are nervous about making pastry, for those who want to avoid high-fat crusts, or just for those who love mashed potatoes.

Makes 6 servings
Crust
1 lb (500 g) Yukon Gold or baking potatoes (about 2), peeled and
       cut in 1-inch (2.5 cm) chunks
¼ cup (50 mL) milk
½ tsp (2 mL) salt
1 tbsp (15 mL) olive oil

Filling
2 cups (500 mL) coarsely chopped cooked broccoli, or
       1 10-oz (300 g) package frozen broccoli florets, defrosted,
       well drained and coarsely chopped
1 cup (250 mL) grated light Cheddar cheese (about 6 oz/175 g)
3 eggs
1 cup (250 mL) milk
½ tsp (2 mL) salt
½ tsp (2 mL) pepper
Pinch ground nutmeg
2 green onions, chopped

PER SERVING

Calories	214
Protein	11 g
Fat	12 g
Saturates	6 g
Cholesterol	117 mg
Carbohydrate	16 g
Fibre	2 g
Sodium	573 mg
Potassium	403 mg

Excellent: Vitamin B12
Good: Vitamin A; Riboflavin; Niacin; Vitamin C; Folate; Calcium

1. Cook potatoes in a large pot of boiling water for about 20 minutes, or until tender. Drain well. Mash with milk and salt. (You should have about 2 cups/500 mL.) Taste and adjust seasonings if necessary.
2. Brush a deep 9-inch (23 cm) pie plate with half the oil. Press in mashed potatoes. Brush with remaining oil.
3. Bake crust in a preheated 375°F (190°C) oven for 25 to 30 minutes, or until potatoes are lightly browned and crusty. Reduce oven temperature to 350°F (180°C).
4. Arrange broccoli and then cheese over bottom of crust.
5. Whisk together eggs, milk, salt, pepper and nutmeg. Pour over broccoli and cheese. Sprinkle with green onions.
6. Bake quiche for 25 to 30 minutes, or until slightly puffed, browned and just set. Allow to cool for 10 minutes before serving.

GOAT CHEESE AND FRESH HERB SOUFFLÉ

Even if you are usually intimidated by soufflés, you shouldn't be by this one. It is baked in a shallow dish, and although it does rise, because it isn't cooked in the traditional shape, nobody is really sure what it is supposed to look like.

You can prepare this ahead, but wait until your guests are in the house before you put the soufflé in the oven, and serve it right away, before it deflates. (It tastes great deflated, too; it just loses some of its panache.) This is great on its own or with a tomato or red pepper sauce.

Makes 8 servings

2 cups (500 mL) cold milk
1/2 cup (125 mL) all-purpose flour
1 clove garlic, minced
1 tbsp (15 mL) chopped fresh thyme, or 1/2 tsp (2 mL) dried
1 tbsp (15 mL) chopped fresh rosemary, or 1/2 tsp (2 mL) dried
2 tbsp (25 mL) chopped fresh parsley
1/2 tsp (2 mL) salt
1/2 tsp (2 mL) pepper
1/4 tsp (1 mL) ground nutmeg
1/4 tsp (1 mL) cayenne
4 egg yolks
3 oz (90 g) soft unripened goat cheese or feta, crumbled
        (scant 1/2 cup/125 mL)
2 oz (60 g) light ricotta cheese, crumbled (scant 1/3 cup/75 mL)
7 egg whites
1 tbsp (15 mL) grated Parmesan cheese

1. In a saucepan, whisk milk into flour until smooth. Add garlic and slowly bring to a boil, stirring often.

2. Stir in thyme, rosemary, parsley, salt, pepper, nutmeg and cayenne. Remove from heat.

3. Beat egg yolks. Beat a little hot sauce into yolks and then add yolk mixture to saucepan.

4. Stir in goat cheese and ricotta. Taste sauce; it should be very well seasoned.

GOAT CHEESE

There are as many different kinds of cheese made from goat's milk as there are made from cow's milk. Most recipes that call for goat cheese, however, refer to the soft creamy variety (also known as chèvre). The taste becomes milder when the cheese is combined with other ingredients, or when it is warmed.

Goat cheese is high in fat, so if you are using it in a spread or a dip, make a lower-fat version by combining it with low-fat cottage cheese, low-fat ricotta or yogurt cheese (page 391).

PER SERVING

Calories	146
Protein	10 g
Fat	7 g
Saturates	4 g
Cholesterol	128 mg
Carbohydrate	11 g
Fibre	trace
Sodium	372 mg
Potassium	179 mg

Excellent: Vitamin B12
Good: Riboflavin; Calcium

5. In a large stainless-steel or glass bowl, beat egg whites until peaks form. Stir one-quarter of whites into sauce base to lighten and then fold sauce gently into remaining whites.

6. Gently spoon soufflé mixture into a shallow, lightly oiled 12- x 8-inch (3 L) gratin dish. Sprinkle with Parmesan. Place in a preheated 425°F (220°C) oven. Immediately reduce oven temperature to 400°F (200°C) and bake soufflé for 20 to 25 minutes, or until browned and puffed. Serve as soon as soufflé comes out of oven.

FRESH HERBS

For years only restaurants had access to fresh herbs, and people wondered why the food sang when they ate out, while at home it just mumbled!

Although many books tell you to use three times the amount of fresh herbs as you would dried, I never follow that rule. When I have leafy fresh herbs, such as parsley, basil, dill, cilantro, mint and sage (fresh sage is much gentler than dried), I use lots, but I am very stingy with dried herbs. (I am also more cautious with more intensely flavoured fresh herbs such as thyme, oregano, tarragon and rosemary.)

Wash fresh herbs gently, dry them well and then wrap them in tea towels and store them in an airtight container in the refrigerator. Use them quickly and add them at the end of a recipe so their delicate flavour doesn't cook away. Some fresh herbs (not all) freeze well, and you can also buy fresh herb pastes, but for me, fresh is best.

BAKED SWEET POTATO HASH

This recipe turns a traditional hash on its ear. Serve it with toasted whole wheat English muffins.

Makes 6 servings

1 tbsp (15 mL) olive oil
1 onion, chopped
2 cloves garlic, finely chopped
1 jalapeño, seeded and finely chopped, or 1 tbsp (15 mL) chipotle
        puree (page 183), optional
1 large sweet potato, peeled and diced (about 3 cups/750 mL)
½ cup (125 mL) water
1 cup (250 mL) corn kernels
¼ lb (125 g) lean smoked ham, smoked turkey or smoked chicken,
        diced
1 tsp (5 mL) salt
½ tsp (2 mL) pepper
6 eggs
½ cup (125 mL) grated smoked mozzarella cheese or Cheddar
        (about 2 oz/60 g)
2 tbsp (25 mL) chopped fresh cilantro or parsley

1. Heat oil in a large, deep non-stick skillet on medium heat. Add onion, garlic and jalapeño and cook for a few minutes, or until fragrant. Add sweet potato and water. Cook for 10 to 15 minutes, or until water evaporates and sweet potato is tender.
2. Add corn, ham, salt and pepper. Cook for a few minutes longer.
3. Spoon mixture into a lightly oiled shallow 6-cup (1.5 L) baking dish or pie dish. (This can also be baked in individual ovenproof dishes.) Break eggs in a single layer over vegetables. Sprinkle cheese on top.
4. Bake in a preheated 350°F (180°C) oven for 15 to 20 minutes, or until cheese has melted and yolks are completely set but are still a bit runny. Sprinkle with cilantro.

PER SERVING	
Calories	213
Protein	13 g
Fat	10 g
Saturates	3 g
Cholesterol	203 mg
Carbohydrate	18 g
Fibre	2 g
Sodium	701 mg
Potassium	260 mg

SCRAMBLED TOFU WITH ONIONS AND MUSHROOMS

Most of my favourite tofu recipes are Asian, so I was really surprised that I liked this, a take-off on scrambled eggs. The recipe comes from my friends Mitchell and Leslie Davis. When they told me it was their favourite tofu recipe, I had to try it because I really trust their taste. If you are looking for a way to love tofu, this may be it.

Makes 4 servings

1 lb (500 g) firm tofu
2 tsp (10 mL) vegetable oil
1 onion, chopped
½ lb (250 g) mushrooms, trimmed and sliced (about 3 cups/
    750 mL)
1 tbsp (15 mL) soy sauce
Pepper to taste
2 tbsp (25 mL) chopped green onions or chives

1. Break tofu into chunks. Place in a strainer and discard any liquid that drains off.
2. Heat oil in a large non-stick skillet on medium-high heat. Add onion and cook, stirring, until well browned, about 8 to 10 minutes. Add mushrooms and cook until pan is dry, about 5 minutes. Remove mushrooms and onion from pan and reserve.
3. Add tofu to pan. Cook, stirring, until tofu releases its liquid and liquid evaporates. This will take about 10 to 15 minutes. Tofu will resemble scrambled eggs.
4. Return onion and mushrooms to pan and sprinkle with soy sauce. Cook for about 5 minutes longer, or until pan is dry and tofu is coloured. Taste and add pepper. Sprinkle with green onions.

PER SERVING	
Calories	110
Protein	8 g
Fat	6 g
Saturates	1 g
Cholesterol	0 mg
Carbohydrate	5 g
Fibre	2 g
Sodium	261 mg
Potassium	450 mg

BREAKFAST PIZZA

This is one of the most spectacular brunch dishes I have ever served.

There are endless variations to this idea; try thinly sliced prosciutto or smoked trout instead of the smoked salmon, or leave out the eggs altogether. Serve this warm or cold.

Makes 8 servings

1 12-inch (30 cm) baked whole wheat or regular pizza crust or
     15- x 8-inch (40 x 20 cm) focaccia
1 cup (250 mL) yogurt cheese (page 391) or
     thick unflavoured low-fat yogurt
1 tbsp (15 mL) honey-style mustard
1/4 cup (50 mL) chopped fresh chives or green onions, divided
2 tbsp (25 mL) chopped fresh dill or parsley
4 eggs
6 egg whites
1/4 cup (50 mL) water
1/2 tsp (2 mL) salt
1/2 tsp (2 mL) pepper, divided
1 tbsp (15 mL) vegetable oil or unsalted butter
6 oz (175 g) smoked salmon, thinly sliced

1. Warm pizza crust in a preheated 350°F (180°C) oven for 10 minutes.
2. Meanwhile, combine yogurt cheese, mustard, 2 tbsp (25 mL) chives and dill.
3. In a separate bowl, whisk eggs, egg whites, water, salt and 1/4 tsp (1 mL) pepper until just mixed.
4. Heat oil in a large non-stick skillet on medium heat. Add egg mixture. Cook and stir gently for a few minutes, or until curds form but mixture is still moist.
5. Spread yogurt mixture over warm pizza crust. Spoon eggs on top. Arrange smoked salmon on eggs. Sprinkle with remaining pepper and chives. Cut into wedges or squares. Serve warm or at room temperature.

PER SERVING	
Calories	255
Protein	18 g
Fat	8 g
Saturates	2 g
Cholesterol	115 mg
Carbohydrate	27 g
Fibre	2 g
Sodium	700 mg
Potassium	279 mg
Excellent: Vitamin B12	
Good: Riboflavin	

**10 LOWER-FAT
SANDWICH SPREADS**

- pesto (page 166)
- salsas
- yogurt cheese
  (page 391), plain or
  mixed with salsa
  or pesto
- salad dressings, such
  as Creamy Roasted
  Garlic Dressing
  (page 121)
- hummos
- dips and spreads
- peanut sauce or Faux
  Peanut Sauce
  (page 125)
- pureed roasted red
  peppers (page 146)
- chutney
- cranberry sauce
  (page 275)

PER SANDWICH

Calories	413
Protein	28 g
Fat	12 g
Saturates	5 g
Cholesterol	222 mg
Carbohydrate	51 g
Fibre	8 g
Sodium	910 mg
Potassium	467 mg

Excellent: Riboflavin;
Niacin; Vitamin B12;
Folate; Iron
Good: Thiamine;
Vitamin B6

BREAKFAST SANDWICH

Grilled sandwiches are so popular now and very easy to make at home. Another one of my ultra-easy favourites is light cream cheese spread on a bagel and then grilled.

Makes 1 sandwich

1 whole wheat bagel
1 egg
¼ tsp (1 mL) pepper
1 slice smoked turkey or Black Forest ham
2 tbsp (25 mL) grated light Cheddar or smoked mozzarella cheese
Hot red pepper sauce to taste

1. Slice bagel in half crosswise.
2. Break egg into a lightly oiled non-stick skillet on medium heat. Cook for about 2 minutes per side, or until white is opaque but yolk is barely cooked through. Sprinkle with pepper. Cover with a lid if necessary while cooking, so egg white firms up but yolk stays just a little runny.
3. Place egg on bottom half of bagel. Top with smoked turkey and sprinkle with cheese and hot pepper sauce. Top with remaining bagel half.
4. Grill sandwich in a sandwich maker, grill pan or non-stick skillet, pressing sandwich flat with a heavy spatula to allow cheese to melt. Turn sandwich and press again. Cook for 1 to 2 minutes per side, or until cheese melts and sandwich browns.

BREAKFAST BRÛLÉE

If you love crème brûlée, try this breakfast version. To brûlée, place the custard dishes under the broiler or use a mini blowtorch. For each serving, place about ¼ cup (50 mL) fresh raspberries or blueberries in the bottom of a custard cup or ramekin. Spread with about ½ cup (125 mL) yogurt cheese (page 391). Sprinkle with 1 tbsp (15 mL) granulated sugar. Broil for 1 to 2 minutes, watching carefully, until sugar melts and begins to brown (it burns very easily). Allow to rest for a few minutes until topping is firm, then eat immediately.

PEANUT BUTTER GRANOLA BARS

These peanut butter squares are great for breakfast, brunch or after-school snacks. I adapted this from a recipe I got from Lyane Hutton, pastry chef at Valemount Lodge in British Columbia, where I taught classes at breakfast and in the evening after a day of heli-hiking. It was a very exciting and delicious time.

Makes about 40 bars

¼ cup (50 mL) sesame seeds, toasted
2 cups (500 mL) crispy rice cereal
2 cups (500 mL) large-flake rolled oats, toasted (page 444)
¼ cup (50 mL) shredded coconut
¼ cup (50 mL) sunflower seeds
¼ cup (50 mL) pumpkin seeds
¼ cup (50 mL) sliced almonds, toasted
¼ cup (50 mL) dried cranberries
½ cup (125 mL) honey
½ cup (125 mL) peanut butter
⅓ cup (75 mL) vegetable oil
½ cup (125 mL) brown sugar

1. In a large bowl, combine sesame seeds, rice cereal, rolled oats, coconut, sunflower seeds, pumpkin seeds, almonds and cranberries.
2. In a saucepan, combine honey, peanut butter, oil and sugar and melt over low heat. Pour over dry ingredients and combine well.
3. Press mixture into a 13- x 9-inch (3.5 L) baking dish lined with plastic wrap. Refrigerate for at least 2 hours, or overnight. Cut into bars.

SESAME SEEDS

Sesame seeds will have twice the flavour if you toast them before using, unless they are going to be browned in some way in the recipe. Place them in a heavy dry skillet and cook on medium-high heat, shaking the pan and watching carefully, until they are almost golden and start to pop. You can also toast the seeds in a microwave; place in a glass pie plate and cook on High for 30 to 60 seconds.

Black sesame seeds have an earthy flavour and are used in Japanese dishes. They should not be toasted.

Keep toasted and untoasted sesame seeds in the freezer.

PER PIECE

Calories	99
Protein	2 g
Fat	6 g
Saturates	1 g
Cholesterol	0 mg
Carbohydrate	11 g
Fibre	1 g
Sodium	33 mg
Potassium	70 mg

MINT TEA

Mint tea is soothing and refreshing at the same time, and you can easily drink it all day long. Warm the pot before making any tea. Simply pour hot or boiling water into the pot and allow it to rest for a few minutes. Discard the water and then make tea.

Makes 8 servings

4 tsp (20 mL) Chinese green tea (e.g., gunpowder)
2 tbsp (25 mL) granulated sugar
1 small bunch fresh mint
4 cups (1 L) boiling water

1. Place tea, sugar and mint in a warmed teapot.
2. Pour boiling water into pot. Cover. Allow to steep for 3 to 4 minutes. Strain into cups, or into another teapot if you are not serving it right away.

PER SERVING	
Calories	13
Protein	0 g
Fat	0 g
Saturates	0 g
Cholesterol	0 mg
Carbohydrate	3 g
Fibre	0 g
Sodium	2 mg
Potassium	27 mg

LEMON ROSEMARY HERBAL REMEDY

Whenever anyone gets a sore throat or has a cough or laryngitis, I make this special remedy. (I sometimes add 1 tbsp/15 mL chopped fresh gingerroot.) It tastes wonderful, soothes your throat and contains lots of vitamin C. Sometimes I drink it when I feel fine, and then I feel even better.

Makes 3 to 4 servings

1 lemon
2 sprigs fresh rosemary, or 1 tbsp (15 mL) dried
1/4 cup (50 mL) honey
3 cups (750 mL) water

1. Roll lemon on counter to soften it so that more juice will be released. Cut lemon in half and squeeze out juice. Save juice and put two halves of lemon in a medium saucepan.
2. Add rosemary, honey and water to lemons in saucepan. Bring to a boil and simmer gently for 10 minutes. Strain, discarding lemon halves and rosemary. Add reserved lemon juice.

PER SERVING	
Calories	89
Protein	0 g
Fat	0 g
Saturates	0 g
Cholesterol	0 mg
Carbohydrate	24 g
Fibre	0 g
Sodium	8 mg
Potassium	33 mg

SPICED CHAI

I first had chai on a trip out west. It was served to me as a warm welcome at Vij's modern Indian restaurant in Vancouver. Today many coffee shops serve chai lattes, and you can also buy chai tea bags and syrups, but I love this homemade version the best.

Makes 8 servings

4 Darjeeling tea bags, or 4 tsp (20 mL) loose tea
10 whole cloves
10 whole cardamom pods, bruised
2 cinnamon sticks, broken
1 star anise
2 tbsp (25 mL) honey
2 cups (500 mL) water
2 cups (500 mL) milk

1. Combine tea, cloves, cardamom, cinnamon, star anise, honey and water in a large saucepan. Bring to a boil. Cook gently for 5 minutes.
2. Add milk and heat thoroughly but do not boil. Strain mixture and serve in mugs.

Chai Latte

Use 3 cups (750 mL) water and do not add milk to tea mixture. Heat milk in a saucepan. Froth milk and add to each serving (use a cappuccino machine or hand frother, or you can whip the milk in a blender and then heat it). Dust with a little cinnamon and nutmeg.

PER SERVING	
Calories	49
Protein	2 g
Fat	1 g
Saturates	1 g
Cholesterol	5 mg
Carbohydrate	8 g
Fibre	0 g
Sodium	38 mg
Potassium	184 mg

STRAWBERRY LEMONADE

This refreshing drink can be made with fresh or frozen berries. Blueberries, blackberries and raspberries also work well. Use freshly squeezed lemon juice.

Makes 6 to 8 servings

2 cups (500 mL) strawberries
1 cup (250 mL) granulated sugar
1 cup (250 mL) lemon juice
3 cups (750 mL) sparkling mineral water
2 cups (500 mL) ice cubes

1. In a saucepan, combine strawberries and sugar. Bring to a boil and cook gently for 5 minutes. Strain through a strainer, pushing through as much pulp as possible. Cool.
2. In a pitcher, combine strawberry puree with lemon juice, sparkling water and ice.

PER SERVING	
Calories	149
Protein	trace
Fat	trace
Saturates	0 g
Cholesterol	0 mg
Carbohydrate	39 g
Fibre	1 g
Sodium	3 mg
Potassium	107 mg
Good: Vitamin C	

HOT SPICED APPLE CIDER

Greet your guests with this warm apple cider on a cold winter night, and they will be yours forever. To make this alcoholic, add $1/3$ cup (75 mL) dark rum, brandy or apple brandy.

Makes 6 to 8 servings

4 cups (1 L) unsweetened apple cider
1 cinnamon stick, broken in half
3 whole cloves
5 whole allspice
4 whole black peppercorns
$1/4$ tsp (1 mL) ground nutmeg
2 tbsp (25 mL) honey

1. In a large saucepan, combine cider, cinnamon, cloves, allspice, peppercorns, nutmeg and honey. Heat gently for about 10 minutes. Taste and adjust seasonings, adding more honey if necessary. Strain if you wish.

PER SERVING	
Calories	104
Protein	0 g
Fat	0 g
Saturates	0 g
Cholesterol	0 mg
Carbohydrate	29 g
Fibre	0 g
Sodium	5 mg
Potassium	201 mg

FARA'S EUROPEAN FRUIT SALAD "DRINK"

This makes a wonderful and cool summer snack, as it is a fruit salad and drink all in one. When Fara was a teenager backpacking through Europe, she would see these colourful and refreshing drinks all lined up in the take-out shops with a spoon for eating and a straw for drinking.

Offer these to your brunch guests when they first arrive. I serve them in wineglasses and sometimes add a tiny bit of orange liqueur or rum.

Makes 8 servings

1/4 seedless watermelon, cut in 1-inch (2.5 cm) chunks (4 cups/1 L)
3 kiwi, peeled and cut in chunks (1 cup/250 mL)
2 cups (500 mL) quartered strawberries
1/2 cantaloupe, cut in chunks (1 1/2 cups/375 mL)
2 cups (500 mL) lemon soda, lemonade or ginger ale

1. In a large bowl, combine watermelon, kiwi, strawberries and cantaloupe.
2. For each serving, fill a glass with about 1 cup (250 mL) fruit. Fill glasses with lemon soda. Place a straw and fork in each glass and allow flavours to mingle for about 10 minutes in refrigerator. Serve cold.

PER SERVING	
Calories	89
Protein	1 g
Fat	1 g
Saturates	0 g
Cholesterol	0 mg
Carbohydrate	22 g
Fibre	2 g
Sodium	13 mg
Potassium	343 mg
Excellent: Vitamin C	

TROPICAL FROZEN SMOOTHIE

This smoothie is so thick that you can serve it as a dessert or a drink. (If you are serving it as a drink right away, add an extra 1/2 cup/ 125 mL juice.) Keep a bag of frozen cubed fruit in the freezer so you can make this any time.

Makes 2 large drinks or 4 dessert servings

PER LARGE DRINK	
Calories	151
Protein	2 g
Fat	1 g
Saturates	trace
Cholesterol	0 mg
Carbohydrate	39 g
Fibre	3 g
Sodium	5 mg
Potassium	482 mg
Excellent: Vitamin C	
Good: Vitamin A; Vitamin B6; Folate	

1 banana
1/2 cup (125 mL) sliced strawberries
1/2 cup (125 mL) cubed mango
1/2 cup (125 mL) orange juice or pineapple juices
1 tbsp (15 mL) honey
1 tbsp (15 mL) lemon juice

1. Cut up banana. Spread banana, strawberries and mango on a baking sheet and freeze until solid, about 2 hours.
2. Place frozen fruit in a food processor or blender. Add orange juice, honey and lemon juice. Puree until smooth.
3. Taste and add more honey if necessary. Serve in dessert dishes with spoons, or in glasses with straws.

COOKING FOR ONE OR TWO

It is a great time to be single if you love good food. Typical family-sized households represent a shrinking market, while the number of couples, unmarrieds, divorcees, widows and widowers and empty-nesters continues to grow. Upscale restaurants that used to ignore single diners are now catering to singles with communal tables, and supermarkets that used to sell only family-sized packages are now offering single servings of prepared meals, as well as packaging fruits and vegetables in smaller sizes. You can even buy mini coffee makers, crock pots and grill pans that encourage cooking in small quantities.

Cooking for one has changed. Here are a few tips:
- Slow-cooked, braised dishes like osso bucco (page 312), shortribs (page 278) and lamb shanks (page 304) take hours to cook, so it makes sense to make lots and freeze leftovers in individual portions to enjoy later.
- Whenever you cook dinner, make twice as much as you need. Eat half the first night. The second night, don't call the remainder leftovers, but turn it into something new. For example, use leftover steak or chicken in a salad, stir-fry or quesadilla, or turn leftover fish steaks or shrimp into a seafood soup or fish taco.
- From time to time, treat yourself by buying a single portion of something special that cooks quickly, such as an expensive tuna steak, big juicy veal chop or filet mignon.

YOGURT FRUIT SHAKE

This makes a delicious quick breakfast if you are in a hurry. For a more leisurely breakfast or brunch, set up a fruit shake bar. Have all the ingredients in separate bowls and let guests make their own concoctions. Any fruit combination can be used. Add sugar only if necessary.

Makes 2 servings

1 ripe banana
$^1\!/_2$ cup (125 mL) halved strawberries
$^1\!/_2$ cup (125 mL) cubed mango
$^1\!/_2$ cup (125 mL) cubed pineapple
$^1\!/_2$ cup (125 mL) unflavoured low-fat yogurt, fruit juice or milk
1 cup (250 mL) ice

1. Peel and break banana into a blender. Add strawberries, mango, pineapple and yogurt and puree.
2. Add ice and blend until ice is very fine and drink is very frothy. Serve in tall glasses with straws.

PER LARGE DRINK	
Calories	148
Protein	4 g
Fat	2 g
Saturates	1 g
Cholesterol	4 mg
Carbohydrate	32 g
Fibre	3 g
Sodium	47 mg
Potassium	540 mg

Excellent: Vitamin C; Vitamin B6
Good: Vitamin A; Riboflavin; Vitamin B12

MANGOES

There are many different kinds of mangoes, though most are not available here. Buy the yellow Alfonso mangoes if you can, as they are sweeter and less fibrous than other varieties.

To cut up a mango, cut a small slice off the top and bottom and stand the mango upright on a cutting board. Cut off the peel from top to bottom, then slice the fruit off the pit (slice off the wide side first) and dice.

YOGURT CHEESE DIP OR SPREAD

Combine 1 cup (250 mL) firm yogurt cheese with 2 minced cloves garlic, 1 tbsp (15 mL) each chopped fresh parsley, chives or green onions and tarragon or dill (if you are using dried herbs, use about ½ tsp/2 mL of each). Season to taste with salt, pepper and hot red pepper sauce. If you are serving this as a dip, add a little milk or regular yogurt.

Makes about 1 cup (250 mL).

YOGURT CHEESE DESSERT TOPPING OR DIP

Combine 1½ cups (375 mL) soft yogurt cheese, 3 tbsp (45 mL) brown sugar, icing sugar, honey or maple syrup. Stir in 1 tsp (5 mL) vanilla or grated orange peel, or ½ tsp (2 mL) ground cinnamon.

Makes about 1½ cups (375 mL).

PER TBSP (15 ML)	
Calories	15
Protein	2 g
Fat	trace
Saturates	trace
Cholesterol	2 mg
Carbohydrate	1 g
Fibre	0 g
Sodium	13 mg
Potassium	46 mg

YOGURT CHEESE

My friend, writer Cynthia Wine, came over when I was making this one day and she couldn't believe how delicious it was. I said it was something you had to taste to believe, and she agreed, saying, "Some recipes just don't taste good in print!"

Many of my students are also surprised by how thick and luscious yogurt cheese is, even when it is made with 1 percent or even non-fat yogurt. It can be used in many recipes instead of sour cream (I think it tastes much better than low-fat sour cream) or whipping cream (it doesn't whip but you can fold it into sauces). And it doesn't weep the way regular yogurt does in salad dressings. Although you can also use the new thick yogurts, yogurt cheese doesn't contain thickeners or gelatin and has, I think, a much more natural taste and texture. Be sure to use natural yogurt containing no stabilizers, gels or thickeners (use the kind that gets watery after you remove some from the container).

Use soft yogurt cheese in place of sour cream in dips or on baked potatoes, as a garnish in soups, in place of mayonnaise in sandwiches or salad dressings or in place of lightly whipped cream in or on desserts; use firm yogurt cheese in place of cream cheese in spreads or on bagels with smoked salmon.

(At the time of this printing, some yogurt manufacturers were making pressed yogurt; this can be substituted for our firm yogurt cheese, but check the fat content.)

Makes 1½ cups (375 mL)

3 cups (750 mL) low-fat natural unflavoured yogurt

1. Line a strainer with cheesecloth, paper towel or coffee filter (you can also use a yogurt strainer—they are fast, non-spill and efficient). Place over a bowl.
2. Place yogurt in strainer and cover with plastic wrap. Allow to rest for 3 hours or up to overnight in refrigerator. After 3 hours, cheese will be medium thick (soft yogurt cheese); if you let it drain overnight, it should be as thick as cream cheese (firm yogurt cheese). Use leftover liquid for cooking rice, as is sometimes done in the Middle East. (Or do what I often do. Save the liquid, label and date the container, and then throw it out two weeks later!) Spoon thickened yogurt cheese into another container. Cover and use as required. Keeps in the refrigerator for about a week.

HEART SMART

BREADS

BLUEBERRY FLAX MUFFINS

Blueberries, flax and oats are so good for you, and these muffins include all three. If you are using frozen blueberries, add them to the batter in their frozen state.

I keep flax seeds in the freezer. You'll need to grind or at least crush them for the full health benefit.

Makes 12 muffins

1 1/2 cups (375 mL) all-purpose flour
1 cup (250 mL) whole wheat flour
1/2 cup (125 mL) ground or crushed flax seeds
1 tsp (5 mL) baking powder
1 tsp (5 mL) baking soda
Pinch salt
1 egg
1/3 cup (75 mL) vegetable oil
1 cup (250 mL) buttermilk
3/4 cup (175 mL) brown sugar
2 cups (500 mL) blueberries

Topping, optional

1/4 cup (50 mL) brown sugar
1/4 cup (50 mL) all-purpose flour
1/3 cup (75 mL) large-flake rolled oats
1/2 tsp (2 mL) ground cinnamon
2 tbsp (25 mL) melted unsalted butter or vegetable oil

1. In a large bowl, combine flours, flax, baking powder, baking soda and salt.
2. In a separate bowl, combine egg, oil, buttermilk and brown sugar.
3. Stir egg mixture into dry ingredients. Stir in blueberries just until blended. Scoop batter into 12 non-stick or paper-lined muffin cups (an ice cream scoop works well).
4. To prepare topping, combine sugar, flour, rolled oats, cinnamon and melted butter. Sprinkle over muffins.
5. Bake in a preheated 400°F (200°C) oven for 25 minutes, or until a cake tester comes out clean.

MIXING DRY INGREDIENTS
When mixing dry ingredients for quickbreads, muffins or cakes, you can sift all the dry ingredients together, but be sure to combine them thoroughly afterwards, as sifting mainly removes the lumps rather than mixing ingredients together. You can also just place ingredients that tend to lump (baking soda, baking powder, icing sugar and cocoa) in a small strainer and sift them into the flour and other ingredients.

PER MUFFIN

Calories	305
Protein	6 g
Fat	11 g
Saturates	2 g
Cholesterol	21 mg
Carbohydrate	47 g
Fibre	4 g
Sodium	185 mg
Potassium	230 mg

Good: Thiamine; Folate; Iron

DRIED FRUITS
Although dried fruits are high in calories, they usually contain no fat, and they can add a lot of taste to dishes because of their concentrated flavour. They are great in muffins, breads and pilafs.

Dried fruits include prunes (now called dried plums, thanks to great marketing), apricots, raisins, dates and figs as well as dried cherries, cranberries, blueberries, apples and pears.

PER SQUARE

Calories	171
Protein	4 g
Fat	7 g
Saturates	1 g
Cholesterol	12 mg
Carbohydrate	28 g
Fibre	5 g
Sodium	170 mg
Potassium	270 mg

Good: Vitamin A; Thiamine

MORNING GLORY MUFFIN SQUARES

These bars are always a great hit, and they freeze well. Of course, you could also bake the batter as 12 large muffins.

Makes 16 squares

1 1/2 cups (375 mL) whole wheat flour
1 1/2 cups (375 mL) bran cereal
1/4 cup (50 mL) sesame seeds, toasted (page 384)
1 tbsp (15 mL) baking powder
1 tsp (5 mL) ground cinnamon
1 tsp (5 mL) ground allspice, optional
1/2 tsp (2 mL) baking soda
Pinch salt
1 egg
1/2 cup (125 mL) brown sugar
3/4 cup (175 mL) buttermilk or unflavoured low-fat yogurt
1/3 cup (75 mL) vegetable oil
2 tbsp (25 mL) molasses or honey
1 1/2 cups (375 mL) grated carrots
1/2 cup (125 mL) chopped dates or raisins

1. In a large bowl, combine flour, bran cereal, sesame seeds, baking powder, cinnamon, allspice, baking soda and salt.
2. In a separate bowl, whisk together egg, sugar, buttermilk, oil and molasses.
3. Stir egg mixture into flour mixture just until moistened. Stir in carrots and dates.
4. Spread mixture in a non-stick or lightly oiled and parchment-lined 9-inch (2.5 L) square baking pan. Bake in a preheated 350°F (180°C) oven for 30 to 35 minutes, or until centre springs back when gently touched. Cool and cut into squares.

CRANBERRY STREUSEL MUFFINS

Cranberries have come a long way since the days when they were only used in cranberry sauce. They are great in muffins, quickbreads and cookies. They are one of the best sources of antioxidants, too.

Makes 12 muffins

1 cup (250 mL) all-purpose flour
1 cup (250 mL) whole wheat flour
1 tbsp (15 mL) baking powder
Pinch salt
1 egg
2/3 cup (150 mL) granulated sugar
1 cup (250 mL) milk
1/4 cup (50 mL) vegetable oil
2 tbsp (25 mL) grated orange or lemon peel
1 1/2 cups (375 mL) cranberries
1/4 cup (50 mL) brown sugar
1 tsp (5 mL) ground cinnamon

1. In a bowl, combine flours, baking powder and salt.
2. In a large bowl, combine egg, granulated sugar, milk, oil and orange peel.
3. Add flour mixture to egg mixture and stir just until combined. Stir in cranberries.
4. Scoop batter into 12 large non-stick, oiled or paper-lined muffin cups.
5. In a small bowl, combine brown sugar and cinnamon. Sprinkle over top of muffins. Bake in a preheated 400°F (200°C) oven for 20 to 25 minutes, or until a cake tester comes out clean.

CRANBERRIES

Cranberries can be fresh, frozen or dried. If you are using frozen cranberries in baked dishes, add them in the frozen state so that they do not bleed too much of their colour into the batter.

Use fresh or frozen cranberries in muffins or cranberry sauce (page 275). Dried cranberries can be eaten as a snack or added like raisins to muffins, breads, cookies and pilafs.

PER MUFFIN

Calories	195
Protein	4 g
Fat	6 g
Saturates	1 g
Cholesterol	16 mg
Carbohydrate	34 g
Fibre	2 g
Sodium	83 mg
Potassium	118 mg

BLUEBERRY BRAN MUFFINS

I met my friend Evelyn Zabloski when she had the busiest coffee shop in all of Banff. She still bakes the most delicious homemade muffins, scones, cookies, pies and cakes at her new ice cream parlour (Evelyn's Memory Lane) in High River, Alberta.

This recipe reminds me of the muffins she sells at her shop. They travel well, whether you are in the car on the way to the mountains or on the subway on the way to work. If you are using frozen berries, add them to the batter while they are still frozen.

Makes 18 muffins

2 cups (500 mL) all-purpose flour
3/4 cup (175 mL) whole wheat flour
1 1/2 cups (375 mL) wheat bran
3/4 cup (175 mL) brown sugar
4 tsp (20 mL) baking powder
2 tsp (10 mL) baking soda
1 egg or 2 egg whites
1/2 cup (125 mL) molasses
1/4 cup (50 mL) vegetable oil
2 cups (500 mL) buttermilk or unflavoured low-fat yogurt
1 1/2 cups (375 mL) blueberries

PER MUFFIN	
Calories	185
Protein	4 g
Fat	4 g
Saturates	1 g
Cholesterol	13 mg
Carbohydrate	36 g
Fibre	4 g
Sodium	225 mg
Potassium	266 mg

1. In a bowl, combine flours, wheat bran, brown sugar, baking powder and baking soda. Mix together well.
2. In a large bowl, combine egg, molasses, oil and buttermilk. Blend well.
3. Add dry ingredients to large bowl and stir into wet ingredients just until moistened. Quickly stir in berries.
4. Spoon batter into 18 large non-stick, lightly oiled or paper-lined muffin cups. Bake in a preheated 375°F (190°C) oven for 25 minutes, or until a cake tester comes out clean.

MINI BERRY CORNMEAL MUFFINS

These muffins have great texture because of the slight crunch from the cornmeal, which also gives them a bright, sunny look. Instead of fresh or frozen raspberries or blueberries (if you are using frozen berries, use them in the frozen state), you can use fresh or dried cranberries or cherries.

Makes 24 mini muffins or 12 medium muffins

1 1/2 cups (375 mL) all-purpose flour
3/4 cup (175 mL) cornmeal
1/2 cup (125 mL) granulated sugar
1 tbsp (15 mL) grated lemon peel
4 tsp (20 mL) baking powder
Pinch salt
1 cup (250 mL) raspberries or blueberries
2 egg whites or 1 whole egg
1 cup (250 mL) milk
1/4 cup (50 mL) vegetable oil
1 tsp (5 mL) vanilla
2 tbsp (25 mL) coarse sugar

1. In a bowl, combine flour, cornmeal, granulated sugar, lemon peel, baking powder and salt. Combine 2 tbsp (25 mL) of this mixture with berries in a separate bowl.

2. In a large bowl, combine egg whites, milk, oil and vanilla. Blend well.

3. Add dry ingredients to large bowl and stir just until combined. Stir in berries very gently.

4. Spoon batter into non-stick, lightly oiled or paper-lined mini muffin cups. Sprinkle with coarse sugar. Bake in a preheated 400°F (200°C) oven for 15 to 25 minutes (25 to 30 minutes for medium muffins), until lightly browned.

PER MINI MUFFIN	
Calories	94
Protein	2 g
Fat	3 g
Saturates	trace
Cholesterol	0 mg
Carbohydrate	16 g
Fibre	1 g
Sodium	53 mg
Potassium	44 mg

LEMON POPPY SEED MUFFINS

This batter can also be baked in a 9- x 5-inch (2 L) loaf pan for 45 to 50 minutes.

Makes 12 large muffins

2 1/2 cups (625 mL) all-purpose flour
1 tbsp (15 mL) baking powder
3/4 tsp (4 mL) baking soda
1/4 tsp (1 mL) salt
1/4 cup (50 mL) vegetable oil
1/2 cup (125 mL) granulated sugar
2 eggs
1 1/2 cups (375 mL) buttermilk or low-fat yogurt
1/4 cup (50 mL) poppy seeds
2 tbsp (25 mL) grated lemon peel

Syrup

1/3 cup (75 mL) lemon juice
1/3 cup (75 mL) granulated sugar

1. In a bowl, combine flour, baking powder, baking soda and salt. Mix well.
2. In a large bowl, beat together oil, sugar, eggs, buttermilk, poppy seeds and lemon peel.
3. Add dry ingredients to large bowl and stir just until combined.
4. Spoon batter into 12 large non-stick, lightly oiled or paper-lined muffin cups. Bake in a preheated 400°F (200°C) oven for 20 to 25 minutes, or until a cake tester comes out clean.
5. Meanwhile, in a small saucepan, bring lemon juice and sugar to a boil. Cool for a few minutes.
6. Prick hot muffins in a few places with a skewer. Spoon syrup over top and allow to soak into muffins. Cool before removing muffins from pan.

PER MUFFIN	
Calories	232
Protein	5 g
Fat	7 g
Saturates	1 g
Cholesterol	37 mg
Carbohydrate	37 g
Fibre	1 g
Sodium	229 mg
Potassium	117 mg

GIANT WHOLE WHEAT POPOVERS

Popovers are so much fun, but they should be baked just before serving. They are great at dinner or brunch. You can also serve these as Yorkshire pudding. Or you can make small popovers in mini muffin pans and serve them as appetizers. Bake for about 20 minutes and stuff them with hummos or other spreads.

Makes 12 popovers

1 cup (250 mL) all-purpose flour
1 cup (250 mL) whole wheat flour
1 tsp (5 mL) salt
2 cups (500 mL) milk
4 eggs
½ cup (125 mL) grated light Cheddar cheese

1. Preheat oven to 350°F (180°C). Place muffin pan in oven while oven is heating up.

2. In a large bowl, combine flours and salt.

3. In a saucepan, heat milk to 125°F (52°C). In a separate bowl, whisk hot milk into eggs.

4. Whisk milk-egg mixture into flour mixture. Do not overmix or worry about little lumps.

5. When muffin pan is hot, spray with non-stick cooking spray. Pour about ⅓ cup (75 mL) batter into each muffin cup. Sprinkle with cheese. Bake for 30 to 35 minutes, or until puffed and browned. Serve hot.

PER POPOVER	
Calories	132
Protein	7 g
Fat	4 g
Saturates	2 g
Cholesterol	69 mg
Carbohydrate	17 g
Fibre	2 g
Sodium	265 mg
Potassium	140 mg

BANANA BREAD

Here's a delicious lower-fat quickbread that can also be made as muffins. Spoon the batter into 12 muffin cups and bake for about 20 minutes.

You can use only whole wheat flour or only all-purpose flour in this recipe, but I like to combine the two.

Makes 1 small loaf (12 slices)

1 cup (250 mL) very ripe mashed bananas (2 medium)
1/2 cup (125 mL) unflavoured low-fat yogurt
1 tsp (5 mL) baking soda
1 egg or 2 egg whites
3/4 cup (175 mL) brown sugar
1/4 cup (50 mL) vegetable oil
1 tsp (5 mL) vanilla
1 cup (250 mL) all-purpose flour
1/2 cup (125 mL) whole wheat flour
1 tsp (5 mL) baking powder
Pinch salt

PER SLICE	
Calories	178
Protein	3 g
Fat	5 g
Saturates	1 g
Cholesterol	18 mg
Carbohydrate	30 g
Fibre	1 g
Sodium	136 mg
Potassium	182 mg

1. In a small bowl, combine bananas, yogurt and baking soda.
2. In a separate bowl, combine egg, sugar, oil and vanilla. Blend well.
3. In a large bowl, combine flours, baking powder and salt. Mix together well.
4. Combine banana mixture with oil mixture. Add to dry ingredients in large bowl and stir together just until moistened.
5. Spoon batter into a non-stick, lightly oiled or parchment-lined 8- x 4-inch (1.5 L) loaf pan. Bake in a preheated 350°F (180°C) oven for 50 to 60 minutes, or until loaf springs back when gently touched.

CORNBREAD WITH CHEDDAR

Cornbread is so easy that anyone can make homemade bread. The house smells amazing and you are a hero. How can you lose?

You can leave out the Cheddar or use another cheese such as smoked mozzarella. You can also bake the batter in 12 muffin cups. Bake for about 20 minutes.

Leftover cornbread is great in stuffings.

Makes 16 squares

1 cup (250 mL) all-purpose flour
1 cup (250 mL) cornmeal
3 tbsp (45 mL) granulated sugar
1 tbsp (15 mL) baking powder
1/2 tsp (2 mL) salt
3/4 cup (175 mL) grated light Cheddar cheese
2 eggs
1 cup (250 mL) milk
3 tbsp (45 mL) olive oil

PER SQUARE	
Calories	125
Protein	4 g
Fat	5 g
Saturates	1 g
Cholesterol	28 mg
Carbohydrate	16 g
Fibre	1 g
Sodium	182 mg
Potassium	64 mg

1. In a large bowl, combine flour, cornmeal, sugar, baking powder and salt. Stir in cheese.
2. In a separate bowl, combine eggs, milk and oil.
3. Stir milk mixture into flour mixture just until combined.
4. Transfer batter to a non-stick or oiled and parchment-lined 8-inch (2 L) square baking dish. Bake in a preheated 400°F (200°C) oven for 25 minutes, or until golden.

SMOKY CORNBREAD WITH CORN AND PEPPERS

Grilled corn, roasted peppers and smoked cheese make this delicious bread extra special. But it can easily be made with plain corn, raw peppers and plain Cheddar.

To barbecue the corn, remove the husks and silk and place the cobs directly on a hot grill. Keep turning them until they brown. To remove the kernels from the cob, break the cob in half, stand it on a cutting board (cut side down) and slice off the kernels from top to bottom.

Makes 12 servings

1 1/2 cups (375 mL) all-purpose flour
1 1/2 cups (375 mL) cornmeal
3 tbsp (45 mL) granulated sugar
1 tbsp (15 mL) baking powder
1 tsp (5 mL) salt
1/2 tsp (2 mL) baking soda
2 eggs
1 1/4 cups (300 mL) buttermilk or unflavoured low-fat yogurt
3 tbsp (45 mL) olive oil
1 cup (250 mL) grilled corn kernels (2 ears)
1 sweet red pepper, roasted (page 146), peeled and diced
    (about 1/2 cup/125 mL)
1 cup (250 mL) grated smoked mozzarella cheese

PER SERVING	
Calories	233
Protein	8 g
Fat	7 g
Saturates	2 g
Cholesterol	45 mg
Carbohydrate	34 g
Fibre	2 g
Sodium	384 mg
Potassium	152 mg

1. In a large bowl, combine flour, cornmeal, sugar, baking powder, salt and baking soda. Stir well.
2. In a separate bowl, beat eggs with buttermilk and oil. Stir wet ingredients into flour mixture just until combined.
3. Gently stir in corn, red pepper and cheese.
4. Spoon batter into a lightly oiled 12- x 8-inch (3 L) baking dish. Bake in a preheated 375°F (190°C) oven for 40 to 45 minutes, or until cornbread is nicely browned and top springs back when pressed gently. Cool for 10 minutes before cutting into squares.

SOUTHWEST CORNMEAL SCONES

This is a great savoury biscuit. Serve it as a snack, with soup or with a Southwest-theme dinner.

Leftovers can be crumbled and used in stuffings, as a breading for chicken or as a topping for casseroles.

Makes 12 scones

1 cup (250 mL) all-purpose flour
1 cup (250 mL) whole wheat flour
3 tbsp (45 mL) cornmeal
1 tbsp (15 mL) baking powder
1 tbsp (15 mL) granulated sugar
1 tsp (5 mL) ground cumin
$\frac{1}{2}$ tsp (2 mL) salt
$\frac{1}{2}$ tsp (2 mL) pepper
$\frac{1}{4}$ cup (50 mL) soft non-hydrogenated margarine or
       unsalted butter, cold
$\frac{1}{2}$ cup (125 mL) grated smoked mozzarella, Monterey Jack or
       Cheddar cheese
1 jalapeño, seeded and finely chopped, or
       1 tbsp (15 mL) chipotle puree (page 183)
1 cup (250 mL) buttermilk, divided
1 tbsp (15 mL) cumin seeds or caraway seeds

1. In a large bowl, combine flours, cornmeal, baking powder, sugar, ground cumin, salt and pepper. With a pastry blender or your finger-tips, cut in margarine until it is in tiny bits.
2. Stir in cheese and jalapeño. Pour $\frac{7}{8}$ cup (225 mL) buttermilk over mixture. Work dough with your fingers until it comes together.
3. Gently press dough into a non-stick or lightly oiled 8-inch (20 cm) round baking pan and score top to make 12 wedges. Brush surface with remaining 2 tbsp (25 mL) buttermilk and sprinkle with cumin seeds.
4. Bake in a preheated 425°F (220°C) oven for 20 to 25 minutes, or until golden and cooked through. Remove from pan and cool on a wire rack before cutting into wedges.

Sweet Cornmeal Scones

Omit cheese, jalapeño, cumin and pepper. Stir 2 tbsp (25 mL) additional granulated sugar and 1 tbsp (15 mL) grated lemon peel into batter. Sprinkle with 1 tbsp (15 mL) coarse sugar before baking.

BAKING SODA

Baking soda makes baked goods rise by reacting with the acid in ingredients like butter-milk, yogurt, bananas, sour cream and molasses. It keeps for about a year in an airtight container.

Mix baking soda with the other dry ingredi-ents. Combine the dry and wet ingredients just before baking, as the baking soda will lose some of its effective-ness if the mixture is not baked immediately.

Baking soda also has many non-food uses. Read the box for more suggestions.

PER SCONE

Calories	143
Protein	5 g
Fat	5 g
Saturates	1 g
Cholesterol	3 mg
Carbohydrate	20 g
Fibre	2 g
Sodium	259 mg
Potassium	82 mg

BAKING POWDER
Like baking soda, baking powder helps baked goods rise. It keeps for about one year (if it fizzes when it is added to boiling water, it is still active). Use about 1 tsp (5 mL) for each cup of flour in a recipe and bake immediately after adding it to the wet ingredients. Keep it in a dry place in a tightly sealed container.

PER BISCUIT	
Calories	151
Protein	5 g
Fat	6 g
Saturates	2 g
Cholesterol	5 mg
Carbohydrate	21 g
Fibre	1 g
Sodium	240 mg
Potassium	91 mg

ASIAGO DROP BISCUITS

These delicious little drop biscuits are great for brunch, tea time or a snack, and they are so easy to make.

Makes 16 biscuits

2 cups (500 mL) all-purpose flour
1 cup (250 mL) whole wheat flour
2 tbsp (25 mL) granulated sugar
1 tbsp (15 mL) baking powder
1 tsp (5 mL) baking soda
1/3 cup (75 mL) soft non-hydrogenated margarine or
    unsalted butter, cold
2/3 cup (150 mL) grated Asiago, Cheddar or
    smoked mozzarella cheese
1 3/4 cups (425 mL) buttermilk

1. In a large bowl, combine flours, sugar, baking powder and baking soda. Stir together well. (If baking powder or baking soda are lumpy, sift ingredients together.)
2. Cut margarine into flour mixture until it is in tiny bits. Stir in grated cheese.
3. Pour buttermilk over flour mixture and stir until a rough batter is formed.
4. Drop batter in 16 mounds on a baking sheet lined with parchment paper. Bake in a preheated 425°F (220°C) oven for 12 to 15 minutes, or until lightly browned.

BUTTERMILK OAT SCONES

Homemade scones taste very different from the coffee-shop variety. They are tender and light (even when made with whole wheat flour), as long as you eat them the day they are made.

Makes 12 scones

³/₄ cup (175 mL) whole wheat flour
³/₄ cup (175 mL) all-purpose flour
3 tbsp (45 mL) granulated sugar
1 tsp (5 mL) baking powder
¹/₂ tsp (2 mL) baking soda
¹/₂ tsp (2 mL) salt
¹/₃ cup (75 mL) soft non-hydrogenated margarine or unsalted
    butter, cold
1 cup (250 mL) large-flake rolled oats
¹/₂ cup (125 mL) currants or raisins
¹/₂ cup (125 mL) buttermilk
1 tbsp (15 mL) icing sugar, sifted

1. In a large bowl, combine flours, granulated sugar, baking powder, baking soda and salt.
2. Cut margarine into flour mixture until it is in tiny bits.
3. Stir in oats and currants. Drizzle buttermilk over everything and gather into a ball. Do not overknead.
4. Pat dough on a floured work surface to a thickness of about 1 inch (2.5 cm). Cut out 2-inch (5 cm) rounds and place on a baking sheet lined with parchment paper. Gently push excess dough together and cut out more rounds.
5. Bake in a preheated 375°F (190°C) oven for 17 to 20 minutes, or until puffed and golden. Cool on racks. Dust with icing sugar.

Choosing a Healthy Margarine

Different margarines contain different kinds of fats. Here are some guidelines to help you choose the healthiest variety.
- Choose a soft, spreadable margarine sold in a tub, not in stick or brick form.
- Look for margarines that are non-hydrogenated. This product will be lower in saturated fat and will not contain trans-fatty acids.
- Do not buy a margarine that does not include nutrition information on the label.

MARGARINE OR BUTTER?

A minimal amount of fat is used in the recipes in this book, because one of the keys to healthy eating is to eat less total fat, especially less saturated fat. Some of the recipes list butter as an option to soft margarine. Although many people, including me, prefer the taste of butter, if you choose to use butter instead of margarine, you should know that the amount of fat will be the same but the type of fat will vary.

For example, in a 2 tsp (10 mL) serving:

	Soft margarine	butter
Calories	70	70
Total fat	8 g	8 g
Saturates	2 g	5 g

PER SCONE

Calories	170
Protein	4 g
Fat	6 g
Saturates	2 g
Cholesterol	0 mg
Carbohydrate	26 g
Fibre	2 g
Sodium	252 mg
Potassium	141 mg

BUTTERMILK AND
SOUR MILK

Because of its name
and rich texture, many
people think buttermilk
is high in fat. Traditionally it was the milk left
over from making
butter. Commercial
buttermilk has approxi-
mately 1 percent fat, but
it is thick and creamy,
and it tastes and smells
wonderful when used in
baked goods, pancakes
and waffles.

If you do not have
buttermilk, substitute
yogurt, sour cream or
sour milk. To make sour
milk, place 1 tbsp
(15 mL) lemon juice or
vinegar in a measuring
cup and add milk to
make 1 cup (250 mL).
Allow to rest for
10 minutes before using
(it may look curdled, but
don't worry).

PER BISCUIT	
Calories	140
Protein	4 g
Fat	4 g
Saturates	1 g
Cholesterol	1 mg
Carbohydrate	23 g
Fibre	2 g
Sodium	263 mg
Potassium	76 mg

BUTTERMILK BLACK PEPPER BISCUITS

These biscuits are irresistible. Serve them with spreads, soups or saucy dishes like barbecued shrimp. They are wonderful fresh and warm or at room temperature, but they also freeze well.

Makes about 10 biscuits

1 cup (250 mL) all-purpose flour
1 cup (250 mL) whole wheat flour
2 tbsp (25 mL) cornmeal
1 tbsp (15 mL) baking powder
1 tsp (5 mL) granulated sugar
1 tsp (5 mL) coarsely ground black pepper
$1/2$ tsp (2 mL) salt
3 tbsp (45 mL) soft non-hydrogenated margarine or unsalted
       butter, cold
$7/8$ cup (225 mL) buttermilk

Topping

2 tbsp (25 mL) buttermilk
1 tbsp (15 mL) cornmeal
$1/2$ tsp (2 mL) coarsely ground black pepper
$1/2$ tsp (2 mL) granulated sugar
Pinch salt

1. In a large bowl, combine flours, cornmeal, baking powder, sugar, pepper and salt.
2. Cut margarine into flour mixture until mixture resembles fresh breadcrumbs.
3. Sprinkle buttermilk over mixture and gather into a rough dough. Knead gently for about 5 seconds.
4. Pat dough out gently on a floured surface to a thickness of about $3/4$ inch (2 cm). Cut into 3-inch (7.5 cm) rounds. Place on a baking sheet lightly dusted with cornmeal or lined with parchment paper.
5. To prepare topping, brush biscuits lightly with buttermilk. In a small bowl, combine cornmeal, pepper, sugar and salt. Sprinkle on biscuits.
6. Bake in a preheated 425°F (220°C) oven for 15 minutes, or until lightly browned.

BEER BREAD WITH ROSEMARY

Quickbreads made with beer have a wonderful yeasty aroma and taste. I originally made this bread with self-rising flour (which includes baking powder and salt), but it can be hard to find, so I reworked the recipe to include regular flour. Use your favourite drinking beer in the bread.

Makes 1 small loaf

1 1/2 cups (375 mL) whole wheat flour
1 1/2 cups (375 mL) all-purpose flour
3 tbsp (45 mL) granulated sugar
1 tbsp (15 mL) baking powder
1 1/2 tsp (7 mL) salt
1 tbsp (15 mL) chopped fresh rosemary, or 1/2 tsp (2 mL) dried
1 1/2 cups (375 mL) beer

Topping

1 tsp (5 mL) olive oil
1 tsp (5 mL) chopped fresh rosemary, or 1/4 tsp (1 mL) dried
1/4 tsp (1 mL) coarse salt

1. In a large bowl, combine flours, sugar, baking powder, salt and rosemary. Stir in beer until dough comes together.
2. Transfer batter to a non-stick, lightly oiled or parchment-lined 8- x 4-inch (1.5 L) loaf pan.
3. Brush top of loaf with oil and sprinkle with rosemary and coarse salt.
4. Bake loaf in a preheated 350°F (180°C) oven for 80 minutes, or until a thermometer inserted into loaf reaches at least 190°F (88°C).

GARLIC BREAD

Cut a baguette into 1-inch (2.5 cm) slices, but leave the bottoms of the slices attached.

In a small bowl, combine 2 tbsp (25 mL) olive oil, 3 minced cloves garlic, 1 tsp (5 mL) chopped fresh rosemary or thyme (or 1/2 tsp/ 2 mL dried), 1/2 tsp (2 mL) coarse salt and 1/4 tsp (1 mL) pepper. With a pastry brush, brush the seasoned oil on the bread slices. Wrap the bread in foil and bake in a preheated 350°F (180°C) oven for 15 minutes. Unwrap and bake for 5 minutes longer.

PER SLICE	
Calories	98
Protein	3 g
Fat	1 g
Saturates	0 g
Cholesterol	0 mg
Carbohydrate	21 g
Fibre	2 g
Sodium	296 mg
Potassium	67 mg

RED RIVER CEREAL BREAD

Red River cereal was my mother's favourite, so I always think of her when I make this bread. I also feel very patriotic, because Red River cereal is a wonderful Canadian product. You can also use five-grain cereal or rolled oats in this recipe.

This bread is hearty and somewhat heavy, so do not have light and fluffy expectations!

Makes 2 loaves

1 cup (250 mL) Red River cereal
2 cups (500 mL) boiling water
3 tbsp (45 mL) honey
1 tbsp (15 mL) vegetable oil
1 tsp (5 mL) salt
1 tbsp (15 mL) granulated sugar
1/2 cup (125 mL) warm water
2 packages dry yeast (2 tbsp/25 mL)
1 1/2 cups (375 mL) whole wheat flour
3 cups (750 mL) all-purpose flour
1/2 cup (125 mL) wheat bran

1. Combine cereal, boiling water, honey, oil and salt. Allow to rest for 20 minutes, or until lukewarm.
2. Dissolve sugar in warm water and sprinkle yeast over top. Allow to rest for 10 minutes, or until doubled in volume.
3. In a large bowl, combine whole wheat flour, 1 1/2 cups (375 mL) all-purpose flour and bran. Stir well.
4. Stir yeast down and add to cereal mixture. Stir into flour mixture. Add extra all-purpose flour until dough does not stick to your fingers but is still very soft. Knead for 10 minutes by hand, 5 minutes in a mixer or 1 minute in a food processor.
5. Place dough in an oiled bowl and turn until oiled on all sides. Cover with oiled plastic wrap and allow to rest in warm place until doubled in size—about 1 1/2 hours.
6. Punch dough down, divide in half and shape into two loaves. Place in two oiled 9- x 5-inch (2 L) loaf pans and cover loosely with oiled plastic wrap. Allow to rise until doubled, about 1 hour.
7. Bake in a preheated 400°F (200°C) oven for 35 to 45 minutes, or until a thermometer reads 190°F (88°C).

PER SLICE (1/16 LOAF)	
Calories	93
Protein	3 g
Fat	1 g
Saturates	trace
Cholesterol	0 mg
Carbohydrate	19 g
Fibre	2 g
Sodium	74 mg
Potassium	58 mg

IRISH SODA BREAD WITH CARAWAY SEEDS

This quickbread is perfect to serve with a meal or as a snack at tea time. You can use 1 tsp (5 mL) dried rosemary, cumin seeds or anise seeds instead of the caraway seeds.

Makes 16 servings

1 1/2 cups (375 mL) all-purpose flour
1 cup (250 mL) whole wheat flour
2 tbsp (25 mL) granulated sugar
1 1/2 tsp (7 mL) baking powder
1/2 tsp (2 mL) baking soda
1/2 tsp (2 mL) salt
1/3 cup (75 mL) currants or raisins
1 tbsp (15 mL) caraway seeds
1 egg
1 1/4 cups (300 mL) buttermilk
3 tbsp (45 mL) vegetable oil

1. In a large bowl, combine flours, sugar, baking powder, baking soda and salt. Stir together well.

2. Stir currants and caraway seeds into flour mixture.

3. In a separate bowl, combine egg, buttermilk and oil. Pour liquid ingredients over flour mixture and combine very lightly to form a rough dough.

4. Place dough in a 9-inch (2.5 L) springform pan lined with parchment paper. Bake in a preheated 350°F (180°C) oven for 50 to 55 minutes, or until a thermometer inserted into loaf reaches at least 190°F (88°C).

PER SERVING	
Calories	119
Protein	4 g
Fat	3 g
Saturates	trace
Cholesterol	14 mg
Carbohydrate	19 g
Fibre	2 g
Sodium	157 mg
Potassium	108 mg

AMAZING SOUTH AFRICAN SEED BREAD

When I was in Cape Town I noticed that all kinds of seeds were used—in breads, sprinkled on salads and as a garnish. One bread really stood out. After trying to reproduce it without much success, I asked Cape Town cookbook author and food writer Phillippa Cheifitz about it, and she shared this sensational recipe with me.

Makes 1 large loaf

1 tbsp (15 mL) granulated sugar
2 1/2 cups (625 mL) warm water, divided
1 package dry yeast (1 tbsp/15 mL)
1/3 cup (75 mL) molasses
1 tbsp (15 mL) vegetable oil
2 cups (500 mL) whole wheat flour
1 cup (250 mL) large-flake rolled oats
1/2 cup (125 mL) rye flour
1/2 cup (125 mL) wheat bran
1/4 cup (50 mL) wheat germ
1/4 cup (50 mL) sunflower seeds
1/4 cup (50 mL) sesame seeds
1/4 cup (50 mL) poppy seeds
1/4 cup (50 mL) flax seeds, crushed or ground, or a combination
4 tsp (20 mL) kosher salt, or 1 tbsp (15 mL) table salt
3 tbsp (45 mL) mixed seeds

1. In a 2-cup (500 mL) glass measure, combine sugar and 1/2 cup (125 mL) warm water. Sprinkle with yeast and let stand for 10 minutes, or until yeast bubbles up and doubles in volume.
2. Meanwhile, combine remaining 2 cups (500 mL) water with molasses and oil.
3. In a large bowl, combine whole wheat flour, rolled oats, rye flour, bran, wheat germ, sunflower seeds, sesame seeds, poppy seeds, flax seeds and salt.
4. When yeast has risen, stir it into water/molasses mixture. Then stir molasses mixture into flour. Batter should be loose.
5. Turn batter into a buttered 9- x 5-inch (2.5 L) loaf pan lined with parchment paper. Press mixed seeds into top. Cover loosely with plastic wrap and let rise in a warm place for about 1 hour, or until batter has risen to top of pan.
6. Bake in a preheated 350°F (180°C) oven for 1 hour. Remove bread from pan, place on a rack and return to turned-off oven for 15 minutes.

PER SLICE (1/8 OF LOAF)	
Calories	168
Protein	6 g
Fat	6 g
Saturates	1 g
Cholesterol	0 mg
Carbohydrate	26 g
Fibre	5 g
Sodium	201 mg
Potassium	286 mg
Good: Thiamine; Folate; Iron	

MASHED POTATO ROLLS

Potatoes and potato water make a bread very moist and tender and the taste and aroma very yeasty. This recipe was developed by my good friend and colleague Linda Stephen, who teaches the bread-baking classes at my school. For an interesting mellow flavour, try adding 1 tsp (5 mL) anise seeds, cumin seeds, caraway seeds or fennel seeds to the dry ingredients.

Makes 18 rolls

1 lb (500 g) Yukon Gold or baking potatoes (2 large)
1 tsp (5 mL) granulated sugar
2 packages dry yeast (2 tbsp/25 mL)
2 tsp (10 mL) salt
2 tbsp (25 mL) vegetable oil
1/4 cup (50 mL) honey
2 eggs
2 cups (500 mL) all-purpose flour
2 cups (500 mL) whole wheat flour

1. Peel potatoes and cut into large pieces. Place in a saucepan and cover with water. Bring to a boil, reduce heat and cook until tender.
2. Drain potatoes, reserving 1 cup (250 mL) cooking liquid. Mash potatoes and reserve.
3. In a small bowl, dissolve sugar in 1/2 cup (125 mL) warm potato water. Sprinkle with yeast. Allow to rise for 10 minutes, or until doubled in volume.
4. In a large bowl, stir salt and oil into remaining 1/2 cup (125 mL) warm potato liquid. Add honey, eggs and mashed potatoes. Blend until smooth. Add yeast mixture.
5. In a separate bowl, combine flours. Add 2 cups (500 mL) flour to liquid mixture and combine well. Dough should be very sticky. Add remaining flour (more if necessary) to form a dough that is moist but not sticky. Knead dough for 10 minutes by hand, 5 minutes in a heavy-duty mixer fitted with dough hook or 1 minute in a food processor.
6. Place dough in an oiled bowl. Turn until oiled on all sides. Cover bowl with oiled plastic wrap and allow to rise in a warm spot for 1 hour, or until doubled in bulk.
7. Punch dough down. Divide into 18 pieces and roll each piece into a ball. Arrange half the balls in a lightly oiled 9-inch (23 cm) spring-form pan or round baking pan. Repeat, making a second layer with

PER ROLL	
Calories	153
Protein	5 g
Fat	3 g
Saturates	trace
Cholesterol	21 mg
Carbohydrate	29 g
Fibre	3 g
Sodium	269 mg
Potassium	171 mg

remaining balls. Cover loosely with oiled plastic wrap and allow to rise for 40 to 60 minutes, or until doubled in bulk.

8. Bake in a preheated 400°F (200°C) oven for 25 to 30 minutes, or until a thermometer inserted into rolls reads at least 190°F (88°C). Remove rolls from pan and cool on racks. To serve, break rolls apart.

YEAST

Yeast is a living organism, which is probably why so many people are afraid to use it. After all, you could kill it! But it is not so difficult to work with. Just remember that yeast loves warm cozy places, so the temperature of the water it is dissolved in and the rising location should not be too hot or too cold.

Yeast is available in two forms, dry and cake. Dry yeast can be regular or instant-dissolving. One package of yeast is a scant table-spoon and will be enough for about 5 cups (1.25 L) flour in a bread recipe. I prefer cake yeast if available, because it rises a bit faster and I think has a slightly nicer flavour. But it can be hard to find and is very perishable. When I find it I buy extra and freeze it. Always dissolve it in warm water before using.

Although you can combine dry yeast directly with the flour, I always "proof" the yeast first by dissolving it in a little warm sugared water to see if it is active. Warm water between 110°F and 120°F (43°C to 49°C) is perfect. If the yeast does not rise in the warm water, either the water is too hot and killed it, or the yeast is inactive. Do not use inactive yeast; if the yeast won't rise in the water, it won't rise in the bread.

SPICED WHOLE WHEAT CHALLAH WITH HONEY AND RAISINS

My grandmother Jenny Soltz was a great bread baker. She had eleven children and not much money, so she would enter her challah breads in country fair bake-offs each year and always won enough flour to keep her family in bread through the winter. She used to make two braids and bake them side by side in a deep square pan—the top would rise over the edge in a beautiful braided bubble.

Challah is a special-occasion bread in Jewish homes and is served every week for Shabbat. This lightly spiced version will make your house smell wonderful, but to make a plain challah, just omit the spices.

Makes 1 large loaf

1 cup (250 mL) warm water
1 tbsp (15 mL) granulated sugar
1 package dry yeast (1 tbsp/15 mL)
1 egg
¼ cup (50 mL) honey
2 tbsp (25 mL) vegetable oil
1 tsp (5 mL) salt
2 cups (500 mL) whole wheat flour
1 cup (250 mL) all-purpose flour
½ tsp (2 mL) ground cinnamon
Pinch ground nutmeg
Pinch ground cloves
Pinch ground ginger
¼ cup (50 mL) raisins, optional

Glaze

2 tbsp (25 mL) beaten egg
Pinch salt
1 tbsp (15 mL) sesame seeds

PER SLICE (1/16 LOAF)	
Calories	126
Protein	4 g
Fat	3 g
Saturates	trace
Cholesterol	22 mg
Carbohydrate	22 g
Fibre	2 g
Sodium	152 mg
Potassium	91 mg

1. In a small bowl, combine warm water and sugar. Sprinkle yeast over water and allow to rest for 10 minutes. Mixture should bubble up and double in volume.
2. Meanwhile, in a separate bowl, combine egg, honey, oil and salt.
3. In a large bowl, combine whole wheat flour, ½ cup (125 mL) all-purpose flour, cinnamon, nutmeg, cloves and ginger. Stir together well.

4. When yeast mixture has doubled, stir down and combine with egg mixture. Add to flour and mix until a sticky dough forms. Add more all-purpose flour until dough comes together into a ball and is just dry enough to be kneaded. Knead dough on a floured surface for about 10 minutes. (Knead dough in a heavy mixer for 5 minutes or in a food processor for 1 minute.)

5. Place dough in an oiled bowl, cover with oiled plastic wrap and put in a warm place until double in bulk—about 1 hour. Punch dough down and knead in raisins.

6. To braid dough, cut into three equal pieces. Roll each piece into a rope about 12 inches (30 cm) long, pinch three ends together and braid ropes together. You can place braided dough in a loaf pan if you want to use it in sandwiches, or bake free-form on a baking sheet that has been oiled or lined with parchment paper. Tuck ends under.

7. Cover dough loosely with oiled plastic wrap and allow to rise in a warm place until doubled in bulk—about 45 minutes.

8. To prepare glaze, combine beaten egg with salt and brush gently over bread. Sprinkle with sesame seeds.

9. Bake in a preheated 350°F (180°C) oven for 25 minutes. Reduce heat to 325°F (160°C) and continue to bake for 25 minutes longer, or until a thermometer inserted into loaf reads at least 190°F (88°C).

SPICES

Spices are the seeds, bark and roots of certain plants. Use them sparingly until you decide whether you like them in a particular recipe. There are some traditional matches, such as nutmeg with spinach or cinnamon with apples, but don't be afraid to experiment. Spices can also replace some of the flavour that is lost by reducing the fat and salt in a recipe.

Ground spices lose their flavour quickly (within a year of being ground), so buy them in small quantities, or buy them whole and grind them as you need them. The original spice grinder was the mortar and pestle, and they still work well. But you can also buy an electric spice mill, or use a coffee grinder that you reserve only for spices.

Store spices in a cool, dry place.

MULTIGRAIN YOGURT BREAD

If you love different flavours and textures in breads, try this one. I really enjoy the very subtle anise taste and aroma. This dough makes great toast bread and is also wonderful baked as hot dog or hamburger buns (bake for 25 to 35 minutes).

Makes 2 loaves

1/2 cup (125 mL) large-flake rolled oats
1/2 cup (125 mL) cornmeal
1 1/2 cups (375 mL) boiling water
1/4 cup (50 mL) honey or brown sugar
1 1/2 tsp (7 mL) salt
1 tbsp (15 mL) vegetable oil
1/2 tsp (2 mL) ground or whole anise seeds, optional
2 tsp (10 mL) granulated sugar
1/2 cup (125 mL) warm water
2 packages dry yeast (2 tbsp/25 mL)
2 cups (500 mL) whole wheat flour
2 cups (500 mL) all-purpose flour
1/2 cup (125 mL) wheat bran
1/2 cup (125 mL) oat bran
1 cup (250 mL) unflavoured low-fat yogurt

Glaze

2 tbsp (25 mL) beaten egg
1/4 tsp (1 mL) salt

1. In a large bowl, combine rolled oats and cornmeal. Stir in boiling water, honey, salt, oil and anise. Stir to dissolve honey and salt. Allow mixture to cool for 20 minutes, or until lukewarm.
2. Dissolve sugar in warm water. Sprinkle yeast over top. Allow mixture to rest for 10 minutes, or until volume doubles and mixture has bubbled up.
3. In a separate bowl, combine whole wheat flour, 1 cup (250 mL) all-purpose flour, wheat bran and oat bran.
4. When yeast mixture has risen, stir down and add to rolled oats mixture. Stir in yogurt and dry ingredients. Add more all-purpose flour if necessary to form soft but manageable dough that does not stick to your fingers.

BRAN

Wheat bran (insoluble fibre) encourages regularity, whereas oat bran (soluble fibre) helps to control blood sugar and blood cholesterol levels. You can always add a little wheat bran to bread and muffin recipes, as it does not absorb much liquid, but if you want to add oat bran to recipes, reduce the other dry ingredients (e.g., flour) to compensate.

I usually use natural wheat bran in muffins, but bran cereals work well, too.

PER SLICE (1/16 LOAF)	
Calories	93
Protein	3 g
Fat	1 g
Saturates	trace
Cholesterol	5 mg
Carbohydrate	19 g
Fibre	2 g
Sodium	134 mg
Potassium	97 mg

5. Knead dough for 10 minutes by hand, 5 minutes with electric mixer or in a large food processor for 1 minute.

6. Place dough in an oiled bowl and turn dough until it is completely coated with oil. Cover bowl with oiled plastic wrap and allow dough to rise in a warm spot for 1 to 1½ hours, or until dough has doubled in bulk.

7. Punch dough down and divide in half. Shape to fit two 9 x 5-inch (2 L) loaf pans. Place dough in lightly oiled and parchment-lined pans. Cover loosely with oiled plastic wrap and allow to rise for 45 to 60 minutes, or until doubled again.

8. Combine egg and salt and brush on breads. Bake in a preheated 400°F (200°C) oven for 45 to 55 minutes, or until a thermometer inserted into breads reads at least 190°F (88°C). Remove breads immediately from pans and cool on racks.

HONEY EGG BREAD

This is similar to challah but not as rich or eggy. It makes delicious toast, French toast, bread pudding and sandwiches.

Makes 1 large loaf
1 cup (250 mL) warm water
1 tbsp (15 mL) granulated sugar
1 package dry yeast (1 tbsp/15 mL)
1 egg
¼ cup (50 mL) honey
¼ cup (50 mL) vegetable oil
1 tsp (5 mL) salt
2 cups (500 mL) whole wheat flour
2 cups (500 mL) all-purpose flour
½ cup (125 mL) raisins, optional

Glaze

1 egg white
¼ tsp (1 mL) salt
1 tsp (5 mL) sesame seeds

1. In a small bowl, combine water and sugar. Sprinkle yeast over top. Let rest for 10 minutes, or until mixture bubbles up and doubles in volume.
2. Meanwhile, in a separate bowl, combine egg, honey, oil and salt.
3. In a large bowl, combine whole wheat flour and 1 cup (250 mL) all-purpose flour.
4. When yeast has bubbled up, stir it down and combine with egg mixture. Add egg mixture to flour and combine to form a sticky dough. This can be done by hand, in a food processor or in a heavy mixer with a dough hook. Add enough extra flour so that dough comes together in a ball and does not stick to your hands but is not dry. Knead dough for 5 to 10 minutes by hand, 1 minute in a food processor or 3 to 5 minutes with a mixer.
5. Place dough in a large oiled bowl and turn dough until it is completely coated with oil. Cover bowl with oiled plastic wrap and set in a warm spot for 1 to 1½ hours, or until doubled in volume.
6. Punch dough down and knead in raisins. Roll out dough, fold into thirds and then roll up tightly from an open end. (Or, divide dough

PER SERVING (1/18 LOAF)	
Calories	146
Protein	4 g
Fat	4 g
Saturates	trace
Cholesterol	10 mg
Carbohydrate	25 g
Fibre	2 g
Sodium	171 mg
Potassium	86 mg

into thirds, roll into ropes and braid.) Place loaf in a 9- x 5-inch (2 L) loaf pan lined with parchment paper. Cover loosely with oiled plastic wrap and let rise in a warm spot for 1 hour.

7. To prepare glaze, mix egg white with salt. Gently brush on loaf. Sprinkle with sesame seeds. Bake in a preheated 350°F (180°C) oven for 25 minutes. Reduce heat to 325°F (160°C) and bake for 25 minutes longer, or until a thermometer reads at least 190°F (88°C).

FRUIT BUTTERS

Fruit butters make delicious fat-free spreads for toast, rolls or bagels. Use them on their own or with yogurt cheese (page 391).

Apple Butter

Peel and core 6 large apples and cut into chunks (if you have a food mill you can strain out the cores and peel after cooking).

In a large saucepan or Dutch oven, combine apples with $1/4$ lb (125 g) dried apple slices (about $1^1/2$ cups/375 mL), 2 cups (500 mL) apple juice, 1 tbsp (15 mL) ground cinnamon, $1/4$ tsp (1 mL) allspice and $1/4$ tsp (1 mL) ground cloves. Bring to a boil, reduce heat, cover and cook gently for 20 minutes, or until thickened. Uncover and cook until very thick. Puree.

Makes about 2 cups (500 mL).

Pear Butter

Peel and core 8 large pears and cut into chunks (if you have a food mill you can strain out the cores and peel after cooking).

In a large saucepan or Dutch oven, combine pears with $1/2$ cup (125 mL) pear juice and $1/4$ tsp (1 mL) ground nutmeg or cinnamon. Bring to a boil, reduce heat, cover and cook gently for 20 minutes. Uncover and cook until very thick. Puree.

Makes about $1^1/2$ cups (375 mL).

MUESLI ROLLS

I love the muesli rolls from European-style bakeries; they seem to include all kinds of healthful treats. Here's my version. You can also bake the dough in loaves.

Makes 16 rolls

1 tsp (5 mL) granulated sugar
1 3/4 cups (425 mL) warm water, divided
1 package dry yeast (1 tbsp/15 mL)
1 1/2 cups (375 mL) whole wheat flour
1 1/2 cups (375 mL) all-purpose flour
1 tsp (5 mL) salt
1/4 cup (50 mL) honey
2 tbsp (25 mL) vegetable oil
1/2 cup (125 mL) raisins
1/2 cup (125 mL) large-flake rolled oats
1/3 cup (75 mL) chopped walnuts or pecans
1/3 cup (75 mL) sunflower seeds
1 tbsp (15 mL) sesame seeds
1 tsp (5 mL) caraway seeds

Glaze

1 tbsp (15 mL) honey
1 tbsp (15 mL) hot water
1 tbsp (15 mL) large-flake rolled oats

1. Dissolve sugar in 1/2 cup (125 mL) warm water. Sprinkle yeast over top and allow to rest for 10 minutes, or until doubled in volume.

2. Meanwhile, in a bowl, combine whole wheat flour, 3/4 cup (175 mL) all-purpose flour and salt.

3. In a large bowl, combine remaining 1 1/4 cups (300 mL) warm water, honey and oil.

4. Stir yeast mixture down and combine with honey water. Stir in flour mixture and then add all-purpose flour until a very soft dough is formed. Knead for 5 minutes in a mixer, 10 minutes by hand or 1 minute in a food processor.

5. Stir in raisins, rolled oats, walnuts, sunflower seeds, sesame seeds and caraway seeds. Add more flour if necessary. Dough should be soft but not sticky.

PER ROLL	
Calories	179
Protein	5 g
Fat	6 g
Saturates	1 g
Cholesterol	0 mg
Carbohydrate	30 g
Fibre	3 g
Sodium	150 mg
Potassium	161 mg
Good: Folate	

6. Place dough in a large oiled bowl and turn until oiled on all sides. Cover with oiled plastic wrap. Allow to rise in a warm spot for 1 hour, or until doubled.

7. Punch dough down and divide in two. Roll each half into a rope about 2 inches (5 cm) thick, and cut into 3-inch (7.5 cm) lengths. Place on parchment-lined baking sheets. Cover loosely with oiled plastic wrap and allow to rise until doubled, about 45 minutes.

8. To prepare glaze, combine honey with hot water and brush gently on rolls. Sprinkle rolled oats on top. Bake in a preheated 350°F (180°C) oven for 20 to 25 minutes, or until a thermometer inserted into centre reads at least 190°F (88°C).

BREAD-BAKING TIPS

Two bread-baking tips have changed my life. The first is that you do not necessarily need to add all the flour called for in a recipe. The second is to use a thermometer to see whether your bread is ready. I learned the hard way that none of the old tips work (tapping the loaf on the bottom to see whether it sounds hollow, for example—it either never sounds hollow or it always does) when I made a huge challah for Rosh Hashanah, and it was not cooked in the centre, much to my guests' shock. When I told my friend Mitchell Davis about it, he told me about the thermometer tip, and now I always use one. The bread is ready when a thermometer inserted into the centre reads at least 190°F (88°C).

Lemon Palacsinta
Moroccan Sliced Oranges with Dried Fruit
Fresh Pineapple Flambé
Bananas Flambé
Autumn Pear Crisp
Fruit Salad "Margarita"
Chocolate-coated Strawberries
Strawberries with Balsamic Vinegar
Bumbleberry Cobbler
Caramelized Pears with Tiramisu Cream
Pears Poached in Pomegranate Juice
Fruit Yogurt Dip and Peach Salsa
Creamy Rice Pudding
Wild Rice Pudding Brûlée
Ray's Favourite Applesauce
Dried Fruit Compote
Deep Berry Glaze
Phyllo Cake with Toasted Almonds and Cinnamon
Phyllo Nests with Caramelized Winter Fruits
Apple Strudel
Apple Phyllo Pie
Pavlova Roulade with Passionfruit Filling
Pavlova with Berries and Flowers

Almond Angel Food Cake with Cinnamon Apricots
Anna's Angel Food Cake with Berry Berry Sauce
Chocolate Angel Food Cake with Chocolate Sauce
Raspberry Upside-down Cake
Frozen Lemon Meringue Cake
Carrot Tube Cake
Quick Apple Cake
Old-fashioned Cheesecake
Strawberry Meringue Shortcakes
Nick Malgieri's Fudge Brownies
Date Squares
Apricot Oatmeal Cookies
Gwen's Almond Haystacks
Hubert's Twice-baked Hazelnut Meringue Cookies
Chocolate Oatmeal Cookies
Chewy Spice Cookies
Mocha Meringue Kisses
Espresso Biscotti

HEART SMART

SMART

DESSERTS

LEMON PALACSINTA

Palacsinta are thin pancakes or crêpes, and this version makes a wonderful dessert, breakfast or brunch. They are even delicious just filled with jam or fresh berries.

I like to make extra-thin crêpes the way my mom did. I add ½ cup (125 mL) batter to the pan, swirl it in the pan and then pour any that doesn't stick to the pan back into the batter bowl. (That way you get a very thin coating.) But most people just add less batter to the pan in the first place, as described below.

Crêpes can be made ahead and frozen. Stack them as they are cooked, placing a piece of waxed paper between each one if you want to defrost them one or two at a time.

You can buy a special crêpe or omelette pan, but I just use a small non-stick skillet.

Makes 6 servings

Crêpes

3 eggs
³/₄ cup (175 mL) all-purpose flour
³/₄ cup (175 mL) milk
1 tbsp (15 mL) granulated sugar
1 tbsp (15 mL) vegetable oil

Filling

¹/₃ cup (75 mL) granulated sugar
¹/₃ cup (75 mL) lemon juice
2 tbsp (25 mL) Limoncello or orange liqueur, optional
2 tbsp (25 mL) icing sugar, sifted

1. To prepare crêpes, whisk eggs. Whisk in flour and then milk. Beat in sugar. If you have time, cover and allow batter to rest for at least 1 hour in refrigerator.

2. Heat oil in an 8-inch (20 cm) non-stick skillet on medium heat. Whisk oil into batter and return oiled skillet to heat.

3. Add ¹/₄ to ¹/₃ cup (50 to 75 mL) batter to skillet and swirl it around to coat bottom and partway up sides. Cook for a few minutes, or just until you can see first side browning through crêpe. Flip and cook second side for about 30 seconds. (Second side will never look as nice.) Repeat until all batter is used. You should have 6 to 8 crêpes.

PER SERVING	
Calories	190
Protein	6 g
Fat	5 g
Saturates	1 g
Cholesterol	94 mg
Carbohydrate	30 g
Fibre	1 g
Sodium	46 mg
Potassium	112 mg
Good: Vitamin B12; Folate	

4. Arrange crêpes nicest side down. Sprinkle each with granulated sugar and lemon juice. Roll up or fold into quarters. Eat at room temperature sprinkled (or not) with liqueur and dusted with icing sugar. To serve hot, place folded crêpes on a parchment-lined baking sheet and heat at 350°F (180°C) for 10 minutes. Sprinkle with liqueur. Flambé if you wish (page 249). Dust with icing sugar.

MOROCCAN SLICED ORANGES WITH DRIED FRUIT

A stunning platter of oranges, grapefruits and dried fruits makes an easy and refreshing dessert after a big dinner. Slice the oranges and grapefruits or cut them into segments.

You can find orange blossom water in Middle Eastern Stores (I found it at the Ararat Bakery in Toronto). It is very exotic and perfume-like, so use only a tiny bit, and if you can't find it, just omit it.

Makes 8 servings

4 large oranges (about 3/4 lb/375 g each)
2 pink grapefruits (about 3/4 lb/375 g each)
Few drops orange blossom water, optional
3 dried dates, pitted and sliced
3 dried figs, sliced
3 dried apricots, sliced
2 tbsp (25 mL) chopped pistachio nuts

PER SERVING	
Calories	117
Protein	2 g
Fat	1 g
Saturates	trace
Cholesterol	0 mg
Carbohydrate	27 g
Fibre	4 g
Sodium	1 mg
Potassium	417 mg

Excellent: Vitamin C
Good: Thiamine; Folate

1. Cut tops and bottoms off oranges and grapefruits so they will stand up on a cutting board, and cut off peel and pith from top to bottom, exposing sections. Slice oranges into rounds and arrange on a platter. Holding grapefruit in the palm of your hand (over a bowl to catch juices), cut out segments between membranes and arrange segments over centre of oranges. Squeeze juice from membranes into bowl—you should have about 1/2 cup (125 mL).
2. Stir orange blossom water into reserved juices. Drizzle over oranges and grapefruits.
3. Arrange dates, figs and apricots over fruit. Sprinkle with pistachios.

FRESH PINEAPPLE FLAMBÉ

The trick to flambéing is to ignite the alcohol in the rum just as it evaporates from the pan. Try using a long fireplace match, and hold it over the pan just after you add the rum. The less liquid there is in the pan and the higher the heat, the faster the alcohol will evaporate and ignite, so be very careful and stand back (this may trigger your smoke detector, so beware). Even if the alcohol does not flambé, the pineapple will still taste great, so don't keep trying.

Serve the pineapple with a scoop of mango sorbet if you wish.

Makes 8 servings

1 fresh pineapple, peeled, cored and cut in 8 rings
1 tbsp (15 mL) soft non-hydrogenated margarine or unsalted butter
1/2 cup (125 mL) brown sugar
1/4 cup (50 mL) pineapple juice or orange juice
2 tbsp (25 mL) kahlua or strong coffee
2 tbsp (25 mL) dark rum or orange juice

1. Place pineapple on paper towels to dry.
2. Heat margarine in a large non-stick skillet on medium-high heat. Add pineapple and cook for 1 to 2 minutes per side, or until lightly browned.
3. Sprinkle with sugar and allow sugar to melt. Add pineapple juice and kahlua and bring to a boil. Cook for 2 minutes.
4. Standing back, add rum and flambé (page 249).

PER SERVING	
Calories	115
Protein	trace
Fat	1 g
Saturates	trace
Cholesterol	0 mg
Carbohydrate	24 g
Fibre	1 g
Sodium	25 mg
Potassium	116 mg

BANANAS FLAMBÉ

There are many versions of this dessert, but the cinnamon, nutmeg and allspice make this my favourite. I serve it a lot when people drop over on the spur of the moment, because I always have the ingredients on hand.

Serve this over frozen vanilla yogurt or with sweetened soft yogurt cheese (page 391) or thick yogurt if you wish, but it is also great on its own. If you can find the tiny finger bananas, use them whole. They look adorable in this dish.

Makes 6 to 8 servings

1/2 cup (125 mL) brown sugar
1/3 cup (75 mL) pineapple juice
1/2 tsp (2 mL) ground cinnamon
1/4 tsp (1 mL) ground nutmeg
1/4 tsp (1 mL) ground allspice
8 bananas
1/4 cup (50 mL) dark rum

PER SERVING	
Calories	234
Protein	2 g
Fat	1 g
Saturates	trace
Cholesterol	0 mg
Carbohydrate	56 g
Fibre	3 g
Sodium	7 mg
Potassium	689 mg
Excellent: Vitamin B6	

1. In a large, deep non-stick skillet, combine brown sugar, pineapple juice, cinnamon, nutmeg and allspice. Stir well and heat on medium-high heat until mixture is boiling and smooth.
2. Peel bananas and cut lengthwise into halves or quarters. Add to sugar mixture in skillet. Cook for about 3 minutes, or until hot.
3. Add rum. When mixture begins to sizzle, flambé (page 249). If it does not flambé, do not worry. It will still taste great.

AUTUMN PEAR CRISP

Everyone expects apples in a crisp, but this luscious, juicy version made with pears is a bit different, and sensational.

I like to use Bosc or Bartlett pears. I usually buy them a few days ahead so they can ripen. And of course you can use apples in this, or a combination of apples and pears.

Makes 6 servings

4 ripe pears, peeled, cored and cut in chunks
3/4 cup (175 mL) all-purpose flour
1/2 cup (125 mL) brown sugar
1/3 cup (75 mL) soft non-hydrogenated margarine or unsalted
    butter, cold
1 tbsp (15 mL) coarse sugar

1. Spread pears in a lightly oiled 8- or 9-inch (2 or 2.5 L) square baking dish.
2. In a large bowl or food processor, combine flour and sugar. Cut in margarine until it is in small bits.
3. Sprinkle topping over fruit. Sprinkle with coarse sugar. Bake in a preheated 350°F (180°C) oven for 50 to 60 minutes, or until topping is browned and crisp and fruit is very tender.

PER SERVING	
Calories	278
Protein	2 g
Fat	11 g
Saturates	1 g
Cholesterol	0 mg
Carbohydrate	46 g
Fibre	3 g
Sodium	144 mg
Potassium	210 mg

FRUIT SALAD "MARGARITA"

For an alcoholic version of this delicious fruit salad, use tequila instead of ginger ale and orange liqueur instead of orange juice. You can also use other fruits such as raspberries or blueberries.

Leftovers can be pureed to make a great drink!

Makes 8 to 10 servings

3 oranges
4 cups (1 L) strawberries
2 kiwis
1 small pineapple
1 ripe mango
1/3 cup (75 mL) limeade concentrate or non-alcoholic margarita
    fruit mix concentrate
1/3 cup (75 mL) orange juice
1/3 cup (75 mL) ginger ale

PER SERVING	
Calories	126
Protein	2 g
Fat	1 g
Saturates	trace
Cholesterol	0 mg
Carbohydrate	32 g
Fibre	4 g
Sodium	3 mg
Potassium	392 mg
Excellent: Vitamin C	
Good: Folate	

1. Cut tops and bottoms off oranges. Holding orange flat side down on a cutting board, cut off peel from top to bottom, exposing segments. Cut out orange segments from between membranes (do this over a large bowl to catch juices).
2. Hull strawberries and cut each berry in half or quarters depending on size. Peel kiwis and cut each one into 6 to 8 chunks. Peel pineapple and cut into chunks. Peel mango and cut into chunks. Toss all fruit together.
3. Combine limeade, orange juice and ginger ale. Pour over fruit and toss. Marinate for up to 1 hour at room temperature or longer in refrigerator.

COOKING WITH WINES AND LIQUEURS

Wines and liqueurs can be great seasonings in cooking. I usually keep wine, brandy, dark rum and an orange liqueur on hand. The orange liqueur can be used when any fruit liqueur is called for.

Brandy, rum and liqueurs do not have to be refrigerated after opening, but opened bottles of wine should be kept in the refrigerator and used quickly. If you plan to use the wine only for cooking, pour a spoonful of olive oil into the bottle. The oil will float on the surface and block out the air, and the wine should keep, refrigerated, for a month or two.

When you are using wine in cooking, always use the driest wine available, unless the recipe states otherwise.

CHOCOLATE-COATED STRAWBERRIES

These seem very rich and decadent, but there is actually only a bit of chocolate on each berry, making this a great HeartSmart™ treat. They can be served on their own or be used to garnish angel food cake or other desserts. For an extra garnish, drizzle white chocolate over the dipped berries.

Here are some pointers to make the berries even easier to prepare:

- Use the freshest berries and the very best chocolate. I like European. (When a dish contains only two ingredients, it is especially important to use the very best.)
- Berries should be perfectly dry when they are dipped. Pat them dry with tea towels or paper towels.
- If the greens on the berries are nice, leave them on to be used as little handles for dipping. If they look wilted, remove them and dip the fat ends of the berries in the chocolate, leaving the points to be used as handles.
- Chopped chocolate melts more evenly than large pieces.
- Place the melted chocolate in a deep rather than wide vessel to make dipping easier. You will have more chocolate than you need, but it can be used again (no one ever seems to have trouble figuring out what to do with extra melted chocolate!).
- Make sure your utensils and bowls are completely dry when you are handling or melting chocolate. The slightest bit of moisture can cause the chocolate to "seize," or become dull and hard.
- Don't be tempted to add a liqueur or any liquid flavouring to the chocolate. (Professional chocolate makers sometimes add flavoured oils, which do not cause seizing.) Some people inject the berries with liqueur, but I like them plain, especially if you are using great chocolate!
- If your chocolate does seize, warm it with 1 tbsp (15 mL) vegetable oil and stir until smooth.
- Chocolate-coated strawberries should not be made too far in advance, as the greens tend to wilt and dry out and the berries become wet and soggy through the chocolate. Prepare them a few hours before serving.

Makes 20 berries

20 medium strawberries, preferably with hulls
1/2 lb (250 g) bittersweet or semi-sweet chocolate, chopped

CHOCOLATE

I use dark chocolate in cooking—either bittersweet or semi-sweet (they can be used interchangeably). Bittersweet has more intense chocolate flavour and less sugar, and 70 percent bittersweet is now being promoted as a source of antioxidants—very good for you in small quantities. The chocolate should keep in a cool cupboard for about a year.

PER STRAWBERRY	
Calories	32
Protein	1 g
Fat	2 g
Saturates	1 g
Cholesterol	0 mg
Carbohydrate	4 g
Fibre	1 g
Sodium	0 mg
Potassium	60 mg

1. Clean and dry berries.

2. Melt chocolate in a bowl set over gently simmering water or on Medium power in the microwave. To prevent chocolate from burning, remove from heat before it has completely melted and stir to finish melting.

3. Transfer chocolate to a 1 cup (250 mL) measure to make dipping easier. Dip strawberries partway into chocolate and place on a waxed paper-lined baking sheet. Allow to set in refrigerator for about 30 minutes.

STRAWBERRIES WITH BALSAMIC VINEGAR

I never get tired of eating these strawberries with their mysterious ingredient—balsamic vinegar. And you certainly cannot get tired of making this dessert, as it only takes a minute! (Be sure to use a good-quality aged vinegar.)

This recipe also works well with raspberry vinegar or lemon juice. Serve the berries on their own or in small cantaloupe halves.

Makes 6 servings

4 cups (1 L) strawberries
3 tbsp (45 mL) granulated sugar
3 tbsp (45 mL) balsamic vinegar

1. Rinse strawberries and pat dry. Trim and cut into halves or quarters, depending on size.

2. Sprinkle berries with sugar and vinegar. Stir gently and allow to marinate for about 10 minutes before serving.

PER SERVING	
Calories	55
Protein	1 g
Fat	trace
Saturates	0 g
Cholesterol	0 mg
Carbohydrate	14 g
Fibre	2 g
Sodium	1 mg
Potassium	173 mg
Excellent: Vitamin C	

BUMBLEBERRY COBBLER

I first heard the word *bumbleberry* when I was in Prince Edward Island—Anne of Green Gables country—and had bumbleberry pie. Bumbleberry, it seems, is not actually a berry but a mix of different kinds of fruits that can vary according to the season. In winter make it with cranberries, apples and pears. Use fresh or frozen fruit.

Makes 8 to 10 servings

1 lb (500 g) rhubarb, diced (about 4 cups/1 L)
2 apples, peeled, cored and diced (about 3 cups/750 mL)
1 cup (250 mL) raspberries
1 cup (250 mL) blueberries
1/2 cup (125 mL) granulated sugar
3 tbsp (45 mL) all-purpose flour

Topping

1 cup (250 mL) all-purpose flour
1/2 cup (125 mL) whole wheat flour
3 tbsp (45 mL) granulated sugar
2 tsp (10 mL) baking powder
1/3 cup (75 mL) soft non-hydrogenated margarine or
        unsalted butter, cold
1 egg
3/4 cup (175 mL) buttermilk
2 tbsp (25 mL) icing sugar, sifted

1. In a large bowl, combine rhubarb, apples, raspberries, blueberries, granulated sugar and flour. Spoon into a 12- x 8-inch (3 L) baking dish.
2. To prepare topping, in a large bowl, combine flours, granulated sugar and baking powder. Cut in margarine with a pastry blender or fingertips (or use a food processor).
3. Whisk together egg and buttermilk. Stir into flour mixture until a soft dough is formed. Spoon batter on top of fruit in 8 large spoonfuls, leaving room for fruit to bubble up around edges.
4. Bake in a preheated 375°F (190°C) oven for 45 to 50 minutes, or until topping is browned and fruit bubbles. Sprinkle with icing sugar before serving.

Peach Cobbler

Instead of rhubarb, apples and berries, use 8 sliced peaches and 1/2 tsp (2 mL) ground cinnamon.

PER SERVING	
Calories	300
Protein	5 g
Fat	9 g
Saturates	1 g
Cholesterol	28 mg
Carbohydrate	52 g
Fibre	5 g
Sodium	202 mg
Potassium	315 mg

PEARS

Pears, like bananas, are one of the few fruits that ripen after they have been picked. I always try to cook with ripe pears (I prefer Bartlett or Bosc), as unripe ones have little flavour.

You can use pears in most recipes that call for apples. Try pear sauce or pear crisp (page 428) for something a little different.

CARAMELIZED PEARS WITH TIRAMISU CREAM

Tiramisu is a wonderful Italian dessert, but it is almost indecently rich. In this recipe I have put together a creamy mixture reminiscent of tiramisu's flavours and combined it with caramelized pears. To be completely true to the name you should use mascarpone, but here I actually prefer the taste and lightness of ricotta.

Garnish this with sprigs of fresh mint.

Makes 8 servings

4 pears, firm but ripe (preferably Bartlett or Bosc)
²/₃ cup (150 mL) granulated sugar
2 tbsp (25 mL) chopped candied ginger
1 lemon, thinly sliced

Filling

¹/₂ cup (125 mL) light ricotta cheese (drained if necessary)
2 tbsp (25 mL) granulated sugar
2 tsp (10 mL) dark rum, coffee liqueur or extra-strong coffee
¹/₂ tsp (2 mL) vanilla
2 tbsp (25 mL) chopped bittersweet or semisweet chocolate
2 tbsp (25 mL) icing sugar, sifted

1. Cut pears in half lengthwise. Scoop out cores (a melon baller works well).
2. Sprinkle granulated sugar over bottom of a large, deep skillet that will hold pears in a single layer. Cook sugar, uncovered, on medium-high heat, until sugar begins to brown, but be careful not to burn.
3. Add pears to skillet cut side down. Sprinkle with ginger and arrange lemon slices over top. Reduce heat and cook gently for about 10 minutes. Cover. Remove from heat and allow to rest for at least 30 minutes, or until room temperature or cold.
4. Meanwhile, to prepare filling, in a small bowl, combine ricotta, granulated sugar, rum and vanilla.
5. Strain chocolate to remove chocolate dust and prevent ricotta from discolouring. Stir chocolate pieces into filling.
6. To serve, place a pear half, cut side up, on each plate. Top with cheese and a cooked lemon slice. Drizzle pear and plate with any syrup from cooking and dust with icing sugar.

PER SERVING

Calories	179
Protein	2 g
Fat	2 g
Saturates	1 g
Cholesterol	5 mg
Carbohydrate	40 g
Fibre	3 g
Sodium	22 mg
Potassium	226 mg

PEARS POACHED IN POMEGRANATE JUICE

A few years ago, I really had to search for pomegranate juice when I wanted to make this. Now it is sold everywhere.

Pomegranates are high in antioxidants, as well being delicious.

Makes 12 servings

6 pears, firm but ripe
1 cup (250 mL) pomegranate juice
1 cup (250 mL) dry red wine or cranberry juice
1 cup (250 mL) water
1/2 cup (125 mL) granulated sugar
1 stick cinnamon
2 tbsp (25 mL) pomegranate seeds, optional

1. Peel pears. Cut in half and remove cores and seeds (a melon baller works well).
2. In a wide saucepan or deep skillet, bring pomegranate juice, wine and water to a boil. Stir in sugar and cinnamon stick. Add pears and cook gently, uncovered, for 20 to 30 minutes, or until tender. Turn pears halfway through cooking time. Remove pears from pan.
3. Return pan to heat and cook juice, uncovered, on medium-high for about 10 minutes, or until liquid is syrupy and reduced to about 3/4 cup (175 mL).
4. Leaving stem end attached, slice each pear so that it can be fanned out on a dessert plate. Serve with juices spooned on top and sprinkle with pomegranate seeds. Serve warm, at room temperature or cold.

PER SERVING	
Calories	92
Protein	0 g
Fat	trace
Saturates	0 g
Cholesterol	0 mg
Carbohydrate	23 g
Fibre	2 g
Sodium	4 mg
Potassium	112 mg

POMEGRANATES

The pomegranate is one of the foods mentioned in the Bible and, with its many seeds, it is a symbol of fertility. The number of seeds (supposedly 613) matches the number of commandments Jews should obey and represents the number of good deeds we will all do in the coming year.

To open a pomegranate easily (and to help prevent the juice from staining everything in sight), slice off the top and bottom and carefully cut the skin lengthwise into four quarters. Place the pomegranate in a large bowl of water and, under the water, gently pull the fruit apart in quarters. Pull out the seeds. The seeds will sink and the membranes will float.

To make fresh pomegranate juice (about 1/3 cup/75 mL per fruit), you can puree the seeds and then strain the mixture by pressing it firmly through a sieve. Or cut the fruit in half and use a citrus press.

FRUIT YOGURT DIP AND PEACH SALSA

I love serving fruit platters for dessert, but often look for something to make them a little more special. Try serving an array of fresh fruit with one or two dipping sauces—one made with yogurt cheese and the other made with fruit. Be sure to use ripe fruit for the best flavour. This yogurt dip is a great topping for other desserts, too.

For an extra treat, serve biscotti (page 464 and 468) along with the fruit.

Makes 1 cup (250 mL) dip; 2 cups (500 mL) salsa

Fruit Yogurt Dip

1 cup (250 mL) yogurt cheese (page 391) or thick unflavoured low-
   fat yogurt
2 tbsp (25 mL) brown sugar
1 tbsp (15 mL) rum or orange liqueur, optional
1 tsp (5 mL) vanilla

Peach Salsa

2 large ripe peaches, plums or mangoes, peeled and diced
6 strawberries, trimmed and diced, or 1/2 cup (125 mL) raspberries
2 tbsp (25 mL) orange marmalade
1 tbsp (15 mL) rum or orange liqueur, optional
1 tbsp (15 mL) chopped fresh mint, optional
Pinch ground cinnamon
Pinch ground allspice
Pinch ground ginger
Pinch ground nutmeg

1. To prepare dip, whisk together yogurt cheese, sugar, rum and vanilla. (Pureeing may make it watery.)
2. To prepare salsa, combine peaches, strawberries, marmalade, rum, mint, cinnamon, allspice, ginger and nutmeg. Mash lightly with a potato masher until mixture holds together.

PER TBSP (15 ML) (FRUIT DIP)	
Calories	22
Protein	2 g
Fat	trace
Saturates	trace
Cholesterol	2 mg
Carbohydrate	3 g
Fibre	0 g
Sodium	14 mg
Potassium	52 mg

PER TBSP (15 ML) (PEACH SALSA)	
Calories	8
Protein	trace
Fat	0 g
Saturates	0 g
Cholesterol	0 mg
Carbohydrate	2 g
Fibre	trace
Sodium	0 mg
Potassium	24 mg

CREAMY RICE PUDDING

When this recipe was first published, hundreds of people wrote to ask for it. They said that it was the long-lost family heirloom recipe they had always been looking for, that was just like the pudding their husband's mother made—one person even wrote that it had saved her marriage! But I guess that's what comfort food is all about.

Use a large heavy saucepan for this and don't worry—even with all the liquid, it will thicken! Although this pudding works with all kinds of rices, short-grain white rice gives you the creamiest texture. If you use brown rice, make sure you use short-grain, though the pudding may not be quite as soft and creamy. You will need about 1 1/2 cups/ 375 mL water, and it will take about 30 minutes to cook the rice in Step 1.

Makes 8 servings

1 cup (250 mL) water
1/2 cup (125 mL) rice (preferably short-grain)
1/3 cup (75 mL) granulated sugar
1 tsp (5 mL) cornstarch
Pinch salt
5 cups (1.25 L) milk
Pinch ground nutmeg
1/4 cup (50 mL) raisins
1 tsp (5 mL) vanilla
1 tbsp (15 mL) ground cinnamon

1. Bring water to a boil, covered, in a large saucepan. Add rice, cover and return to a boil, reduce heat and simmer gently for 15 minutes, or until water is absorbed.

2. In a bowl, combine sugar, cornstarch and salt. Whisk in 1 cup (250 mL) milk and stir until smooth.

3. Add sugar mixture, remaining milk, nutmeg and raisins to rice and combine well. Stirring, bring to a boil.

4. Reduce heat to barest simmer and cook, covered (but with lid slightly ajar to help prevent boiling over) for 1 to 1 1/2 hours, or until mixture is very creamy and tender. Stir occasionally and watch to make sure mixture does not boil over.

5. Stir in vanilla. Transfer pudding to a serving bowl and sprinkle with cinnamon. Serve hot or cold.

PER SERVING	
Calories	173
Protein	6 g
Fat	3 g
Saturates	2 g
Cholesterol	11 mg
Carbohydrate	31 g
Fibre	1 g
Sodium	77 mg
Potassium	288 mg
Good: Riboflavin; Calcium	

BAIN MARIE

A water bath, or bain marie, acts like a double boiler in the oven. It keeps the cooking temperature even for soft, creamy baked custards. I put the baking pan(s) of food in a larger roasting pan and place the whole thing in the preheated oven. I then pour boiling water from the kettle into the roasting pan until it comes halfway up the sides of the baking pan. (This is easier than the usual technique of transferring the roasting pan full of hot water to the oven.)

PER SERVING

Calories	301
Protein	8 g
Fat	3 g
Saturates	1 g
Cholesterol	83 mg
Carbohydrate	63 g
Fibre	1 g
Sodium	61 mg
Potassium	305 mg
Good: Riboflavin	

WILD RICE PUDDING BRÛLÉE

This is a modern version of rice pudding and a less rich (but no less delicious) version of crème brûlée. If you decide not to brûlée, omit the sugar on top and serve as is or with a berry sauce (page 450) or other fruit sauce. By far the best way to brûlée the top is to use a small blowtorch, but if you do not have one you can broil the pudding very carefully until the sugar melts and browns lightly.

Makes 8 servings

½ cup (125 mL) wild rice
½ cup (125 mL) short-grain brown or white rice
4 eggs
⅓ cup (75 mL) brown sugar
2 tbsp (25 mL) maple syrup
2 tsp (10 mL) vanilla
¼ tsp (1 mL) ground cinnamon
2 cups (500 mL) milk
⅓ cup (75 mL) raisins, dried cherries, cranberries or chopped
       dried apricots

Topping

½ cup (125 mL) brown or granulated sugar

1. Bring a large pot of water to a boil. Add wild rice and brown rice and simmer for 40 to 50 minutes, or until rice is very tender. Brown rice should be soft and wild rice should have opened up. Drain well.
2. In a large bowl, whisk eggs, sugar, maple syrup, vanilla, cinnamon and milk. Stir in rice and raisins.
3. Pour mixture into a lightly oiled 9-inch (2.5 L) square baking dish. Bake in a water bath in a preheated 350°F (180°C) oven for 45 to 50 minutes, or until custard is just set. Pudding can be served warm or cold.
4. Just before serving, sift brown sugar over top of pudding (or sprinkle with granulated sugar). Pat sugar down gently and broil just until sugar melts and browns lightly (or use a blowtorch to melt sugar).

RAY'S FAVOURITE APPLESAUCE

My husband loves applesauce. He used to be addicted to a commercial version but happily he is now addicted to mine. He prefers it mashed with a potato masher rather than pureed.

In cooking, I like to use apples that have a strong apple taste (e.g., Spy, Braeburn, Golden Delicious or Fuji); I usually find crisp eating apples too juicy and tart for cooking.

Makes 6 cups (1.5 L)
6 lb (3 kg) apples (10 to 12)
3/4 cup (175 mL) brown sugar
2 tsp (10 mL) ground cinnamon

1. Peel and core apples and cut into large chunks. Place chunks in a large pot or Dutch oven. Add sugar and cinnamon.
2. Cover and cook on low heat for 15 to 20 minutes, or until apples are almost tender. (Check every 5 minutes or so to make sure apples are not sticking or burning.) Mixture should be very juicy.
3. Uncover and cook gently until liquid evaporates and apples are very tender and thick. Mash with a potato masher.

PER 1/2 CUP (125 ML)	
Calories	154
Protein	0 g
Fat	1 g
Saturates	trace
Cholesterol	0 mg
Carbohydrate	40 g
Fibre	4 g
Sodium	5 mg
Potassium	249 mg

SUBSTITUTES FOR WINES AND LIQUEURS

You can almost always substitute another ingredient for an alcoholic product. Remember, though, that different substitutes are used for different reasons, and that a substitute will never give you exactly the same taste as the original.

- white wine: substitute chicken stock or vegetable juice in savoury dishes and white grape juice or other light-coloured fruit juices (apple, orange or pineapple) in desserts
- red wine: substitute beef stock or tomato juice in savoury recipes and red grape juice or other red fruit juices in desserts
- Marsala, Madeira or Port: substitute stock or vegetable juice in savory recipes and fruit juice concentrates in desserts
- fruit liqueurs: substitute fruit juice concentrate, citrus peel or pure vanilla extract
- Cognac, brandy or rum: substitute fruit juice concentrates or concentrated stocks in savoury recipes and fruit purees or concentrated juices in desserts

MARSALA

Marsala is a fortified wine that keeps well for a month or two after opening. Use the driest one you can find, although they are all quite sweet. You can also use other fortified wines in its place, such as Vin Santo, ice wine (if you can afford it!), Madeira, Port or even a liqueur.

PER 1/2 CUP (125 ML)	
Calories	375
Protein	3 g
Fat	trace
Saturates	0 g
Cholesterol	0 mg
Carbohydrate	90 g
Fibre	9 g
Sodium	28 mg
Potassium	1273 mg
Excellent: Iron	
Good: Vitamin A; Vitamin B6	

DRIED FRUIT COMPOTE

Prunes have always been popular in France and Italy, but they have never caught on here, perhaps because of their medicinal image. Now that they have been renamed dried plums, maybe people will finally realize how delicious they really are.

This compote can be served on its own or with yogurt cheese (page 391). It can also be served on top of plain cakes, in meringues or phyllo cups (page 63), rolled in crêpes or used as a base for a crisp or cobbler. The flavours are spicy and rich, and all kinds of dried fruits can be used.

Makes about 2 cups (500 mL)

1 cup (250 mL) dried plums (prunes)
1 cup (250 mL) dried apricots
1/4 cup (50 mL) dried cherries
1/4 cup (50 mL) chopped candied ginger
1 cup (250 mL) Marsala or orange juice
1/4 cup (50 mL) lemon juice
1/2 cup (125 mL) maple syrup, honey or brown sugar
1 cup (250 mL) water

1. In a saucepan, combine dried plums, apricots, cherries, ginger, Marsala, lemon juice, maple syrup and water. Bring to a boil.
2. Reduce heat and simmer gently, uncovered, for 10 to 15 minutes, or until fruit is tender. Serve warm or cold.

DEEP BERRY GLAZE

When I ordered berry yogurt for breakfast at the Kingfisher Spa in Courtenay on Vancouver Island, I was served a ramekin of silky smooth plain yogurt spread with a glistening purple-red sheet of an intensely berry-flavoured glaze. When I dipped my spoon in, the white and red mixtures melded together in artistic swirls and it was so delicious that I ordered it again at dinner for dessert. They told me the berry glaze was a commercial product, so I made up my own. I also eat it on ice cream, pancakes, French toast, angel food cake, meringues and with a spoon. It is a real winner.

Makes about 2 cups (500 mL)

4 cups (1 L) strawberries
1 1/2 cups (375 mL) blueberries
1 cup (250 mL) raspberries
1/4 cup (50 mL) cranberry or pomegranate juice
2 tbsp (25 mL) granulated sugar

1. In a saucepan, combine strawberries, blueberries, raspberries, cranberry juice and sugar. Bring to a boil. Reduce heat and simmer gently for 5 minutes.

2. Strain mixture through a food mill and return to saucepan. (If you do not have a food mill, puree in a blender or food processor and then strain through a sieve to remove seeds if you wish.) Bring to a boil again, reduce heat and cook gently for 10 minutes longer, or until mixture is thick but not sticky. You should have about 2 cups (500 mL).

3. Refrigerate or freeze glaze. It will keep in the refrigerator for at least 2 weeks.

PER TBSP (15 ML)	
Calories	16
Protein	0 g
Fat	1 g
Saturates	0 g
Cholesterol	0 mg
Carbohydrate	4 g
Fibre	1 g
Sodium	1 mg
Potassium	45 mg

BERRIES

Fresh berries should be handled gently and used quickly. Store them in flat, wide containers to avoid crushing and to prevent them from becoming mouldy. Overripe berries lose their pectin or thickening potential, so do not use them in jams. Instead, poach or bake them, or use them in sauces.

Freeze berries in a single layer on a waxed paper-lined baking sheet, freeze and then pack them into bags or containers. This way the berries stay separate and can be removed as you need them. Use frozen berries in cooked or pureed dishes. You can buy berries frozen in syrup, but I prefer the individual quick-frozen ones.

If you are adding frozen berries to baked goods such as muffins and cookies, add them in their frozen state.

PHYLLO CAKE WITH TOASTED ALMONDS AND CINNAMON

This beautiful Moroccan phyllo cake is a luscious, crispy dessert. You can make the phyllo layers ahead, but add the yogurt cheese just before serving so the phyllo remains crispy.

Makes 12 servings

3/4 cup (175 mL) whole almonds, toasted (page 464)
1/3 cup (75 mL) granulated sugar
1/4 cup (50 mL) unsalted butter, melted
2 tbsp (25 mL) water
8 sheets phyllo pastry (about 1/2 lb/250 g)
1/2 tsp (2 mL) ground cinnamon
2 cups (500 mL) yogurt cheese (page 391)
1/2 cup (125 mL) icing sugar, sifted
2 tsp (10 mL) vanilla

Garnish

1 tbsp (15 mL) icing sugar, sifted

1. Chop almonds and combine with granulated sugar in a small bowl. Combine melted butter and water in a second small bowl.
2. Unwrap phyllo sheets and cover with plastic wrap and a damp tea towel. Place one sheet of phyllo on a baking sheet, brush with butter and sprinkle with almonds and sugar. Place another sheet of phyllo on top, and top with butter and almond mixture. Repeat three times until you have four separate phyllo stacks on four baking sheets (or do this in batches). Bake stacks in a preheated 375°F (190°C) oven for 5 to 8 minutes, or until crisp and browned.
3. Add cinnamon to remaining almond and sugar mixture.
4. In a separate bowl, combine yogurt cheese, icing sugar and vanilla.
5. Arrange one phyllo stack on a large serving platter. Spread with one-third of the yogurt filling. Sprinkle with one-quarter of the almond/sugar/cinnamon mixture. Repeat until all ingredients are used and top with almond mixture.
6. To serve, cut cake into squares with a large chef's knife. Dust with sifted icing sugar before serving.

PER SERVING	
Calories	237
Protein	7 g
Fat	11 g
Saturates	4 g
Cholesterol	14 mg
Carbohydrate	29 g
Fibre	1 g
Sodium	150 mg
Potassium	277 mg
Good: Riboflavin; Vitamin B12; Calcium	

PHYLLO NESTS WITH CARAMELIZED WINTER FRUITS

This is a version of one of my recipes that was published in a *Bon Appétit* article featuring desserts created by North American cooking teachers. It looks amazing and tastes fabulous. You can serve the dessert warm or at room temperature.

Leftover fruit can be served on its own or on oatmeal for breakfast. It can also be served as a condiment with roast pork or duck, or it can be pureed or chopped finely and used as a jam. The fruit can also be served on top of frozen yogurt, angel food cake or in phyllo cups (page 63).

Makes 8 servings

Phyllo Nests

8 sheets phyllo pastry (about 1/2 lb/250 g)
1/4 cup (50 mL) unsalted butter, melted
1/4 cup (50 mL) water
1/3 cup (75 mL) dry breadcrumbs
1/4 cup (50 mL) granulated sugar

Caramelized Winter Fruits

1 cup (250 g) granulated sugar
2 apples, peeled, cored and sliced
2 pears, peeled, cored and sliced
1 1/2 cups (375 mL) dried fruits (combination of apricots, prunes,
        figs, cherries, cranberries, etc.)
2 tbsp (25 mL) diced candied ginger
1 cup (250 mL) Port, sherry, sweet wine, orange juice or apple juice
1 cup (250 mL) strong tea (regular or herbal)
2 tbsp (25 mL) lemon juice

Topping

1/2 cup (125 mL) yogurt cheese (page 391) or
        thick unflavoured low-fat yogurt
1 tsp (5 mL) vanilla, or 1 tbsp (15 mL) dark rum or orange liqueur

1. To prepare phyllo nests, line two baking sheets with parchment paper. Unwrap phyllo pastry and cover with plastic wrap (could be a clean plastic bag opened up) and a damp tea towel.

PER SERVING	
Calories	428
Protein	5 g
Fat	8 g
Saturates	4 g
Cholesterol	17 mg
Carbohydrate	84 g
Fibre	5 g
Sodium	175 mg
Potassium	477 mg
Good: Iron	

2. In a small bowl, combine melted butter and water. Combine bread-crumbs and sugar in a separate bowl.

3. Place one sheet of phyllo on work surface. Brush lightly with butter mixture. Dust with breadcrumbs and sugar. Fold in thirds length-wise. Brush again with butter mixture and sprinkle with bread-crumbs.

4. To form nests, hold about one quarter of phyllo in place on a baking sheet to make a base. Wrap remaining strip around base to form a nest. It can look ragged and uneven, so don't worry (or you can bake the first nest just to see what it looks like). Repeat until you have made eight nests.

5. Bake nests in a preheated 400°F (200°C) oven for 8 minutes. Reduce heat to 350°F (180°C) and bake for 5 to 8 minutes longer, or until pastry is crispy and browned. Cool.

6. Meanwhile, to make fruit mixture, place sugar in a large, deep, heavy skillet on medium-high heat. Cook, watching closely but not stirring, until sugar starts to brown.

7. Add apples and pears. Cook for 5 to 8 minutes, or until juicy. Do not worry if caramel becomes sticky—it will melt. Add dried fruits, ginger, Port, tea and lemon juice. Bring to a boil and simmer gently for 10 to 15 minutes, or until fruit is tender. Juices should be thick.

8. To make topping, in a small bowl, combine yogurt cheese and vanilla.

9. To serve, drizzle a little juice from fruit onto a dessert plate, top with phyllo nest and spoon filling into centre. Spoon a small amount of topping on each serving.

Phyllo Nests with Mango Ice

Fill phyllo nests with a scoop of mango ice cream. Dust with sifted icing sugar and garnish with fresh strawberries.

APPLE STRUDEL

For a nuttier oat taste, spread the rolled oats on a baking sheet and bake at 350°F (180°C) for 10 minutes before using. The apple mixture can also be used as a pie filling.

This can be made ahead and frozen (for up to one month) either baked or unbaked. To reheat the frozen baked strudel, bake at 375°F (190°C) for 40 to 45 minutes. To bake the frozen unbaked strudel, double the baking time (if the top becomes too brown, cover with foil and reduce the heat to 350°F/180°C).

Serve this with sweetened yogurt cheese (page 391), vanilla ice cream or frozen yogurt.

Makes 8 to 10 servings

4 apples, peeled, cored and chopped
1 cup (250 mL) large-flake rolled oats, toasted
½ cup (125 mL) brown sugar
¼ cup (50 mL) chopped candied ginger or dried cranberries
1 tsp (5 mL) ground cinnamon
Pinch ground nutmeg
Pinch ground allspice
2 tbsp (25 mL) unsalted butter, melted
3 tbsp (45 mL) water
⅓ cup (75 mL) dry breadcrumbs
2 tbsp (25 mL) finely chopped toasted walnuts
2 tbsp (25 mL) granulated sugar
6 sheets phyllo pastry

1. In a large bowl, combine apples, rolled oats, brown sugar, ginger, cinnamon, nutmeg and allspice.
2. In a small bowl, combine melted butter and water. In a separate bowl, combine breadcrumbs, nuts and granulated sugar.
3. Arrange a sheet of parchment paper on a large, heavy baking sheet. Place one sheet of phyllo on parchment. (Keep remaining phyllo covered with plastic wrap and a damp tea towel.) Brush with butter/water mixture and sprinkle with crumbs. Repeat until all 6 sheets are stacked.
4. Spoon apple mixture along long side of pastry. Roll up strudel. Cut shallow diagonal slices through top layer so that cutting and serving will be easier after strudel is baked. Brush top with any extra butter.
5. Bake in a preheated 375°F (190°C) oven for 40 to 45 minutes, or until apples are very tender and pastry is brown and flaky.

APPLES

Everyone has their favourite eating apple, but when you cook, you want an apple with a strong apple taste (rather than an apple that is just crisp and tart) that keeps its shape when baked. McIntosh, for example, are great for eating but tend to turn into mush when cooked, whereas Golden Delicious, which are not my favourite for eating (because they lack crispness), are great for cooking. I also like to cook with Spy, Empire, Ida Red, Fuji, Braeburn and Royal Gala apples.

PER SERVING

Calories	273
Protein	4 g
Fat	6 g
Saturates	2 g
Cholesterol	8 mg
Carbohydrate	52 g
Fibre	3 g
Sodium	131 mg
Potassium	354 mg

Good: Thiamine; Iron

APPLE PHYLLO PIE

This was one of the most popular recipes in *Simply HeartSmart*—
the pie looks and tastes sensational, and it is perfect for anyone who
has a fear of traditional pastry. If you want to make sure the bottom
of the pie is crisp (though it doesn't bother me if it isn't), you can
place a pizza stone or baking sheet in the oven while it is preheating
and place the pie pan on the hot sheet before baking.

Makes 10 to 12 servings

6 apples (about 3 lb/1.5 kg), peeled, cored and sliced
1/2 cup (125 mL) brown sugar
1/4 cup (50 mL) all-purpose flour
1/2 tsp (2 mL) ground cinnamon
Pinch ground nutmeg
1/4 cup (50 mL) dry breadcrumbs
2 tbsp (25 mL) granulated sugar
10 sheets phyllo pastry
1/3 cup (75 mL) soft non-hydrogenated margarine or unsalted
    butter, melted
2 tbsp (25 mL) icing sugar, sifted

1. Combine apples, brown sugar, flour, cinnamon and nutmeg.
2. In a small bowl, combine breadcrumbs and granulated sugar.
3. Working with one sheet of phyllo at a time (keep remaining sheets
covered with plastic wrap and a damp tea towel), brush pastry lightly
with melted margarine and dust with breadcrumb mixture. Fold
pastry in half lengthwise and brush again. Place pastry in a 10-inch
(3 L) springform pan with one short end in centre of pan and other
end hanging over edge. Sprinkle with breadcrumb mixture.
4. Repeat with remaining sheets of phyllo, overlapping each slightly
when arranging in pan. Leave a lot of pastry hanging over edge.
Bottom of pan should be covered.
5. Spoon apple mixture into pastry. Fold pastry back over filling so
filling is completely covered and pastry is somewhat ragged looking.
Brush top of pie with remaining margarine.
6. Bake in a preheated 400°F (200°C) oven for 15 minutes. Reduce
heat to 350°F (180°C) and bake for 50 to 55 minutes longer, or until
apples are tender when pie is pierced with a sharp knife. Cool for at
least 15 minutes before removing from pan. Dust with icing sugar
before serving.

PER SERVING	
Calories	257
Protein	3 g
Fat	7 g
Saturates	1 g
Cholesterol	0 mg
Carbohydrate	47 g
Fibre	3 g
Sodium	267 mg
Potassium	186 mg

PAVLOVA ROULADE WITH PASSIONFRUIT FILLING

It is hard to believe you can roll up a meringue, but trust me—it works. Tart, juicy passionfruit tastes wonderful in this recipe, but if you cannot find fresh passionfruit, use kiwi. In either case, cut the fruit in half and scoop the pulp over the filling. Sometimes you can find passionfruit pulp frozen or in cans (in South Africa it is called grenadilla); use about 1/4 cup (50 mL).

Makes 10 servings

5 egg whites
3/4 cup (175 mL) granulated sugar
1 tbsp (15 mL) white vinegar
1 tsp (5 mL) vanilla
2 tbsp (25 mL) cornstarch
1 tbsp (15 mL) sifted icing sugar
1 cup (250 mL) yogurt cheese (page 391)
1/4 cup (50 mL) icing sugar
2 passionfruit or kiwi
2 cups (500 mL) fresh strawberries, sliced
Sprigs of fresh mint

1. In a large stainless-steel or glass bowl, beat egg whites until light. Slowly add granulated sugar and continue to beat until whites are stiff and shiny. Beat in vinegar and vanilla. Sift cornstarch on top of egg whites and fold in.

2. Spread meringue over a 15- x 10-inch (40 x 25 cm) baking sheet lined with parchment paper. Bake in a preheated 325°F (160°C) oven for 10 to 12 minutes, or until puffed and lightly browned. Cool. Dust top with 1 tbsp (15 mL) icing sugar. Run a knife around edge to prevent sticking and then invert onto another piece of parchment.

3. To prepare filling, combine yogurt cheese and 1/4 cup (50 mL) icing sugar. Spread over meringue.

4. Cut passionfruit in half and scoop pulp over yogurt cheese. Roll cake up lengthwise using parchment paper as a guide.

5. Refrigerate roulade until ready to serve. Cut roll into serving pieces and garnish with strawberries and sprigs of mint.

PER SERVING	
Calories	129
Protein	5 g
Fat	1 g
Saturates	trace
Cholesterol	2 mg
Carbohydrate	27 g
Fibre	1 g
Sodium	63 mg
Potassium	200 mg
Good: Vitamin B12; Vitamin C	

PAVLOVA WITH BERRIES AND FLOWERS

This dessert is too beautiful to believe and, as a bonus, it is low in fat. The trick to making a great pavlova is beating the egg whites properly, adding vinegar to the meringue at the last moment and baking it just to the point where the meringue is crunchy on the outside and marshmallowy on the inside.

If berries are not in season, try using mangoes, passionfruit, kiwi, bananas or caramelized apples or pears (page 433). You can make individual pavlovas or shape the meringue into baskets. You can also use softened frozen yogurt or sorbet as a topping instead of yogurt cheese, but be sure to serve the dessert right away.

Makes 8 servings
4 egg whites
1 cup (250 mL) granulated sugar
2 tsp (10 mL) white vinegar
1 ½ cups (375 mL) yogurt cheese (page 391)
2 tbsp (25 mL) honey or icing sugar
1 tsp (5 mL) vanilla
4 cups (1 L) fresh berries
Fresh edible flowers

PER SERVING	
Calories	189
Protein	7 g
Fat	2 g
Saturates	1 g
Cholesterol	5 mg
Carbohydrate	39 g
Fibre	2 g
Sodium	68 mg
Potassium	291 mg

Excellent: Vitamin C
Good: Riboflavin; Vitamin B12

1. In a large stainless-steel or glass bowl, beat egg whites until light.
2. Gradually add granulated sugar to egg whites and continue to beat until firm. Beat in vinegar.
3. Outline a 12-inch (30 cm) circle on a piece of parchment paper and place on a baking sheet. Spoon egg whites inside circle shape and spread in loose waves. Bake in a preheated 275°F (135°C) oven for 2 hours. Remove from oven and cool. Freeze if not using immediately.
4. Meanwhile, in a small bowl, combine yogurt cheese, honey and vanilla.
5. Just before serving, spoon yogurt mixture over meringue. Top with berries and scatter flowers over top. Serve immediately.

ALMOND ANGEL FOOD CAKE WITH CINNAMON APRICOTS

Angel food cake is a mainstay of healthy eaters who love dessert. It is old-fashioned and comforting but low in fat and completely natural. Warming the egg whites gives the cake a fluffy texture and allows you to use fewer egg whites. If you don't have a heavy-duty mixer, make friends with someone who has one, or just use a hand mixer.

You can easily substitute other nuts for the almonds, or omit the nuts entirely. The cake can be served with winter fruits (page 442) instead of the apricots, and the apricots on their own can be served on top of sorbets, in phyllo cups (page 63) or with yogurt.

Makes 12 to 16 servings
1 cup (250 mL) cake and pastry flour
1 1/2 cups (375 mL) granulated sugar, divided
1/4 cup (50 mL) finely chopped toasted almonds
1 1/2 cups (375 mL) egg whites (about 12)
1 tsp (5 mL) cream of tartar
Pinch salt
1 tsp (5 mL) vanilla
1/2 tsp (2 mL) almond extract
1 tsp (5 mL) grated lemon peel

Cinnamon Apricots
2 cups (500 mL) water
2/3 cup (150 mL) honey or granulated sugar
2 cinnamon sticks, broken up
1/4 cup (50 mL) Amaretto, orange liqueur or
      orange juice concentrate
1 1/2 cups (375 mL) dried apricots (about 40)
1 tbsp (15 mL) lemon juice

Yogurt Drizzle, optional
1/2 cup (125 mL) yogurt cheese (page 391) or
      thick unflavoured low-fat yogurt
1 tbsp (15 mL) honey
1 tbsp (15 mL) Amaretto, orange liqueur or orange juice concentrate

PER SERVING	
Calories	271
Protein	5 g
Fat	2 g
Saturates	trace
Cholesterol	0 mg
Carbohydrate	61 g
Fibre	2 g
Sodium	55 mg
Potassium	309 mg

1. Sift flour and $3/4$ cup (175 mL) sugar into a large bowl. Stir in almonds.

2. In large bowl of an electric mixer, combine egg whites, cream of tartar and salt. In a medium saucepan, heat a few cups of water to a simmer and place bowl of egg whites over water, stirring, until egg whites feel a little warm. This takes 3 to 5 minutes. Immediately start beating egg whites with mixer until frothy and opaque. Gradually beat in remaining $3/4$ cup (175 mL) sugar. Beat until soft peaks form. Beat in vanilla and almond extract.

3. Gently fold flour mixture into egg whites in three additions. Fold in lemon peel. Gently spoon batter into a 10-inch (4 L) tube pan, preferably one with a removable bottom.

4. Bake in a preheated 350°F (180°C) oven for 40 to 45 minutes, or until a cake tester comes out clean and dry and top of cake springs back when gently touched. Turn cake upside-down on a rack and cool for 1 hour. To remove cake from pan, use a thin knife to loosen sides. Use a spatula or knife to loosen bottom (if pan has a removable bottom, remove sides and then loosen bottom with a knife).

5. Meanwhile, to prepare apricots, in a large saucepan, combine water, honey and cinnamon and bring to a boil. Add liqueur and cook for 5 minutes. Add apricots and cook for 15 to 20 minutes, or until soft and tender. Add lemon juice and cook for 1 minute longer. Remove cinnamon sticks or warn guests not to eat them (they do make a great-looking garnish). If syrup becomes too thick when it cools, just add a little hot water.

6. To prepare drizzle, combine yogurt cheese, honey and Amaretto in a small bowl. If mixture is too thick to drizzle, thin with a little milk. (You can put yogurt in a squeeze bottle to drizzle or just use a spoon.) Serve cake with apricots, juices and yogurt drizzle.

Chocolate Chip Angel Food Cake

Add $1/2$ cup (125 mL) chopped milk chocolate or dark chocolate to batter with almonds. Omit lemon peel.

ANNA'S ANGEL FOOD CAKE WITH BERRY BERRY SAUCE

This is my daughter's very favourite cake. She not only loves to eat it, she even loves to make it.

This cake freezes well, and you can serve it with the berry sauce or with plain fresh fruit, sweetened yogurt cheese (page 391) or sorbet. You should use a traditional tube or angel food cake pan, and remember that the trick to making a high, light cake is to beat the egg whites properly.

The berry sauce makes a fabulous dessert as well as a sauce—just use more berries. You can serve it with meringues or in bowls with a bit of sweetened yogurt cheese on top. I often use frozen raspberries for pureeing, as fresh ones are so precious that I'd rather eat them whole. A food mill (a relatively inexpensive old-fashioned gadget) will puree the raspberries and strain out the seeds at the same time. If you puree the raspberries in a blender or food processor, you will have to strain the mixture afterwards if you want to remove the seeds.

If you use unsweetened frozen berries, you may want to add a little sugar to the sauce.

Makes 12 to 16 servings

1 1/2 cups (375 mL) granulated sugar, divided
1 cup (250 mL) cake and pastry flour
1 1/2 cups (375 mL) egg whites (about 12)
1 tsp (5 mL) cream of tartar
Pinch salt
1 tbsp (15 mL) lemon juice or orange juice concentrate
1 tsp (5 mL) vanilla
1 tsp (5 mL) grated lemon or orange peel

Berry Berry Sauce

1 10-oz (300 g) package frozen raspberries
2 tbsp (25 mL) orange or raspberry liqueur, optional
2 cups (500 mL) fresh strawberries, trimmed and quartered
1 cup (250 mL) fresh raspberries
1 cup (250 mL) fresh blueberries

FOOD MILL
The old-fashioned food mill is one of my favourite pieces of kitchen equipment. It's the original food processor. I use it when I want to strain and puree at the same time (tomato sauce, applesauce or raspberry puree), or for mashing potatoes without over-processing.

PER SERVING

Calories	182
Protein	5 g
Fat	trace
Saturates	0 g
Cholesterol	0 mg
Carbohydrate	41 g
Fibre	4 g
Sodium	50 mg
Potassium	221 mg

Good: Vitamin C

1. Sift 1/2 cup (125 mL) sugar with flour.

2. In large bowl of electric mixer, combine egg whites, cream of tartar, salt and lemon juice.

3. In a medium saucepan, heat a few cups of water and place bowl of egg whites over water. Stir egg whites until they feel a little warm. This should take 3 to 5 minutes. Immediately start beating egg whites with electric mixer. Slowly add remaining 1 cup (250 mL) sugar, beating constantly. Egg whites should be very light and stiff. Beat in vanilla and lemon peel.

4. Gently fold in flour mixture in three additions. Do not overfold so as not to deflate egg whites.

5. Spoon or pour batter very gently into a 10-inch (4 L) tube pan. Bake cake in a preheated 350°F (180°C) oven for 40 to 45 minutes, or until a cake tester comes out clean and dry and top of cake springs back when lightly touched.

6. Meanwhile, to prepare sauce, defrost frozen raspberries. If they come in a syrup, strain them. Reserve juices and puree berries through a food mill or in a blender or food processor. Add enough reserved juices to make a medium-thick sauce. Add liqueur and gently stir in fresh strawberries, raspberries and blueberries.

7. Invert cake pan on rack and cool for 1 hour. To remove cake from pan, use a long, thin knife to loosen edges. If pan has a removable bottom, remove sides and then loosen bottom with a knife. If you are using a one-piece pan, use a spatula or knife to loosen bottom. Do not worry if cake seems crushed—it usually springs back into shape. Serve cake with berry sauce.

Cappuccino Angel Food Cake

Add 1 1/2 tbsp (20 mL) crushed instant coffee powder and 1/4 tsp (1 mL) ground cinnamon to flour mixture. Add 1/4 tsp (1 mL) almond extract to beaten egg whites with vanilla.

Angel Food Cake with Tiramisu Cream

Cut baked cake in half horizontally. Spread tiramisu cream (page 433) over bottom half of cake. Replace top half of cake and spread cream over top. Dust with sifted icing sugar.

CHOCOLATE ANGEL FOOD CAKE WITH CHOCOLATE SAUCE

This cake has a light but very satisfying chocolate flavour. Serve it with or without the sauce. It can also be served with raspberry sauce. For a mocha-flavoured cake, add 1 tbsp (15 mL) crushed instant coffee powder to the flour mixture.

Makes 12 to 16 servings

1 ³/₄ cups (425 mL) granulated sugar, divided
1 cup (250 mL) cake and pastry flour
¹/₃ cup (75 mL) cocoa
1 ¹/₂ cups (375 mL) egg whites (about 12)
1 tsp (5 mL) cream of tartar
Pinch salt
1 tsp (5 mL) vanilla

Chocolate Sauce

6 oz (175 g) bittersweet or semisweet chocolate, chopped
2 tbsp (25 mL) cocoa
3 tbsp (45 mL) corn syrup
¹/₂ cup (125 mL) water
1 tsp (5 mL) vanilla

1. Sift ³/₄ cup (175 mL) sugar with flour and cocoa.
2. Place egg whites in large bowl of electric mixer with cream of tartar and salt. In a medium saucepan, heat a few cups of water and place bowl of egg whites over water. Stir egg whites for 3 to 5 minutes, or until they feel just a little warm. Immediately start beating egg whites with mixer. Gradually beat in remaining 1 cup (250 mL) sugar. Beat in vanilla.
3. Fold reserved flour mixture into egg whites in three additions. Do not overfold, but make sure there are no pockets of flour in batter.
4. Gently turn batter into a 10-inch (4 L) tube pan. Bake in a preheated 350°F (180°C) oven for 40 to 45 minutes, or until a cake tester comes out clean.
5. Meanwhile, to prepare chocolate sauce, combine chocolate, cocoa, corn syrup and water in a saucepan on medium heat and cook gently, stirring, until smooth. Remove from heat and stir in vanilla. Cool.
6. Invert cake pan on rack and allow to cool for 1 hour. Remove gently from pan by running a knife around inside edge of pan and centre tube. Slice cake and serve drizzled with sauce.

RASPBERRY SAUCE

Serve this with cakes, meringues, sorbet or ice cream.

Defrost two 10-oz (300 g) packages frozen raspberries and drain, reserving juices. Puree with 2 tbsp (25 mL) granulated sugar. Strain out seeds if you wish (this is a good time to use a food mill). Stir in 2 tbsp (25 mL) orange or raspberry liqueur (or 1 tbsp/15 mL frozen orange juice concentrate) and enough reserved juice to make a sauce. (If you use sweetened frozen berries, omit the sugar and/or add a little lemon juice.)

Makes about 2 cups (500 mL).

PER SERVING

Calories	255
Protein	6 g
Fat	7 g
Saturates	4 g
Cholesterol	0 mg
Carbohydrate	49 g
Fibre	2 g
Sodium	80 mg
Potassium	1 mg

RASPBERRY UPSIDE-DOWN CAKE

You can make upside-down cakes with many different fruits, but fresh berries say summer best. Use raspberries, blackberries, blueberries or a combination. In winter, use cranberries. The little bit of butter in the topping goes a long way.

Makes 8 servings

2 tbsp (25 mL) unsalted butter
2/3 cup (150 mL) brown sugar
2 cups (500 mL) fresh raspberries
1/3 cup (75 mL) vegetable oil
1 cup (175 mL) granulated sugar
1 egg
2 egg whites
1 tbsp (15 mL) grated orange peel
1 tsp (5 mL) vanilla
1 1/2 cups (375 mL) all-purpose flour
1 1/2 tsp (7 mL) baking powder
1/2 tsp (2 mL) baking soda
1 cup (250 mL) buttermilk or unflavoured low-fat yogurt

PER SERVING	
Calories	373
Protein	5 g
Fat	13 g
Saturates	3 g
Cholesterol	35 mg
Carbohydrate	60 g
Fibre	2 g
Sodium	174 mg
Potassium	188 mg
Good: Folate	

1. Place butter in an 8-inch (1.5 L) baking dish and place in a preheated 350°F (180°C) oven for 3 to 5 minutes, or until melted. Sprinkle butter with brown sugar and pat down. Sprinkle berries over sugar.
2. In a large bowl, beat together oil, granulated sugar, egg, egg whites, orange peel and vanilla.
3. In a separate bowl, combine flour, baking powder and baking soda.
4. Stir flour mixture into egg mixture alternately with buttermilk just until combined.
5. Spoon batter over berries and spread evenly. Bake for 35 to 40 minutes, or until cake springs back when lightly touched in centre. Cool on a wire rack for 5 minutes. Invert onto a serving plate.

FROZEN LEMON MERINGUE CAKE

This looks spectacular garnished with frozen grapes. When frozen, the grapes take on a frosted look. They have about 15 minutes of fame and then start to defrost, so take them out of the freezer just before serving.

Makes 10 to 12 servings

1 1/2 cups (375 mL) granulated sugar, divided
2 tbsp (25 mL) cornstarch
6 egg whites
1/4 tsp (1 mL) cream of tartar
1 tsp (5 mL) vanilla

Lemon Filling

1/3 cup (75 mL) cornstarch
1 1/4 cups (300 mL) granulated sugar
2 eggs
1 cup (250 mL) lemon juice
2/3 cup (150 mL) orange juice
2 tbsp (25 mL) grated lemon peel
2 cups (500 mL) light ricotta cheese, pureed

Garnish

Sifted icing sugar

1. Trace four 8-inch (20 cm) circles on two baking sheets lined with parchment paper.
2. Prepare meringues by combining 3/4 cup (175 mL) sugar and cornstarch in a small bowl. Reserve.
3. Combine egg whites and cream of tartar in a large stainless-steel or glass bowl. With an electric mixer, whip egg whites until they start to turn opaque. Beat in remaining 3/4 cup (175 mL) sugar until white, opaque and firm. Beat in vanilla. Fold in cornstarch/sugar mixture.
4. Spoon or pipe meringue onto parchment paper to fill circles. Smooth tops and bake in a preheated 300°F (150°C) oven for 1 hour, or until dry. Cool completely.
5. Meanwhile, to prepare filling, in a large saucepan, combine cornstarch and sugar. Whisk in eggs, lemon juice, orange juice and lemon peel. Bring to a boil and cook gently, stirring, until thick. Transfer to a large bowl and cool. (If you put filling over a large bowl filled with

PER SERVING	
Calories	330
Protein	9 g
Fat	4 g
Saturates	2 g
Cholesterol	58 mg
Carbohydrate	67 g
Fibre	trace
Sodium	108 mg
Potassium	166 mg
Good: Vitamin B12	

ice and water, it will chill more quickly.) Fold in pureed ricotta.

6. To assemble, place one meringue in a 9-inch (23 cm) springform pan. Trim it to fit if necessary (meringues can expand when baked). Spread with one-third of the filling. Place another meringue on top, spread with another one-third of the filling. Top with third meringue and spread with the remaining filling. Take the fourth meringue, break it into pieces and sprinkle over top. Freeze for at least a few hours.

7. Remove cake from springform and place on a serving platter about 30 minutes before serving. Dust with icing sugar.

BEATING EGG WHITES

- To beat egg whites properly, the bowl and the beaters must be absolutely clean and grease free (even a little oil or egg yolk in the bowl will stop the whites from reaching their greatest volume when beaten). When you separate the eggs, make sure no egg yolk gets into the whites. If there is a bit of yolk in the whites, try scooping it out using half an eggshell; it seems to work like a magnet to attract the yolk.

- Separate each egg in a clean small bowl, adding yolks to yolks and whites to whites in larger bowls.

- Although you do not need a copper bowl for beating egg whites (I seldom use one), copper works well because it reacts with the beater to stabilize the whites. Clean the inside of the bowl with a little vinegar or lemon juice and salt just before you use it.

- If you do not have a copper bowl, use glass or stainless steel, as plastic bowls can trap grease. Adding $1/4$ tsp (1 mL) cream of tartar or 1 tsp (5 mL) lemon juice for every four egg whites will also help stabilize the whites. If you are adding sugar, start to beat it in slowly just after the egg whites turn opaque.

- Bring egg whites to room temperature before beating.

- Do not overbeat egg whites. They should be light and fluffy but not dry.

- When you are folding beaten egg whites into a heavier mixture, always stir about one-quarter of the whites into the base first, to lighten it. Then gently fold in the remaining whites. It doesn't matter whether you fold the whites into the base or the base into the whites; just use the larger bowl.

- Egg whites are also sold in cartons in the dairy section of some supermarkets and specialty stores. I don't think they beat up as well as fresh egg whites but because they are pasteurized, they are good for dishes that contain uncooked egg whites (e.g., mousses).

CARROT TUBE CAKE

Carrot cake is always a favourite. The batter can also be baked in layers or a single layer (use two 8-inch/20 cm round cake pans or one 10-inch/25 cm cake pan) and bake for 25 to 30 minutes. Add a cream cheese frosting, dust with icing sugar or top with Ricotta Drizzle.

Makes 16 servings

4 eggs
1 1/2 cups (375 mL) brown sugar
2/3 cup (150 mL) vegetable oil
1 cup (250 mL) all-purpose flour
1 cup (250 mL) whole wheat flour
2 tsp (10 mL) baking powder
1/2 tsp (2 mL) baking soda
1 tsp (5 mL) ground cinnamon
1/4 tsp (1 mL) ground nutmeg
Pinch salt
2 cups (500 mL) finely grated carrots (about 4), packed
3/4 cup (175 mL) drained crushed pineapple
3/4 cup (175 mL) raisins or chopped nuts

1. In a large bowl, beat eggs and sugar with an electric mixer until very light. Beat in oil.
2. In a separate large bowl, combine or sift flours with baking powder, baking soda, cinnamon, nutmeg and salt. Stir flour mixture into egg mixture just until combined. Stir in carrots, pineapple and raisins.
3. Spoon batter into a 10-inch (4 L) tube pan or bundt pan that has been lightly oiled or sprayed with non-stick cooking spray. Bake in a preheated 350°F (180°C) oven for 45 to 50 minutes, or until a cake tester comes out clean. Cool for 10 minutes. Remove from pan.

RICOTTA DRIZZLE
Combine 1/4 lb (125 g) light ricotta cheese (about 1/2 cup/125 mL) with 3 cups (750 mL) sifted icing sugar and 1 tsp (5 mL) vanilla. Blend until smooth.
Makes about 2 cups (500 mL).

CREAM CHEESE FROSTING
Beat 1/4 lb (125 g) light cream cheese with about 2 1/2 cups (625 mL) sifted icing sugar, 1 tsp (5 mL) vanilla and 1 tbsp (15 mL) grated orange peel. Add more icing sugar if necessary until you have a spreadable consistency.
Makes about 1 cup (250 mL).

PER SERVING	
Calories	276
Protein	4 g
Fat	12 g
Saturates	1 g
Cholesterol	47 mg
Carbohydrate	41 g
Fibre	2 g
Sodium	103 mg
Potassium	221 mg
Excellent: Vitamin A	

QUICK APPLE CAKE

Although some cakes are time-consuming to make, this one is quick enough for a last-minute dessert. It is a dense cake with great flavour. Make it first, and by the time you have prepared the rest of the meal and eaten, the cake will be ready to serve.

Makes 12 pieces

1 egg
1/2 cup (125 mL) granulated sugar
1/3 cup (75 mL) vegetable oil
3 tbsp (45 mL) orange juice or apple juice
1 tsp (5 mL) vanilla
3/4 cup (175 mL) all-purpose flour
1 tsp (5 mL) baking powder
Pinch salt
1/3 cup (75 mL) brown sugar
1 tsp (5 mL) ground cinnamon
3 apples, peeled and sliced

PER PIECE	
Calories	165
Protein	1 g
Fat	7 g
Saturates	1 g
Cholesterol	18 mg
Carbohydrate	26 g
Fibre	1 g
Sodium	29 mg
Potassium	76 mg

1. In a large bowl, beat together egg and granulated sugar until thick and light. Beat in oil, juice and vanilla.

2. In a separate bowl, combine flour, baking powder and salt. Stir into egg mixture and combine just until blended.

3. Combine brown sugar and cinnamon.

4. Arrange apples in bottom of a lightly oiled 8-inch (2 L) square baking dish. Sprinkle with half the brown sugar mixture. Smooth batter on top. Sprinkle with remaining brown sugar mixture.

5. Bake in a preheated 350°F (180°C) oven for 35 to 40 minutes, or until cake slightly comes away from sides of pan. Cool for 10 minutes before serving from the pan.

OLD-FASHIONED CHEESECAKE

People still love cheesecake, but this version is less guilt-inducing than most. It is plain, but I love it that way the best.

Makes 24 squares

Crust

1 cup (250 mL) Graham cracker crumbs
¼ tsp (1 mL) ground cinnamon
¼ cup (50 mL) soft non-hydrogenated margarine or
    unsalted butter, melted

Filling

12 oz (375 g) light cream cheese
12 oz (375 g) light ricotta cheese
1 cup (250 mL) granulated sugar
3 eggs
½ cup (125 mL) low-fat sour cream
2 tbsp (25 mL) all-purpose flour
1 tsp (5 mL) vanilla

Topping

1 cup (250 mL) low-fat sour cream
2 tbsp (2 mL) granulated sugar
½ tsp (2 mL) vanilla
12 fresh strawberries, halved

1. To prepare crust, combine Graham crumbs, cinnamon and melted margarine. Press into a 12- x 8-inch (3 L) baking dish.

2. To prepare filling, in a large bowl, beat cream cheese, ricotta and sugar until light. Beat in eggs, sour cream, flour and vanilla until smooth. Pour over crust. Bake in a preheated 350°F (180°C) oven for 30 to 35 minutes, or until set.

3. Meanwhile, to prepare topping, combine sour cream, sugar and vanilla. Spread over hot cake and return to oven for 5 minutes. Cool completely.

4. Refrigerate cake until firm. Cut into squares and garnish with strawberry halves.

PER SQUARE	
Calories	143
Protein	6 g
Fat	6 g
Saturates	2 g
Cholesterol	32 mg
Carbohydrate	16 g
Fibre	trace
Sodium	180 mg
Potassium	45 mg

STRAWBERRY MERINGUE SHORTCAKES

Perfect meringues are supposed to be crisp and crunchy, but this dish actually works better when the meringues are slightly chewy. In other words, whichever way they turn out is great.

If you leave the meringues in the oven overnight, put a sign on the oven door to remind you that they're in there!

Makes 6 servings

Meringues

3 egg whites
1/4 tsp (1 mL) cream of tartar
1/2 cup (125 mL) granulated sugar
1/2 tsp (2 mL) vanilla

Filling

2 cups (500 mL) sliced strawberries
3 tbsp (45 mL) granulated sugar, divided
1 1/2 cups (375 mL) yogurt cheese (page 391) or thick unflavoured
        low-fat yogurt
1 tbsp (15 mL) orange liqueur or rum, optional

Garnish

2 tbsp (25 mL) sifted icing sugar
6 whole fresh strawberries
6 sprigs fresh mint

PER SERVING	
Calories	185
Protein	8 g
Fat	2 g
Saturates	1 g
Cholesterol	6 mg
Carbohydrate	35 g
Fibre	1 g
Sodium	80 mg
Potassium	318 mg

Excellent: Vitamin C; Vitamin B12
Good: Riboflavin; Calcium

1. To prepare meringues, in a large bowl, beat egg whites and cream of tartar until light. Gradually beat in 1/2 cup (125 mL) granulated sugar until stiff peaks form. Beat in vanilla.

2. Trace 12 3-inch (7.5 cm) circles on parchment-lined baking sheets. Spread meringue inside circles. Using back of a wet spoon, make an indentation in centre of each meringue.

3. Place meringues in a preheated 375°F (190°C) oven and turn off heat immediately. Allow to rest in oven for 6 hours or overnight.

4. To prepare filling, combine sliced berries with 1 tbsp (15 mL) granulated sugar and allow to marinate for 30 to 60 minutes.

5. Just before serving, combine yogurt cheese, remaining 2 tbsp (25 mL) sugar and liqueur.

6. Set one meringue on each serving plate. Top with yogurt cheese and sliced berries. Place remaining meringues on top and dust with icing sugar. Garnish with whole berries and fresh mint. Serve immediately.

NICK MALGIERI'S FUDGE BROWNIES

Nick Malgieri, author of *Chocolate* and many other wonderful dessert cookbooks, has fabulous recipes. Although I have been known to say that if you want a brownie, just eat half of the real thing rather than a bunch of low-fat ones, these are truly satisfying. They freeze very well.

Makes 16 squares

1 cup (250 mL) all-purpose flour
1/2 cup (125 mL) cocoa
1 tsp (5 mL) baking powder
1/2 tsp (2 mL) salt
2 tbsp (25 mL) unsalted butter, at room temperature
1 1/2 cups (375 mL) granulated sugar
2 egg whites
1/2 cup (125 mL) unsweetened applesauce
1 tsp (5 mL) vanilla

1. Sift flour, cocoa, baking powder and salt into a bowl.
2. In a large bowl, beat together butter and sugar. Whisk in egg whites, applesauce and vanilla.
3. Stir flour mixture into butter/applesauce mixture just until combined.
4. Line bottom of an 8-inch (2 L) square baking pan with parchment paper. Pour batter into pan. Bake in a preheated 350°F (180°C) oven for 35 to 40 minutes, or until firm. Cool in pan. Cut into squares.

Fudge Brownies with Dried Cherries
Add 1/2 cup (125 mL) dried cherries to batter.

COCOA

Cocoa is unsweetened powdered chocolate with much of the cocoa butter removed. While it can't be substituted for regular chocolate in all cases, in some recipes it can add a deep, rich chocolate flavour, with only a small amount of fat.

PER SQUARE	
Calories	129
Protein	2 g
Fat	2 g
Saturates	1 g
Cholesterol	4 mg
Carbohydrate	27 g
Fibre	1 g
Sodium	116 mg
Potassium	40 mg

DATE SQUARES

Wonderful old-fashioned treats like these are making a big comeback. They freeze perfectly, so don't think you have to eat them all at once!

Makes 25 squares
Filling
1 lb (500 g) dates
¼ cup (50 mL) granulated sugar
1½ cups (375 mL) water
1 tbsp (15 mL) lemon juice

Base and Topping
½ cup (125 mL) soft non-hydrogenated margarine or
     unsalted butter
¾ cup (175 mL) brown sugar
3 tbsp (45 mL) granulated sugar
1 cup (250 mL) all-purpose flour
1 cup (250 mL) large-flake rolled oats
¼ tsp (1 mL) baking soda

PER SQUARE	
Calories	151
Protein	1 g
Fat	4 g
Saturates	1 g
Cholesterol	0 mg
Carbohydrate	29 g
Fibre	2 g
Sodium	63 mg
Potassium	160 mg

1. Chop dates (the easiest way is to cut them up with kitchen scissors). You should have about 3 cups (750 mL).

2. To prepare filling, in a saucepan, combine dates, granulated sugar, water and lemon juice. Bring to a boil, reduce heat and simmer gently, stirring often, for 10 to 15 minutes, or until thickened. Cool.

3. To prepare base and topping, in a large bowl, combine margarine and sugars and beat well.

4. In a separate bowl, combine flour, rolled oats and baking soda and stir well. Stir flour mixture into margarine mixture. Mixture should be a little crumbly.

5. Pat two-thirds of flour mixture into bottom of a lightly oiled or parchment-lined 9-inch (2.5 L) square baking dish. Spread date mixture on top. Sprinkle with remaining flour mixture.

6. Bake in a preheated 350°F (180°C) oven for 25 to 30 minutes, or until top is lightly browned. Cool and cut into squares.

APRICOT OATMEAL COOKIES

I tasted a cookie like this at the Granville Market in Vancouver and then rushed right home to make my own.

Makes 36 cookies

3/4 cup (175 mL) soft non-hydrogenated margarine or
        unsalted butter, at room temperature
3/4 cup (175 mL) brown sugar
1/2 cup (125 mL) granulated sugar
1 egg
2 tbsp (25 mL) water
1 tsp (5 mL) vanilla
3/4 cup (175 mL) whole wheat flour
3/4 tsp (4 mL) baking soda
1/4 tsp (1 mL) salt
3 cups (750 mL) large-flake rolled oats
1 1/2 cups (375 mL) chopped dried apricots

1. Cream margarine until light. Beat in sugars. Add egg, water and vanilla and mix in.

2. In a large bowl, combine flour, baking soda and salt. Stir in rolled oats.

3. Stir flour mixture into egg mixture. Stir in apricots.

4. Drop batter in 1 1/2 tbsp (20 mL) mounds on a parchment-lined baking sheet. Flatten cookies and bake in a preheated 350°F (180°C) oven for 12 to 15 minutes, or until cookies are crispy around edges and chewy in middle. Cool on racks.

PER COOKIE	
Calories	123
Protein	2 g
Fat	5 g
Saturates	1 g
Cholesterol	5 mg
Carbohydrate	20 g
Fibre	2 g
Sodium	99 mg
Potassium	169 mg

GWEN'S ALMOND HAYSTACKS

This cookie, from my Montreal friend Gwen Berkowitz, is perfect—really delicious, low in fat, rich with almonds and good for Passover, or any time at all.

Makes about 30 cookies

2 egg whites
½ cup (125 mL) granulated sugar
½ tsp (2 mL) vanilla, optional
3 cups (750 mL) sliced almonds

1. In a large bowl, mix (don't whip) egg whites with sugar and vanilla. Stir in almonds.
2. With a teaspoon, place small mounds of mixture on a parchment-lined baking sheet. Bake in a preheated 350°F (180°C) oven for about 20 minutes, or until golden brown. Turn off oven and leave cookies in oven with door open for 10 minutes longer.

PER COOKIE	
Calories	71
Protein	2 g
Fat	5 g
Saturates	1 g
Cholesterol	0 mg
Carbohydrate	5 g
Fibre	1 g
Sodium	5 mg
Potassium	76 mg

HUBERT'S TWICE-BAKED HAZELNUT MERINGUE COOKIES

This is an unusual biscotti-style cookie that chef Hubert Aumeier introduced me to a few years ago.

Makes 36 cookies

4 egg whites
3/4 cup (175 mL) granulated sugar
3/4 cup (175 mL) all-purpose flour
3/4 cup (175 mL) ground toasted hazelnuts

1. In a large bowl, beat egg whites until light. Gradually beat in sugar.
2. In a separate bowl, combine flour and nuts. Fold into egg whites.
3. Spoon batter into a 9- x 5-inch (2 L) loaf pan lined with parchment paper. Bake in a preheated 300°F (150°C) oven for 35 minutes. Cool for 1 hour.
4. Remove loaf from pan. Slice as thinly as possible and place cookies in a single layer on parchment-lined baking sheets. Bake in a preheated 300°F (150°C) oven for 10 to 12 minutes, turning once, until browned and crisp.

PER COOKIE	
Calories	38
Protein	1 g
Fat	1 g
Saturates	0 g
Cholesterol	0 mg
Carbohydrate	6 g
Fibre	trace
Sodium	6 mg
Potassium	20 mg

NUTS

Although nuts do not contain cholesterol, most are very high in fat, so they should be used sparingly. Nuts go rancid, so freeze any that you are not using right away. Walnuts go rancid particularly quickly. (I use Californian walnuts whenever possible because they are harvested efficiently, kept refrigerated and are well packaged. If I can't find them, I often substitute pecans.)

Many people are allergic to nuts, so always warn guests if dishes contain them. If you can't use nuts in cooking or don't want the extra fat, try using crunchy cereals in cookies, etc., or use raisins, dried cherries or dried cranberries instead.

You can double the flavour of nuts by toasting them before using— you won't need to use so many. Spread the nuts on a baking sheet in a single layer and toast in a preheated 350°F (180°C) oven for 5 to 10 minutes, or until lightly coloured. Chop or grind the nuts after toasting.

CHOCOLATE OATMEAL COOKIES

These cookies taste much richer than they really are. You can process the oatmeal in a food processor or blender.

Makes about 34 cookies

¹/₂ cup (125 mL) soft non-hydrogenated margarine or unsalted
     butter, at room temperature
¹/₂ cup (125 mL) granulated sugar
¹/₂ cup (125 mL) brown sugar
2 egg whites
¹/₂ tsp (2 mL) vanilla
¹/₂ cup (125 mL) all-purpose flour
¹/₂ cup (125 mL) whole wheat flour
1 ¹/₄ cups (300 mL) large-flake rolled oats, ground into a flour
¹/₂ tsp (2 mL) baking powder
¹/₂ tsp (2 mL) baking soda
1 cup (250 mL) dried cherries or raisins
¹/₂ cup (125 mL) grated milk chocolate (about 2 oz/60 g)

PER COOKIE	
Calories	92
Protein	2 g
Fat	4 g
Saturates	1 g
Cholesterol	0 mg
Carbohydrate	14 g
Fibre	1 g
Sodium	62 mg
Potassium	76 mg

1. In a large bowl, cream margarine with sugars until light. Beat in egg whites and vanilla.

2. In a separate bowl, combine flours, ground oats, baking powder and baking soda. Stir together well.

3. Stir flour mixture into margarine mixture. Stir in cherries and chocolate.

4. Drop batter by the tablespoon onto parchment-lined baking sheets and press down. Bake in a preheated 325°F (160°C) oven for 12 to 14 minutes, or until lightly browned. Cool on racks.

CHEWY SPICE COOKIES

This was adapted from a recipe by Marianne Saunders, who used to have a fabulous bakery in Calgary. It is the best gingerbread cookie I have ever tasted.

Makes about 64 cookies

½ cup (125 mL) soft non-hydrogenated margarine or unsalted
      butter, at room temperature
1 cup (250 mL) granulated sugar
1 egg
¼ cup (50 mL) molasses
1½ tbsp (20 mL) strong liquid coffee
1 cup (250 mL) all-purpose flour
1 cup (250 mL) whole wheat flour
1 tsp (5 mL) baking soda
1 tsp (5 mL) ground cinnamon
1 tsp (5 mL) ground ginger
½ tsp (2 mL) ground cloves
½ cup (125 mL) raisins
½ cup (125 mL) chopped dried apricots
¼ cup (50 mL) chopped candied ginger
2 tbsp (25 mL) granulated sugar

1. In a large bowl, cream margarine and sugar until light. Beat in egg, molasses and coffee.
2. In a separate bowl, combine flours, baking soda, cinnamon, ground ginger and cloves.
3. Stir dry ingredients into egg mixture. Stir in raisins, apricots and candied ginger. Knead dough together and refrigerate for 1 to 2 hours.
4. Divide dough into 8 equal pieces. Roll each piece into a log about 1 inch (2.5 cm) in diameter. Each log should be about 16 inches (40 cm) long.
5. Place logs on baking sheets lined with parchment paper. Press flat. Bake in a preheated 350°F (180°C) oven for 8 to 10 minutes. Logs should still be soft. (Do not overbake or cookies will not be chewy.)
6. Sprinkle cookies with sugar. Cut on diagonal into 1-inch (2.5 cm) slices. You should have about 7 or 8 cookies per strip. Cool cookies on racks.

PER COOKIE	
Calories	53
Protein	1 g
Fat	2 g
Saturates	trace
Cholesterol	3 mg
Carbohydrate	10 g
Fibre	1 g
Sodium	39 mg
Potassium	69 mg

MOCHA MERINGUE KISSES

These meringues should be dry and crisp. If you make them for Passover, omit the cornstarch. Sometimes we even sneak in a little chopped chocolate.

Makes about 60 cookies

3 egg whites
1/4 tsp (1 mL) cream of tartar
2/3 cup (150 mL) granulated sugar, divided
1/2 tsp (2 mL) vanilla
2 tsp (10 mL) cornstarch
1 tbsp (15 mL) crushed instant coffee powder
1/4 cup (50 mL) finely chopped toasted hazelnuts or almonds

1. In a large stainless-steel or glass bowl, beat egg whites and cream of tartar until frothy. Gradually add 1/3 cup (75 mL) sugar and beat until stiff. Beat in vanilla.

2. Combine remaining 1/3 cup (75 mL) sugar with cornstarch, coffee powder and nuts. Fold into beaten egg whites.

3. Spoon meringue mixture onto parchment-lined baking sheets or transfer mixture into a large piping tube fitted with a star nozzle and pipe in 1 1/2-inch (4 cm) mounds.

4. Bake in a preheated 300°F (150°C) oven until dry, about 25 to 30 minutes. Turn off oven and allow cookies to cool in oven. Tops should be dry and only slightly browned.

PER COOKIE	
Calories	13
Protein	trace
Fat	trace
Saturates	0 g
Cholesterol	0 mg
Carbohydrate	2 g
Fibre	0 g
Sodium	3 mg
Potassium	8 mg

ESPRESSO BISCOTTI

Biscotti—twice-baked cookies—are very hard, dry Italian treats that are meant to be dipped into coffee, tea or Vin Santo so that they soften slightly. This recipe is a variation of one given to me by Nick Malgieri, one of New York's leading baking and dessert instructors, who teaches at my school each year.

Makes about 60 cookies

2 cups (500 mL) all-purpose flour
2/3 cup (150 mL) granulated sugar
1/2 cup (125 mL) finely ground almonds
1 tbsp (15 mL) instant espresso powder
1/2 tsp (2 mL) baking powder
1/2 tsp (2 mL) baking soda
1/2 tsp (2 mL) ground cinnamon
1/2 cup (125 mL) whole unblanched almonds
1/3 cup (75 mL) honey
1/3 cup (75 mL) strong coffee, hot

Dipping Sugar
1/4 cup (50 mL) granulated sugar
1/2 tsp (2 mL) ground cinnamon

1. In a large bowl, combine flour, sugar, ground almonds, espresso powder, baking powder, baking soda and cinnamon. Stir together well. Stir in whole almonds.

2. In a small bowl, combine honey and coffee. Stir into flour mixture until a stiff dough forms.

3. Divide dough in half. Shape each half into a log about 15 inches (40 cm) long.

4. Place logs at least 2 inches (5 cm) apart on a non-stick or parchment-lined baking sheet. Bake in a preheated 350°F (180°C) oven for 30 minutes, or until well risen, firm and golden. Be sure to bake them fully.

5. Cool logs for about 15 minutes and place on a cutting board. Cut on diagonal into 1/2-inch (1 cm) slices.

6. Combine sugar and cinnamon. Dip each cookie into cinnamon sugar. Return cookies to pan, cut side down, and bake for 15 minutes, until dry and lightly coloured.

PER COOKIE	
Calories	45
Protein	1 g
Fat	1 g
Saturates	trace
Cholesterol	0 mg
Carbohydrate	8 g
Fibre	trace
Sodium	12 mg
Potassium	25 mg

INDEX